The Development and Disorders of Speech in Childhood

The Development and Disorders of Speech in Childhood

MURIEL E. MORLEY
D.Sc., F.C.S.T., F.A.C.S.T. (Hon.)

Formerly Speech Therapist-in-Charge of the Speech Therapy Unit, the United Newcastle-upon-Tyne Teaching Hospitals and the Newcastle-upon-Tyne Hospital Management Committee Group

Foreword by

PROFESSOR S. D. M. COURT
C.B.E., M.D., F.R.C.P., D.C.H., F.C.S.T.(Hon.)

The James Spence Chair of Child Health, University of Durham

Third Edition

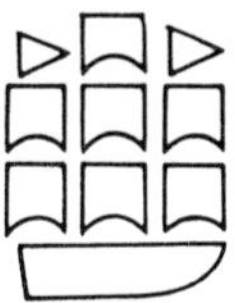

CHURCHILL LIVINGSTONE
EDINBURGH AND LONDON 1972

ISBN 0 443 00895 7

First Edition *1957*
Second Edition *1965*
Reprinted *1967*
Third Edition *1972*

PRINTED IN GREAT BRITAIN BY MORRISON AND GIBB LTD.,
LONDON AND EDINBURGH

Foreword

THE significance of speech in human affairs is self-evident. It is the most complicated, flexible and exciting instrument that man has created in his long social development. We take our ability to speak for granted, but the deep importance we attach to it is widely reflected in the anxiety of parents when a child fails to speak at the expected time. Yet we are still largely ignorant of the mental processes involved in speech. It is with this keen sense of its biological complexity and everyday importance that Miss Morley handles her subject. She writes as a speech therapist and a teacher, and she writes for speech therapists, specialist and family doctors, and teachers.

She has avoided pretentious classification and been content to consider the main developmental disorders of speech in broad categories—categories which are consistent with accepted neurological concepts and of proven value in treatment and prognosis.

But her experience and outlook are not bounded by the walls of the clinic; she has extended her clinical observation to the homes and schools and relevant institutions of the local community. And on the journey she has drawn parents, paediatricians, neurologists, psychologists, statisticians, health visitors and teachers into her company. The result is a fine balance of observation and judgment; a practical handbook which increases our understanding and should improve the management of the disorders in question.

DONALD COURT

DEPARTMENT OF CHILD HEALTH,
KING'S COLLEGE, NEWCASTLE-UPON-TYNE

Preface to the Third Edition

'THE therapists of to-day', says Margaret Eldridge[1] (1967), 'have inherited the investigations, the experiences, the aspirations, the successes and the failures of their predecessors. It is their privilege to build on the foundations which have been laid down for them, and to make their own contribution to their profession in this century.'

Some of these early foundations are described by James Hunt[2] in 1854 and by his son, also James Hunt, in 1870. 'Dyslalia', they say, 'consists either in the impossibility or difficulty of correctly forming and enunciating certain articulate sounds for the purpose of distinct utterance.' They described speech as 'articulated voice', reported on the treatment of 1700 stammerers, and said, 'all the muscles supplied by these nerves must act in harmony in the production of speech; and a want of control over the emission of voluntary power to one of these muscles may affect a number of other muscles with which they are in the habit of acting conjointly'. And also, 'This perfect mechanism, by which most complicated acts are executed, is not subject to the will. The muscles by which articulation is effected are, at first, only partially subject to the will. Thus we have control over the movements of the lips, the cheeks, and the greater part of the muscles of the tongue, but over the muscles of the pharynx, the soft palate and those muscles of the tongue which carry its root upwards and downwards, our power is not so complete.'

When John Wyllie,[3] a physician in Edinburgh, published his book Disorders of Speech (1894), he was one of the first to demonstrate the developing interest in the subject of speech disorders as a science with a medical background, rather than as conditions which would respond to the teaching of those trained in the artistic use of the voice and speech.

[1] Eldridge, Margaret (1967). A History of the Treatment of Speech Disorders. Edinburgh: E. & S. Livingstone Ltd.

[2] Hunt, James (1854). Stammering and Stuttering (7 editions). Facsimile of 1861 edition and Introduction by Elliott J. Schaffer (1967). New York and London: Hafner Pub. Co.

[3] Wyllie, John (1894). Disorders of Speech. Edinburgh: Oliver & Boyd.

Since then increasing interest in the subject has led to its academic and clinical study in Universities and special training schools, and the reporting of the results in many, many articles and books on the varying types and aspects of disorders of spoken language.

This book was first written to place on record (a) the results of an investigation into the development of speech in a community, with comparisons between those whose speech development was considered to be within the normal limits, and those who had some failure of speech development; (b) clinical information based on observations during treatment, reactions to treatment, results of treatment, and a follow-up over a number of years in order to gain greater understanding of varying types of speech disorders and their prognosis. This was greatly assisted by close and regular co-operation with members of the Hospital Staff in the departments of paediatrics, neurology, otolaryngology, plastic surgery, psychiatry and psychology; (c) as the results of these investigations over a period of ten years a simple, tentative classification of speech disorders in childhood emerged and was described, with suggestions for diagnosis and the possibilities of prognosis. Suggestions for treatment were also included, based on intensive therapeutic procedures, over a period of 25 years, with an average of approximately 100 individuals a week, three-quarters of whom were children.

One learns intuitively through such experience, but also through the discipline of trained, accurate observation, and scientific evaluation of the observations made. Such study is possible to all clinicians who have an interest in their work. Whilst there is a need for continuing investigations within a scientific and statistical framework, some of this work would seem to be too mechanistic, sometimes failing to consider the many simple and variable factors which are an essential part of human nature, many of which are difficult to control, and which may modify and even pervert the findings.

Because much that is contained in this book is an account and description of clinical observations, these cannot be changed, but their implications can be modified in the light of further knowledge. There is no single way of viewing reality, so that what is described must be to some extent subjective, relating to personal experiences, as well as objective considerations based on investigation, observations and findings.

In the second edition there were certain additions as the result of further study. A diagramatic representation of the functions, receptive and expressive, at various developmental levels of speech was included, also indicating where break-downs in such functions can occur. This was first presented at the International Conference of Logopaedics in London, 1959, and subsequently published under the title Defects of Articulation in Folia Phoniatrie Vol. 11. Nos. 1–3 (1959).

Further experience of the condition described as Developmental Receptive Aphasia led to the publication in Speech Pathology and Therapy, October, 1960, of an article on this subject giving details of five children with this condition who had all been observed over a number of years. Much of the information in this paper has also been incorporated into this second edition.

A study of dyspraxia in children, described as clumsy children, has been carried out by Walton, Ellis and Court,[1] demonstrating how this condition affects learned skills requiring movement and muscle co-ordinations, in particular the more complex. We have continued to find the term articulatory dyspraxia useful as describing the failure or limited ability to control and direct the movements and co-ordinations of the respiratory, laryngeal and oral muscles for articulation when muscle tone and movement is otherwise adequate, and as differentiated from dysarthria.

In this edition, I have referred to many of the more recent theories and findings of others to indicate the development of ideas during the last decade. In a book such as this, on such a wide subject, one cannot hope to present all that one would wish to include, but ideas have been presented briefly, and references given, to assist the student to further reading. The references to articles by many writers will again provide further references to lead the student to a more intensive study of any particular aspect of the subject.

In recent years the study of Linguistics has given a new

[1] Walton, J. N., Ellis, E., & Court, S. D. M. (1962). Clumsy Children: A Study of Developmental Apraxia and Agnosis. *Brain*, **85**, 602.

perspective to the understanding of the development of speech in early childhood, its disorders and abnormalities, and to the modification of therapeutic clinical methods. Linguistics is concerned with discovering, analysing, describing and explaining the rules which govern the use of language, that is, what a speaker must know in order to speak and to understand his language. This is his linguistic competence. References have been included to these developing ideas in this edition, and to their application to the study of speech in childhood.

In Great Britain, clinical training has always been of first importance, and with the increasing interest in clinical training in the United States for the Certificate of Clinical Competence, it is hoped that the clinical descriptions and suggestions given will continue to prove useful to all students in training, and to clinicians.

Since the first edition of this book was published I have found it interesting that further clinical experience, and observation when visiting other countries, particularly the United States, Australia and New Zealand, has tended to confirm that the occurrence, type and incidence of speech disorders is similar, at least among English speaking peoples. Such experience has helped to clarify, and to confirm the usefulness of, the descriptions of speech disorders in childhood as presented in 1957 in the first edition of this book.

In conclusion, I should like to thank many friends, in Great Britain, Australia, New Zealand and in the United States, who have helped me to 'keep in touch' since retirement from my own hospital appointments in 1964. I wish to thank the Council of the College of Speech Therapists, London, for inviting me to edit the British Journal of Disorders of Communication, with the professional contacts this implies; for an invitation from the University of Queensland, the Australian College of Speech Therapists and the Department of Education in New Zealand to teach and to lecture in 1963; also Professor Ken Shank, Ph.D., for an invitation in 1968 to teach as Visiting Professor at the University of Indiana, and to Professor Charles Parker, Ph.D., to teach at the University of Montana—interesting experiences which I remember with pleasure; also many other friends, including Dr. Van Riper of Western Michigan University, and Dr. Ruth Lencione of Syracuse, and those in other

Universities where I have visited and had recent stimulating opportunities to teach, lecture and talk to staff and students. I found the same types of speech disorder and the same response to treatment as at home. Such experiences have helped me to revise this book with, I hope, advantage to its readers. My interest has never been allowed to lapse, and 'retirement' has proved to be one of the most interesting periods of my professional life.

MURIEL E. MORLEY

1972

Preface to First Edition

DURING the last quarter of a century the value of speech therapy has been increasingly recognised. Yet we are still largely in ignorance as to the mental processes involved in this aspect of human behaviour which we call speech, and of the reason why in some there is failure to develop and use normal speech.

Disorders of speech may be developmental or acquired, and elaborate classifications have been evolved to describe the varying symptoms. It was felt that a classification based on aetiology and on accepted neurological terminology might form a basis for future development. During the last eight years, therefore, a group consisting of a paediatrician, a neurologist, a psychologist and a speech therapist has carried out clinical observations on children with developmental disorders of speech who were attending for speech therapy at hospital clinics in Newcastle-upon-Tyne.

It was also possible to see a representative sample of young children of the City between the ages of three and eight years of age in their own homes in order to gain knowledge and experience concerning the development and use of speech in such children.

A detailed survey was also undertaken of the incidence and type of speech disorder in children of school age, that is between five and fifteen years, in a local urban community.

In these three ways we have studied the development and disorders of speech in childhood within the context of the local community. As we have done so the children we have seen have fallen naturally into four broad categories: those who have normal speech, those who do not understand speech and do not speak, those who understand but do not speak, and those who both understand speech and speak, but in whom articulation or speech is defective.

This book presents a classification of developmental disorders of speech. The findings relating to various types of speech disorder are given and principles of treatment described. In arranging the material it was necessary to decide whether this should be done in terms of the underlying conditions and within the accepted neurological terminology, or in relation to the variety of symptoms met with in everyday practice. With our present limited knowledge it was thought wise to use both these approaches where most appropriate.

The first chapter is introductory, presenting a general picture, and outlining conditions which are considered in more detail in later chapters.

The material has been divided into six parts dealing with:—

I. The pattern of speech development as it emerged from a detailed investigation of the speech of children in 1000 families in Newcastle-upon-Tyne.
II. The delayed development of speech.
III. Defective articulation.
IV. Stammering.
V. Speech disorders in twins.
VI. Lateral dominance and disorders of speech.

Each part is subdivided into chapters, but forms a unit in itself, a list of pertinent references being found at the end of each chapter. Where a part commences with an introductory chapter this is included to present the picture as a whole before discussing the various points in greater detail. In order that each part might be complete some repetition was inevitable, but may be useful in that it emphasises important points and the interdependence of varying types of speech disorder.

The findings described relate to work carried out in the Royal Victoria Infirmary, the Fleming Hospital for Sick Children, and the General Hospital, Newcastle-upon-Tyne. This has been possible chiefly because the Department of Speech Therapy in the Royal Victoria Infirmary has, for the last ten years, been closely associated with the Children's Department and the University Department of Child Health.

I am greatly indebted to the late Sir James Spence for his helpful guidance. I owe much to the opportunity to work in a department where one was constantly aware of his ideas, and was stimulated by his questions and conversation to think, and to reassess developing opinions. To him I largely owe my appreciation of the mother-child relationship as something to be accepted as a whole in dealing with the young child. Therapy is not then limited to the child alone but involves both mother and child.

To Professor S. D. M. Court of the University Department of Child Health and the Children's Department of the Royal Victoria Infirmary I am indebted for his help in our attempt to gain further understanding of disorders of speech in children. Without his interest, advice and encouragement this book would not have been written. During the last eight years we have held regular consultations for the observation and study of children in whom speech had failed to develop normally. In this work we were assisted by Dr. H. G. Miller who carried out the neurological examinations, and Mr. R. F. Garside of the Department of Psychological Medicine to whom we are indebted for an estimation of the intelligence of these children. So we have gained further insight into, and have extended our knowledge and understanding of, the child with a speech disability.

I also wish to express my thanks to Professor Court for suggestions concerning this book, and also to those speech therapy and medical colleagues who have kindly read the text in manuscript and have given me useful criticisms and suggestions, namely Miss Muriel Ferrie, Dr. Henry Miller, Mr. F. McGuckin, Mr. Fenton Braithwaite, and Dr. G. Knox. I am also indebted to Dr. R. Errington Ellis, and the physiotherapists and speech therapist of the Percy Hedley School for children with cerebral palsy. With their co-operation the study of speech disorders in these children was made possible. The study and assessment of hearing disorders was greatly assisted by Mr. W. Wearmouth of the Northern Counties School for the Deaf and those Members of his staff who advised concerning the assessment of speech attainment in the children in this school. I wish to thank Dr. G. McCoull, Medical Superintendent of the Prudhoe and Monkton Hospital and of Earl's House Hospital, Durham, for the opportunity to assess the speech of the mentally defective, and also Mrs. F. Thompson, Headmistress of the Hospital School. For an invitation to take part in the survey of One Thousand Families I am grateful to the late Sir James Spence and Dr. F. J. W. Miller, and also to the Secretary, Miss M. F. Thompson, and the Health Visitors who formed part of the group of people engaged in this work. I also wish to acknowledge my appreciation of the work of the

King's College Department of Photography, Newcastle, under its Director, Mr. H. Duncan, who reproduced the diagrams, graphs and illustrations in this book originally executed by Miss D. Mustart. I should also like to record my gratitude for the assistance given to me by my sister, Miss Joan W. Morley, and for the care she exercised in reading the proofs.

In conclusion I wish to express my gratitude to the United Newcastle-upon-Tyne Teaching Hospitals, the Newcastle Regional Hospital Board, and the Department of Education, King's College, Durham University, for permission to take the greater part of my time from clinical work for one year with full pay in order to collect and arrange the material in this book, and in addition for a financial grant towards expenses from the Royal Victoria Infirmary, Newcastle-upon-Tyne.

Finally, I express my appreciation of the assistance and co-operation of the publishers, Messrs. E. and S. Livingstone of Edinburgh.

NEWCASTLE-UPON-TYNE,
February, 1957

Contents

Part II

THE DELAYED DEVELOPMENT OF SPEECH

Part III

DEFECTIVE ARTICULATION

Part IV
STAMMERING

Part V
SPEECH DISORDERS IN TWINS

Part VI
LATERAL DOMINANCE AND SPEECH

Appendix
Tables I-V

THE AGE OF SPEECH DEVELOPMENT

Tables VI-VIII

ASSESSMENT OF LANGUAGE ABILITY

Tables IX-XIII

ARTICULATION

Tables XIV-XV

THE DEVELOPMENT OF SPEECH AND SEX

Tables XVI-XVIII

DEFECTIVE ARTICULATION AND SEX

Tables XIX-XXI

THE DEVELOPMENT OF SPEECH AND POSITION IN FAMILY

Tables XXII-XXV

SOCIAL STATUS AND THE DEVELOPMENT OF SPEECH

Tables XXVI-XXVIII

DYSARTHRIA IN CEREBRAL PALSY

Tables XXIX-XXXVII

LATERAL PREFERENCE AND SPEECH DISORDERS

DEVELOPMENTAL DISORDERS OF SPEECH

A Simple Classification

I. DISORDERS OF LANGUAGE

1. Aphasia - (a) Mainly receptive.
   (b) Mainly executive.
2. Alexia.
3. Agraphia.
4. Delayed development of speech associated with -
   (a) General mental retardation.
   (b) Mental illness.
   (c) Hearing deficiency.

II. DISORDERS OF ARTICULATION

1. Anarthria.
2. Articulatory apraxia.
3. Dyslalia.
4. Defective articulation due to -
   (a) Hearing defects.
   (b) Structural abnormalities -
      (i) Inadequate intra-oral air pressure (e.g. cleft palate).
      (ii) Abnormalities of the tongue.
      (iii) Dental irregularities.
      (iv) Other anatomical conditions.

III. DISORDERS IN THE UTTERANCE OF SPEECH

(a) Stammering.
(b) Defects in the rhythm of speech as in cluttering, or hesitant speech.

IV. DISORDERS OF VOICE (Aphonia).

In certain conditions A- denotes the neurological defect. The prefix A- may be used for a complete, and Dys-for a partial failure of the symptom.

I. Speech

MAN is essentially a social being, and of all human activities the desire to communicate with others is one of his most important characteristics. Our social system is based largely on this aspect of human behaviour, whether such communication be by means of mime, gesture, music or painting, by the inarticulate cry of the infant, or through spoken or written words, conveyed directly or by means of the various electronic devices of modern civilisation.

Communication occurs at varying biological levels between most animate creatures and is an integral part of human behaviour whether it be verbal or non-verbal. Non-verbal communication takes place in many ways, from the physical contact of the infant with his mother through touch, visual impressions of facial expression, gesture, and other movements and sensations. Perhaps one of the most important to his later adjustment to life is the sense of security he receives from his mother's arms, of being cared for and wanted. Verbal communication is an extension and development of such behaviour by the use of sounds produced by muscle movements. These are signals, but become recognised as symbols or signs when they become part of a linguistic system, and, as phonemes, are arranged in sequences and categories to convey information through spoken language. The symbols used are augmented by varying intonation, facial expression and gesture, all of which add considerably to the meaning of the words and phrases used. Facial, and general immobility whilst speaking would be unnatural and conspicuous.

By means of speech we are able to describe our thoughts, so that not only may we share them with each other but that in the process we may also discover more clearly our own ideas. Although our thoughts influence and direct the words we use, these words may also influence our thought. Speech arises in the mind of the speaker, but the process of communication also involves the transference of thoughts to others and is complete only when the words written or spoken arouse ideas in the mind of another. Thought may be in the form of mental pictures and exist in the absence of language, but it is facilitated by the formulation of such thoughts into words, spoken or unspoken.

Speech is an integrated function involving the reception of words by the ear or the eye, their interpretation and synthesis as language within the brain and the expression of this language response in further spoken or written words. It includes the whole of this receptive, formative and expressive activity. Words are composed of sequences of sounds. They are symbolic and have a consistent range of meaning.

In complete or embryonic form they are constructional units of thought and language, and in terms of the movements of speech are heard and understood, arranged and rearranged, articulated and spoken. Language is both the word library of speech and the sum of those meaningful associations of words current in the life and literature of any society (Morley *et al.*, 1955).

Language is the term used to denote the means by which thought is formulated into a linguistic system as a basis for the conveyance of thought. Both the receptive and expressive aspects are involved, requiring processes of decoding and encoding, both dependant upon cortical activity. Knowledge of the system is gained through learning, the listener and the speaker sharing a common store of linguistic knowledge, without which neither could understand the other. Use of language requires the selection and organisation of certain language units, made audible, in order that meaningful ideas may be communicated to another, whilst the listener, or receiver, having received the acoustic cues, organises the information perceived in order to comprehend the ideas conveyed. Communication through use of language is dependant upon the use of symbols which may be spoken or written.

Reading requires the ability to associate printed or written symbols with meaning. Normally, an association develops between the verbal appreciation of symbols and the visual symbols and meaning, but may be based on visual appreciation of symbols where the auditory system has failed to develop, as in the severely deaf child. In written language the muscle movements involved are those of the fingers, hands and arm. Normally, use of spoken language develops before written language, and under certain conditions, written language may be retained when ability to use the verbal symbols adequately is lost. Some children may communicate more easily through writing and typing when hand movements are better than those required for articulation, as in some children with cerebral palsy. This implies that language may be adequate for both the encoding and decoding processes when muscle movements are inadequate to produce accurately the verbal or written symbols essential to convey information.

Articulation is the process by which words are expressed through muscular movements controlled by complex neuromuscular changes, with the production of vocal and articulate sounds. In standard received English there are approximately 47 phonetic sounds, 15 vowels, 23 consonants and 9 diphthongs, although there are some consonant and many vowel variations occurring in local dialects. The number of different sounds which it is possible to produce in the restricted space of the human mouth is limited, and so we find the same phonetic sounds, with some additions and omissions, occurring in most of the languages of the various countries of the world, but the sequences in which they are used to produce words, with their symbolic meaning, varies according to the language of each society of human beings.

The parts of the body used for speech have, as their original function, the processes of respiration, sucking, chewing and swallowing. By a process of modification and development such primitive reactions have been gradually adapted by man for the complex neuromuscular function of articulate speech. Visual, auditory, tactile and kinaesthetic sensations play a part in the processes involved in the reception of the sounds of speech, and in their recall for the purpose of expressive speech. We do not yet understand by what mental processes we are enabled to interpret the meaning of the thoughts expressed by others through articulate sounds, nor in what way our thoughts are formulated into language, but the articulate and vocal sounds we make are based on the general neurophysiological principles of muscle movement. In speech such movements are so rapid that they probably approach the limit of speed possible to muscular movement in man.

Communication through speech requires then that through complex mental processes thoughts are formulated into language and that language is transmitted through the activity of the motor nerves, the resulting muscular movements producing articulate sounds forming recognisable symbols. Such sounds are carried through the air to the hearer by a process which is dependent on the physical characteristics of the conduction of sound waves in air, and are received by and react on the tympanum of the ear. They are transmitted through the middle ear to the cochlea and from thence by way of the auditory nerve to the cortex, producing those complex central and cortical processes by which we attend to, recognise and understand the meaning of the spoken symbols of speech.

In recent years much thought has been directed to the study of languages in relation to their structure within the field of linguistics. Whilst linguistics describes the nature of language, psycholinguistics describes its relationship to society, and such studies have provided new and meaningful ways of viewing normal language acquisition and its general use.

Basic work on the study of spoken language was chiefly concerned with single speech sounds, phonetics, or single words. More recently, interest has been directed towards the study of connected speech and word sequences. The linguist is concerned with sounds as the medium by which information is conveyed, and with the analysis of speech as an orderly sequence of specific sounds and sequences of sounds.

Phonetics, according to Pit Corder (1968) deals with the surface phenomena of language and he describes articulation as the *last* stage in language *production* and the *first* stage in *understanding* language. Whilst the phonetic structure of speech is primarily associated with positions and movements, the *phoneme* represents the smallest change which can convert one word into another. Phonemes, therefore, are the basic elements of a language of which there are a certain number in each language. Linguists suggest about 40 in English. 'Run', 'fun', 'sun', 'pun', and 'bun' differ from each other by one phoneme which is phonemically distinct because thereby the meaning is changed. As such they may be described as phonetic distinctions used to convey meaning, but are not units of meaning in themselves.

The *phonemic system* of any language is described by Fry (1968) as the basis for all the higher order linguistic structures.

The phonological field includes the phonemic units, the rules governing the combination of phonemes and the possibilities of phonemic sequences, the rules linking acoustic cues in the phonemic categories, phonemes with articulation and articulation with acoustic cues. Phonemes are the basic units for analysis, but also correspond to the fact of behaviour in the muscular movements for articulation.

Linguists recognise three levels or processes involved in speaking; the phonological system, the grammatical or syntactic, and the semantic levels in communication.

Chomsky (1957) suggests that syntax or grammar, as a whole, can be regarded as a device for pairing phonetically represented signals with semantic interpretations, semantics being described as the use of linguistic rules to express thought.

Gleason (1955) described language as an arbitrary, prearranged set of signals requiring a channel by means of which such signals may be conveyed. The use of this channel to express meaning is described as *encoding*, whilst *decoding* is the interpretation and understanding of this meaning. Language operates with (*a*) sounds, (*b*) ideas and meanings, and the patterning of utterances according to the sequences recognised in any particular language. For example, one can say 'a little dog', but not 'little a dog'. Such sequences involve phonological patterning, dependant upon the use of certain *phonetic sound units*, and their sequential use as *phonemes* in words and sentences.

The sounds we use in speech are physical signals, and, as Cherry (1957) reminds us, it is the orderly selection of these sounds in linguistic sequences which conveys the thought which initiated the utterance, this being controlled by the rules of the language, or syntax. There may be wide variability within which there is recognition and understanding, and which is not essentially affected by changes of pitch, volume of vocal tone, dysphonia, when the voice is breathy or husky, or in singing.

Whilst the positions for the production of sounds in isolation are known, the articulatory muscles are moving almost continuously during speech, and the positions for the production of sounds in sequence are not necessarily identical nor constant for each individual. In rapid speech there are approximations, yet the ear appears to be able to assess these variations, recognise the essential elements, and the meaning they convey. Understanding is, however, completely affected if there is no voice and no laryngeal air for articulation of sounds, as in post-laryngectomy before compensatory air pressure is achieved, and severely, if articulatory movements are inadequate.

Haas (1968) has suggested that the speech therapist concerned with understanding the development of verbal behaviour and its disorders, may acquire and use the theories, methods and descriptions of the linguist in describing both the required verbal behaviour, the deviations from it, and also in planning, and in monitoring progress during treatment. Articulation would be seen in the framework of the patterning of a language operating at varying linguistic levels, and the factors essential for the required movements and co-ordinations which are recognised acoustically.

However Teuber (1960) stresses our ignorance of the neural basis of speech. 'We simply do not know how the listener manages to analyse the stream of speech, structure it into phonemes and morphemes, and comprehend strings of sentences according to syntactic rules.' However whilst the central mechanisms for speech may present problems, increasing understanding of the in-put and out-put aspects of speech through observations of behaviour of the sensory and motor processes involved tends to lessen the gap between them.

The Development of Speech

In slightly more than two years, children acquire full knowledge of the grammatical system of their native tongue. The process behind this stunning intellectual achievement is essentially one of invention (McNeill, 1966).

The development of speech in a child is not an instinctive process. It is dependent on neurological development and is the result of imitation, which again would seem to be the result of an inborn urge to be like those around him. Because he sees others walking in the upright position he endeavours to pull himself up into a similar position and eventually learns to balance himself and to control the movements of his feet and legs in walking. In the same way the child develops the use of certain muscle groups during the gradual process of mental growth and neuromuscular maturation for the imitation and use of the sounds of speech he hears around him.

The growth and development of speech requires firstly that there should be full functional activity of the peripheral and central processes by which the child hears and *imitates sounds* accurately, and secondly that he should gradually learn to *associate these sounds with objects and with meaning.* This requires that his general intelligence and mental development should be such that he is able to recognise, associate, recollect and reproduce the sounds of speech with or without meaning. Such processes may be illustrated by a child of three years who, hearing an elder brother repeating, 'Amo, amas, amat', reproduced it as 'Amo, amas, a carpet'. Brain (1961) also describes how a word can exist independantly of its meaning. A child can correctly utter a word whilst unaware of its meaning.

'It is difficult to appreciate that these developmental processes in early childhood, which so seldom fail, and are so effortless, are so exceedingly complicated (Sheridan, 1959). We are still only at the beginning of understanding the biological, otological, neurological, psychological, emotional and educational implications. Intelligence, auditory capacity, visual localisation, kinaesthetic awareness, motor control and personality are all important.'

Many agree with Lenneberg (1967) that this process could only be accomplished if the systematic sequence of events which occurs during the development of speech were based on innate physiological prerequisites for language acquisition. As McNeill (1966) states, this process occurs in spite of racial differences in conditions of learning, as children apparently share an inborn capacity for language. So deeply rooted is this ability that children with severe handicaps, and those living under the worst social conditions and neglect (Lenneberg, 1967) will yet acquire language, and what Chomsky (1959) describes as 'the linguistic knowledge which is his linguistic competence.' Teuber (1960) also believes that the tasks facing the child are so complex that some important aspects of language could not be learned were they not innate and dependant, therefore, upon maturation. He also points out that certain essential features of all human languages, such as the patterning of phonemes in terms of distinctive features, and the organising of syntax, are universal features of all human languages and therefore must be innate.

The child's phonological system develops simultaneously along two lines, the perceptive and the motor, but the child's ability to receive acoustic cues and appreciate speech is normally in advance of his ability to use speech. At the phonetic and phonemic level, perception of a distinctive feature precedes its production. The child then proceeds from broad contrasts to finer distinctions, and through approximations and variations in the appreciation and production of articulate sounds. Comprehension as well as the production of speech, 'entails the use of generative rules which every child discovers for himself for his own mother tongue during the optimal period for first language learning (Chomsky and Katz, 1964), even though no child, and very few adults, can describe these rules.'

The development of speech must therefore be dependant upon maturation, and whilst some think that the child will learn when he is ready, and that intensive instruction may modify but will not accelerate speech development, Luria and Yudovich (1959) suggest that there is evidence that maturation may be stimulated or retarded by environmental influences although the direction is predestined.

Whilst increasingly linguists are beginning to specify what it means to have language, to perceive it and produce it, through analysis based on observation of its production, it is essentially dependant upon neurosensory and neuromuscular processes, including integration at the cortical level, which gradually develops during pre-natal and post-natal life.

Behaviour

Three forms of behaviour are evident during the development of speech, reflex, spontaneous and imitative.

Reflex behaviour. At birth the infant is able to breathe, cry, and swallow, and, soon after, the complicated reflex activity of sucking is established. Although the same muscles are concerned in the co-ordinated movements of respiration, phonation and articulation, speech does not develop at this early age. This acquired function of human behaviour develops later, being determined partly by inherent imitative tendencies and stimulated by the individual's essential need to communicate with others, to express his feelings and his desires.

Sherrington (1947) has described the difference between reflex and acquired behaviour, and how exhaustive tests bear out the assertion that any animal under certain conditions following transection of the spinal cord may still execute certain acts but is devoid of mind. 'Thoughts, feelings, memory, percepts, conations, etc., of these no evidence is forthcoming or to be elicited.' 'Yet the animal remains a motor mechanism which can be touched into action in certain ways so as to exhibit pieces of its behaviour.' In defining such reflex actions he states that ' the conception of a reflex therefore embraces that of at least three separate structures—an effector organ, e.g. gland cells or muscle cells; a conducting nervous path or conductor leading to that organ; and an initiating organ or receptor whence the reaction starts.' He also described how such 'involuntary movements can sometimes be brought under subjection to the will. From this subjection it is but a short step to the acquisition of co-ordinations which express themselves as movements newly acquired by the individual. The controlling centres can pick out from an ancestrally given motor reaction one part of it, so as to isolate that as a new separate movement, and by enhancement this can become a skilled adapted act added to the powers of the individual.' So the early reflex movements of the muscles used for speech and their use in the first and spontaneous production of sounds may be co-ordinated for use by higher cortical processes when thought is formulated into language. Habit then plays a part in the stabilisation of this learned behaviour, and again Sherrington states that 'as life develops it would seem that in the field of external relation conscious behaviour tends to replace reflex, and conscious acts to bulk larger and larger. Along with this change and indeed as part of it, would seem an increased role of habit.' 'Habit arises always in conscious action; reflex behaviour never arises in conscious action. Habit is always acquired behaviour, reflex behaviour is always inherent and innately given.'

As involuntary movements can sometimes be brought under subjection to the will, acquired volitional movements, even if achieved at an early age with little conscious effort, may also become involuntary, and both processes are probably involved in the development and use of speech.

Reflex sounds uttered by the child begin with the first inspiration and the birth cry. Later, sounds appear indicative of hunger, a reaction to comfort, or to pain. Such sounds involve the use of respiration and its co-ordination with movements of the laryngeal muscles to produce variations of vocal tone associated from the beginning with sensory feedback.

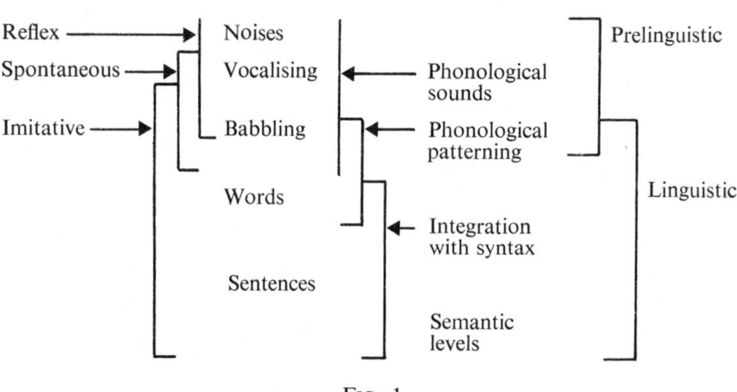

FIG. 1

The development of behaviour, utterances and linguistic competence.

Thus are the foundations laid for the use of voice in speech as the child, beginning with primitive movements, proceeds to those which become increasingly differentiated.

Spontaneous behaviour succeeds the early reflex behaviour as the child produces sounds apparently for the pleasure and satisfaction of so doing. These sounds appear to arise independantly of any acoustic information and include vocalising and babbling. This is an egocentric stage, based mainly on autostimulation, although the appearance of another individual may increase the stimulation and cause increased and intensified reactions, perhaps the first indications of verbal communication. This stage evolves into an increasing awareness of surrounding speech sounds, leading to imitative behaviour.

Imitative behaviour. This would seem to be innate and perhaps genetically determined. Vygotsky (1934, trs. 1962) has described how when the child is only a few months old there is evidence that he is responding to the world around him and even to the verbalisations of his environment. However, the child does not at first respond with understanding, but rather to the broad acoustic variations of intensity, duration of stimulus, pitch and tonal quality which characterise speech. He also begins to discriminate between the noises around him, such as the door opening, the dog barking, and so forth.

The child also becomes interested in watching facial and lip movements. The fact that a child can watch his mother's lips as she says 'ma ma' and, in response, attempt to move his own lips in a similar way, is evidence of his ability to imitate. How does the child know what movement to make and how to make it? He cannot see himself. He does not experiment by moving other structures. Environmental reinforcement may encourage him to continue, but does not account for the fact that such imitation is universal in children, regardless of environment (Morley and Fox, 1969).

Imitative verbal behaviour would seem to arise only after the child has had sufficient sensorimotor experience during the reflex and spontaneous phases of speech development. It emerges during the spontaneous stage of speech development and continues at increasing levels of complexity until full linguistic competence is achieved, and, in fact, throughout life. Such imitation is not, however, conscious reproduction of behaviour, but rather the result of social facilitation, when the performance of a pattern of behaviour apparently leads to the release of similar behaviour by others. Luria and Vinograd (1959) also describe how, with increasing mental development, linguistic association systems progress from those based on superficial sound similarities to the stage when semantic systems predominate.

Imitative behaviour, at whatever level of speech development, is based upon sensorimotor processes, whether it be self imitation, or the imitation of others. Motor impulses result in movements which produce sounds, which are appreciated through the various sensory processes. So a control, or monitoring system is established through sensorimotor experience. Thus the child develops a form of automatic control through feedback in a closed loop circuit.

Such a closed loop circuit is one in which the action of a machine is dependant upon performance, as, for example, an automatic electric toaster. In human physiology respiration is regulated by the amount of carbon dioxide in the blood; fluid balance, thermal equilibrium of body temperature and hormonal balance are also examples of the closed loop system of control whereby homeostasis is maintained. Bodily movements and balance, in standing and walking, and so forth, also develop through sensory control acquired through experience. Motor and sensory functions work in close co-operation with one another, forming a single functional process. Such a principle of feedback is universal in the operation of the nervous system, and forms the basis for the highly complex integration of the neurological processes which are essential for speech. Mysak (1966) also describes the speech mechanism as a complex multiple closed loop system and suggests that closed loop activities of the human organism are the basis of learned skills which then become stabilised through experience, making it possible for the higher centres of the brain to engage in more intellectual pursuits.

Walshe (1948), describing the sensorimotor control for speech, defines the *motor*, or pyramidal system, as a common pathway by which the *sensory* system initiates and continuously directs in willed movements the activities of the nervous motor mechanisms, and that 'receptor activity including both distance receptors (auditory in-put) and proprioceptive and tactile sensory processes, is so essentially correlated with motor function that the physiology of the latter cannot be comprehended apart from the recognition of this correlation'. The effector system for speech can therefore be considered as being dependant upon, and continuously controlled and monitored by the receptor processes through sensory feedback. Repeated sensorimotor experience, involving constant interplay between the receptor and effector functions, determines the development and use of all reflex actions and learned motor skills including that of articulation, phonological development and the integration of phonological into linguistic competence.

The part that imitation plays may develop early in life.

Bühler and Hetzer (1928) have described the response of 27 children in the first 14 days of life to the crying of another child. A crying child was brought near to a silent one, and in 84 per cent of the attempts the silent child also began to cry. The experiment was carried out 30 times for each of the 27 children. This may indicate imitative behaviour but is more probably a sympathetic emotional reaction. However, it may demonstrate the child's awareness of, and ability to respond to the sounds heard, even at this early stage.

Miller (1951) described primitive imitative, or echoic behaviour, as creating an internal circular reaction which provides the first real guidance of motor development by perceptive development, and Fraser, *et al* (1963) suggest that imitation is a perceptual skill which can be used without evidence of understanding. Imitation also involves verbal memory. Whilst the child may be able to reproduce a single sound, or the same sound in a repetitive series, he will have greater difficulty both in perceiving clearly and in reproducing a longer series of varying sounds in linguistic sequences.

Whilst the child uses acoustic information and other sensory processes he may frequently produce sounds, or sequences of sounds, which are not part of the linguistic system of his environment. These arise spontaneously, as described. Later, those occurring in the phonological system tend to appear more frequently, and would seem to be selected. However, most children experiment to some extent for themselves. The use of the phonological system may develop through a series of approximations, the ultimate result being dependant upon the maturation of sensorimotor skills. Other children, however, develop use of the phonological system accurately with little or no individual variation. However, whilst acquiring the use of syntax most children use utterances which they could not have heard in their environment. Wingfield (1969) suggests that the child's errors indicate his attempts to use the rules of his environment. Such expressions as 'take it to part' compared with 'take it to pieces', or 'put it *to* gether', or 'foot' and 'feet' may produce 'foots' and 'feets', indicating early attempts, without conscious awareness, to apply syntactical rules.

At the end of the first four weeks there may be response to a familiar voice indicated by a cessation of crying. At seven to eight weeks the child may turn towards the sound of a voice and at three to four months he may respond to the speech of others by attempting to make vocal or articulate sounds.

Development of *recognition* for sounds, associated with understanding for their meaning, is a stage in the growth of language which normally develops with growing experience of life.

Thus speech patterns become increasingly important, and environmental stimulation and re-inforcement helpful to the child's acquisition of any particular language system through imitation. From his environment he learns *what* to produce, but the environment does not teach him *how* to produce it. This he does for himself with very little effort, based on the phonological skill which he has been gradually developing since birth.

Utterances

Progression from vocalising to speech

Prelinguistic

Vocalising. Occurs during the reflex period of speech development. During this period the child acquires the use of the laryngeal muscles in association with respiration and develops the varying co-ordinations of the muscle changes involved. Through early vocalisation, crying, cooing, with varying contours of intonation, volume and pitch, he is acquiring control and experience, both motor and sensory. Such sounds involve little movement of the tongue and lips, although varying modifications occur in the oral cavity, including use of the soft palate as initial nasal sounds are replaced by oral sounds. Interruptions and constrictions of the air stream in the mouth eventually produce sounds with the properties of stop and continuant non-vowel sounds, which may be voiced or unvoiced according to use of a vibrating or non-vibrating air stream, and in association with vowel sounds in simple syllabic sequences.

Babbling. Much has been written on this subject, but whatever part it plays, or does not play, in phonological and linguistic development, it is a stage which is common to almost all children during the normal development of speech. At this stage contours of intonation patterns are more important to the child than the production of individual phonemes.

Myklebust (1957) has said, that with the onset of babbling, the behaviour of the human becomes characteristic and essentially unique, and he defines babbling as the pleasurable use of vocalisation by the child in the preverbal period. It forms a basis for language development which in general consists in acquiring symbols to represent experiences. Babbling is described by Mowrer (1950) as the means whereby the child begins to relate to others in his environment and he believes that it assists the development and integrity of the peripheral and central nervous systems for speech. Early sounds, including babbling, are described by Watts (1944) as apparently aimless vocal activity 'which is an indispensable preliminary to the articulate speech which comes later'. Cruttendon (1970) defines it as the emergence of pulmonic-lingual sounds, and describes babbling, as observed in his own twin daughters, as showing a general drift towards the mother-tongue in preparation for speech. To him, it seemed to provide the children with a first approximation to early words, whilst with increasing awareness of linguistic contrasts, the approximations to adult usage became closer. He suggests that babbling may be divided into pre-language babbling and post-language babbling, that is babbling persisting when the child is also using meaningful utterances after the emergence of the first words.

The most important aspect of babbling is the development of the circuitry which links auditory feedback and auditory memory with proprioceptive and kinaesthetic feedback and memory (Fry, 1968). The child is learning through *experience* to connect the auditory impressions of the sounds he is making with patterns of the motor activity which give rise to the sounds. He learns what acoustic changes will follow when he changes movements. and how to change the movement to produce a particular sound, all without conscious awareness. This is a once-for-all-time operation.

When these associations are firmly established the child has an effective means for learning new articulations. He has a readily available technique for modifying his articulation in any required direction, for matching the sounds he utters with those he hears from others, and for continuously monitoring his own production of speech sounds, all based on experience.

Fry also describes how the child's use of phonemic categories is closely bound up with his ability to articulate sounds. As the motor and sensory aspects of articulation develop simultaneously, and the number of phoneme units used by the child increases, so will the number of acoustic cues. With increasing appreciation of acoustic distinctions, the child passes through a series of developmental levels of skill and complexity, and it is the interaction between the developing articulatory skill and the phonemic system which is vital to the language learning process. Although phonology and articulation are not identical, there is a close link between them. Again such learning is below the level of conscious thought, and is through experience rather than conceptual.

Thus babbling would seem to be firstly, an exercise in motor co-ordination of the muscle movements upon which articulation depends. Secondly, it stimulates and develops the processes of sensory feedback for the simultaneous development of perception for speech and motor activity including association of the various sensory processes involved, auditory, tactile and kinaesthetic. Perception of speech would seem to be closely linked with sensory stimulii, and is the means whereby the movements are produced in order that sounds heard may be imitated. Liebermann *et al* (1952) believed that their observations provided support for the assumption that the perception of speech depends in any final analysis on the proprioceptive stimulii which arise from the movements of articulation. Hence, the normal development of the essential neurological processes is stimulated through experience, learning and maturation.

So far, development of speech can be described as prelinguistic, but it proceeds to the linguistic stage without any clear line of demarcation. Single words make their appearance whilst babbling still persists, but with the emergence of the more mature stages of speech development activity of the earlier, prelinguistic stages decreases.

However, the first identifiable words occur at a time when articulation may still lack fine control, whilst the child's lack of concern for phonetic accuracy indicates a fundamental principle in the development of language, that *what* is acquired are patterns and structures, rather than constituent elements. The child reproduces words and phrases as a whole sequence, shorter sequences being easier to reproduce accurately than longer sequences, and not as a sequence of isolated successive sounds.

Linguistic development

The child's first interest is in persons and their names, followed by action words concerning what people do. His first use of expressive speech is therefore usually limited to single words, and involves the recollection and use of the required sound sequences. His first attempt at phrases may be just two or three words as 'Mummy—cake' or 'Bobby get down'. Vocabulary increases throughout life and continues to develop with each new experience and with the need to express new ideas.

During the prelinguistic period of experience and learning, the child has acquired control of articulation and has developed the ability to imitate sound sequences. As the child's babble sequences increasingly approach those in the phonological system of his environment his use of linguistic sequences with meaning appears. Sounds, which earlier he did not differentiate acquire distinctness, and he begins increasingly to organise his utterances in phoneme categories. The phonetic sounds he has learnt to use appear in phoneme clusters of increasing length and variety, and verbal approximations become active attempts to communicate with others. There may be differences from the adult language models, but the child is organising the sounds he hears and is using phoneme sequences in words, phrases and sentences in association with objects, activities and with meaning. Eventually, using the acquired experience which has given him automatic control of the phonological system, he is able to integrate his phonemic utterances with linguistic sequences without conscious awareness of the individual sounds he is using.

Echolalia is normally a transient stage, but may persist in certain cases of mental retardation or abnormality. It tends to disappear as the child increasingly formulates his thoughts into concepts expressed through language.

During the early stages of language usage children vary in

their ability to incorporate accurately their phonological system into their linguistic system. Sounds which have been used accurately in babbling may not be correctly incorporated into linguistic sequences. Use of /k/ and /g/ may be heard in babbling but may not be used in phonemic sequences in words and phrases, /t/ and /d/ being substituted. Another child, aged 2 years 4 months, with advanced speech development, used 'kʌndi sku:l' for several weeks, when obviously able to use a normal /s/ in other words and in a blend. Without any known correction he changed to 'sʌndi sku:l' and probably without being aware that he had done so.

Similarly, the child is not consciously aware of linguistic rules governing syntax, yet he gradually acquires the ability to use language structure. Berko (1958) has shown that children can apply their developing appreciation of structure to such nonsense words as 'One is a Wug, now there are two, they are —? Wugs', and so forth.

The ability to tell a story or recount happenings, involving the description of events occurring in order of time sequence, marks a further stage in the development of speech, whilst Watts (1944) states that the ability to state clearly what follows logically from certain types of statement and to outline the pros and cons of an argument about familiar problems does not usually appear before the age of 14 years. True use of speech requires always that some meaning should be expressed, no matter how simple the form it may take, as in the expression of a simple need and as a means of communication with others.

The receptive and expressive aspects of spoken language may perhaps be illustrated by a diagram (Fig. 2a) representing some of the functions involved in speaking (Morley, 1959). This has been suggested by and deduced largely from clinical experience of breakdowns in the ability to use speech in children and adults, or of failure to develop spoken language in childhood.

At level I the child produces sounds, a cry or vocalisation. This is the level of basic sensation and primitive movements. Auditory, tactile and kinaesthetic sensory processes are involved in addition to movements of the muscles of the mouth, pharynx and larynx, the control of the movements being through the lower end of the motor cortex, pyramidal tract, upper and lower motor neuron pathways. So the child utters a sound, and, through the receptor processes, a feed-back circuit is established. At this level also the child may hear incoming sounds from another child or adult, a cry, vocalising and so forth, and may imitate these sounds which he hears, at the same time associating these sounds with his own sensory and motor experience.

At level II the child is beginning to discriminate and to recognise sounds, associating such sounds with objects—the door bell, the dog barking, or mother's voice. He is also developing the use of consonant sounds which he uses in babbling, and will do this spontaneously and imitate himself, or will respond to similar sounds made by others, again building up associations between what he hears from others and his own receptive-expressive behaviour. During this stage he is using a variety of vowel and consonant sounds, and is developing receptor and executive patterns, some of which will be required later for use in words, together with increasing control of the muscle movements and co-ordinations required in speech.

At level III the sounds used by others begin to have meaning for the child as the receptor processes for increasing comprehension for language gradually develop. Almost simultaneously use of words may occur, sometimes used with meaning and sometimes in the form of echolalia, but based on the previously acquired sensori-motor experience and acquired patterns of utterance. This stage is succeeded by the use of meaningful sequences of sounds to meet the developing need for expression of wants and thoughts through the processes involved in executive speech.

At Level IV the developing thought processes influence the knowledge acquired through receptor activity and the ever increasing expression of ideas through executive language. General intelligence is an important factor for this further stage of development of spoken language. It is probable that direct imitation at levels I and II occurs in children with subnormal intelligence, and to a limited extent at Level III. Direct imitation of sounds and words heard, or echolalia, whilst it is a stage in the normal development of speech, usually indicates some degree of mental retardation if it persists. Language is used to express thought, and where intelligence is limited both comprehension for spoken language and the use of expressive

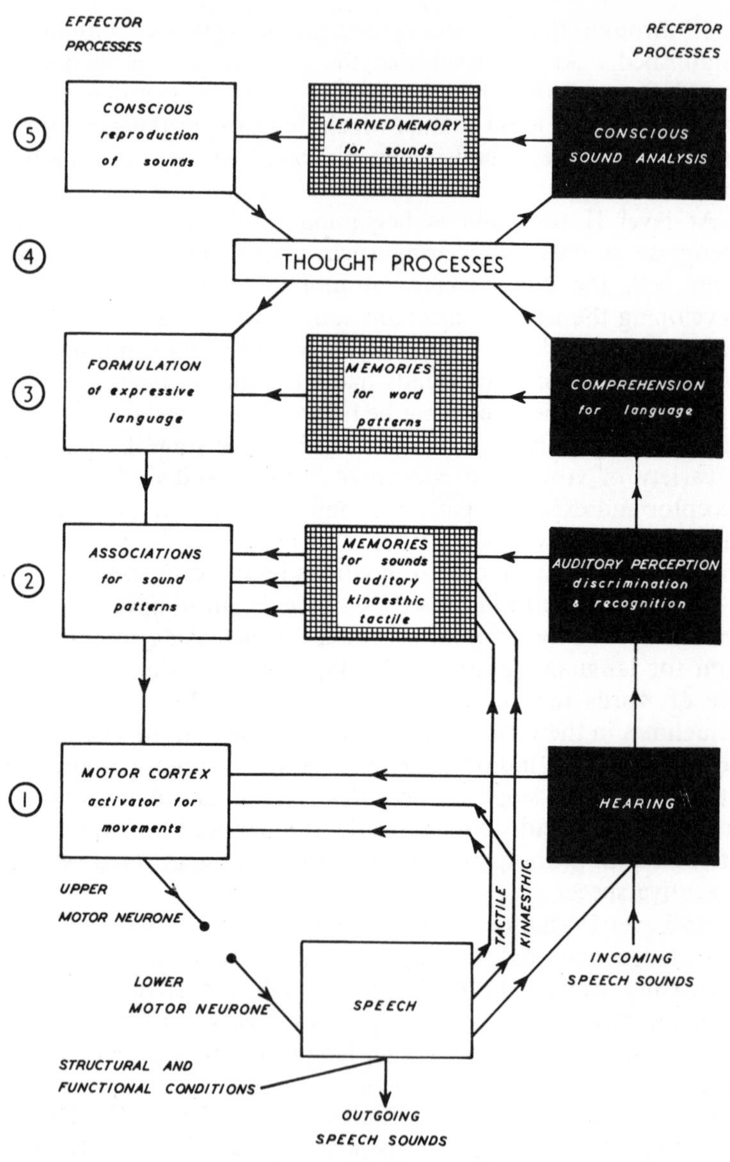

FIG. 2a

Some processes involved in speech.

Level I: Basic sensation and movements.

Level II: Receptor-effector processes for articulate sounds. Basic articulation.

Level III: Receptor-effector processes for integration of articulation with language.

Level IV: Mental processes associated with the reception and expression of thought through spoken language.

Level V: Involves conscious sound analysis and synthesis.

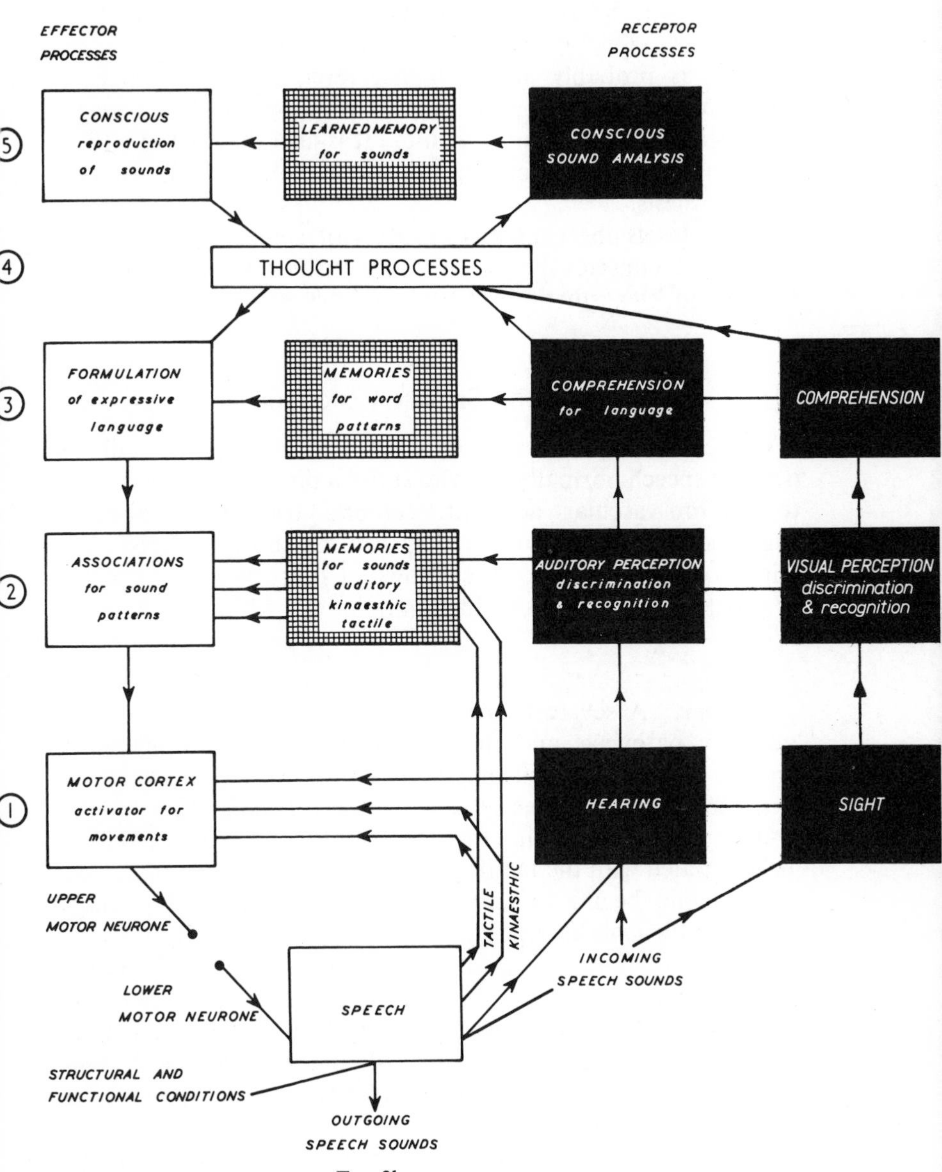

FIG. 2b

As Fig. 2a, but showing additional pathways.

language will be correspondingly limited in quality and in quantity.

There is probably also a higher level, Level V, which is dependant upon intelligence, and at which we learn a foreign language in school, or in later life. It is also the level at which one would study phonetics, using conscious sound analysis and synthesis.

At all levels the expressive aspects of spoken language are monitored consciously or subconsciously through auditory, tactile and kinaesthetic feed-back sensory processes.

Disorders of Spoken Language

Clinical experience with children and adults who fail to develop speech normally, or who suffer a disorder of speech due to cerebro-vascular accident, cerebral trauma or disease, suggests that such a disorder of speech may be considered as a failure of development or breakdown of function at some point or points indicated on the diagram.

Level I.

Sensory. A severe hearing loss would effectively block the auditory pathways and prevent the normal development of speech. The visual sensory pathway, shown on the diagram (Fig. 2b), would be used as a substitute for the auditory pathway or jointly with it, and these sensory impressions would then be associated with the tactile and kinaesthetic afferent pathways as the child begins to understand some speech and perhaps to speak through lip-reading.

Motor. A failure here would affect the basic muscle movements and co-ordinations for articulation, and in severe cases, for sucking and swallowing. Due to brain damage or neurological disease muscle tone is affected, and there may be degrees of spasticity, flaccidity, athetosis affecting not only the muscles of the tongue, lips and soft palate, but also those of the larynx for phonation and those for respiration, with their complex co-ordinations. Ability to reproduce vocal and articulate sounds may be normal apart from the ability to make the requisite movements at the speed required for conversational speech.

The resulting speech disorder is then described as anarthria or dysarthria.

Level II.

Sensory. A partial hearing loss would cause some degree of defective auditory discrimination and recognition for the sounds used in speech. This will affect comprehension and articulation. The child will hear the sounds of speech in a distorted way, and will imitate them as he hears them.

It is also possible that there may be some degree of auditory imperception when hearing for pure tones on audiometric assessment is normal, and that this may contribute to a disorder of articulation. However, it is difficult to prove this in the young child, the tests requiring a certain level of intellectual development, and training in the processes involved in testing, which are not normal to the young child. It may be that this condition is the result of some limitation of auditory memory rather than of discrimination.

Motor. A defect of articulation at this level is one of failure to reproduce accurately, in the correct sequence, the articulate sounds as used in speech. In the developmental condition in children it chiefly affects the use of consonant sounds, but vowel sounds may also be defective. In the adult with the acquired disorder, vowel sounds tend to return before consonant sounds, use of vowel sounds being associated mainly with Level I and consonants with Level II. In the developmental condition there may be limitation of the consonant sounds acquired with omissions and substitutions. These may be consistent or erratic. There may also be failure to use vowel and consonant sounds in correct sequence in words, when the individual sounds can be produced normally, e.g. 'bilikses' for 'bicycle'. This disorder of speech has been described as dyspraxia, or articulatory dyspraxia. In the acquired condition in adults or children it may be found in isolation, but is more usually associated with some degree of expressive dysphasia. Where it is found as a developmental disorder in children there is frequently some delay in the initial onset of the use of language, and also a limitation of vocal play and babbling.

Level III.

Sensory. A failure to develop normal understanding for spoken language in childhood, or developmental receptive aphasia, is rare, but when it occurs it is a severe condition, limiting the use of spoken language, in our experience, throughout life. The expressive speech used is limited, and is frequently jargon, perhaps because it cannot be monitored adequately, resulting in expressive aphasia. Articulation may be normal in the speech used, indicating that there may be no failure of auditory perception, or there may be mispronunciation of words in consecutive speech when reproduction of isolated words is normal. In the acquired condition there is again a limitation of understanding for spoken language. The extent of the condition varies according to the underlying damage, and again executive speech is frequently jargon.

Motor. A developmental expressive aphasia is found in children when understanding for language would appear to be adequate. It is possible that in some children there may have been some delay in understanding in the first two years of life, and the mother's story sometimes indicates that these children were at first thought to be deaf. However, the normal range for speech development is wide, from eight months for the first use of words to three and a half years for the first use of simple phrases (ref. p. 45). A failure to use expressive language by the age of four and a half years therefore constitutes a delay. If the use of language is developing by six years of age the condition may be described as a transient expressive aphasia, but if there is further delay beyond this age the diagnosis of some degree of expressive aphasia is probable, if intelligence and hearing are normal. (See p. 155).

Because intelligence is adequate these children can usually learn in school, although ability to express themselves in spoken and written language will be delayed and limited. In the acquired condition, in childhood or adult life, an expressive aphasia is usually associated with some degree of receptive aphasia, and perhaps with dyspraxia or dysarthria as some speech returns.

Each of these conditions has been briefly described in isolation, but as they result from cerebral damage or dysfunction the effect on the use of spoken or written language will be dependant upon the extent of the underlying condition and may cause more than one type of speech disorder.

Structural conditions and defects, such as cleft palate, interfere with ability to produce the articulate sounds clearly and normally in the mouth and are due to peripheral conditions not necessarily related to cerebral dysfunction. However, it must be remembered that a child may have a disorder of speech such as dysphasia or dyspraxia in addition to a structural abnormality, and that a speech defect in a child with abnormal nasopharyngeal occlusion, or a successfully operated cleft palate, may not always be the result of the anatomical condition.

Dyslalia. We have reserved this term for those defects of articulation occurring in early childhood, and which resolve spontaneously as use of language progresses, or where function is normal but there has been imitation of defective articulation of another child or adult.

Emotional states may affect the whole of the receptive and expressive aspects of speech at any or all levels, causing an effective barrier to comprehension for speech, and inhibition for the use of expressive speech, perhaps causing retardation of speech development. The speech of the child with autistic behaviour is affected because he lacks desire to make contact with others in any way, including speech, whilst the pre-psychotic child may use incomprehensible speech. Neurotic and psychotic conditions also affect the speech used by adults. Communication with others is impaired, including the use of speech as a means of communication. In some there may be hysterical aphonia, or there may be maluse of voice, resulting in dysphonia due to generalised strain or nervous tension.

Non-fluency or stammering may be evident temporarily, or may be more prolonged if environmental stresses are present. The developing co-ordinations for speech are unstable, and anything affecting neuromuscular tensions and control may affect use of speech in its formative stages. Such a disorder is not essentially a disorder of language nor of articulation, but there is some evidence to suggest that stammering may be associated with some delay in the establishment of normal articulation in some children (see p. 69), possibly relating to some delay in establishment of the neuromuscular mechanisms for speech.

Retarded mental development affects the understanding for speech, and the thought processes involved in the acquisition of an ever increasing vocabulary related to learning and experience. Intelligence also determines the use of spoken language to express increasingly complicated and abstract ideas, or the ability to learn and to use a foreign language.

The use of written language and the ability to read are not represented here to avoid over complication of the diagram. But at Level I there would be vision and on the motor side ability to use the hand for making marks and to use a pencil or crayon for scribbling or simple drawing.

At Level II visual discrimination for symbols develops and there is visual memory for the symbols used in writing and ability to copy. Levels III and IV would represent comprehension for written language through reading, and ability to express thoughts in writing. Spelling would be dependant upon auditory and visual memory for the sequences of sounds or written symbols in words.

This diagram must represent an over simplification of the complexities of the varying conditions affecting use of spoken language, although it may be a useful guide in diagnosis. There are also many individual differences and it must be remembered that it is the patient with the speech disorder who must be considered and his difficulty in communicating with others through the use of spoken language.

If, therefore, there should be delay or failure of development at some point in the neurophysiological processes required for speech, there will be some form of speech disorder which will interfere with the ability to communicate with others. The extent of these disorders will vary at different age levels and in different communities.

Reynell (1969) also describes the development, and the conditions essential for the development of language. First, there must be adequate experience of the mode of communication through speech; secondly, an intact sensory channel by which the experiences may reach the child, visual, tactile, auditory or other senses; thirdly, there must be ability to appreciate meaningful patterns in the stimulus which may be spatial or temporal; fourthly, the incorporation of meaningful patterns of stimulii into existing concepts: generalisation, classification and other modes of interrelation of concepts occur. These four stages complete the processes involved in the reception of language to the incorporation of receptive language into thought. Stages five to seven are directly involved in language expression. At stage 5, thought processes are encoded into a symbolic form. Stage 6 involves the peripheral aspects of expression, that is the co-ordinated movements for articulate speech, whilst stage 7 is concerned with opportunities for communication (Fig. 3 and Fig. 4). Figure 5 shows the

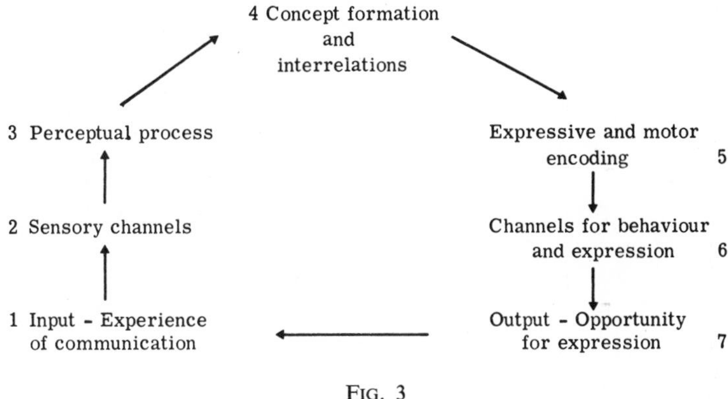

FIG. 3

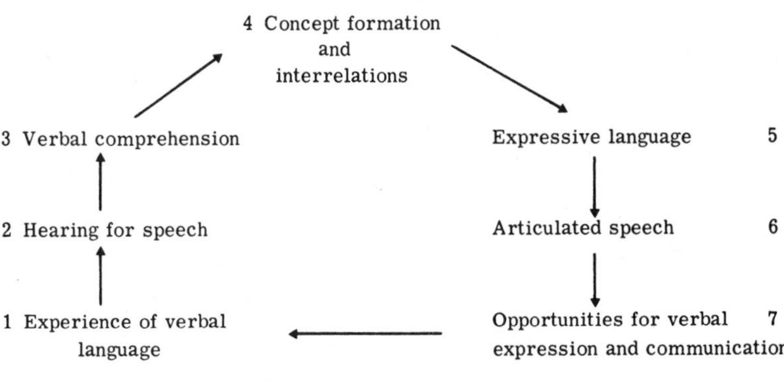

FIG. 4

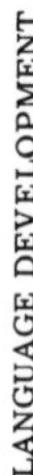

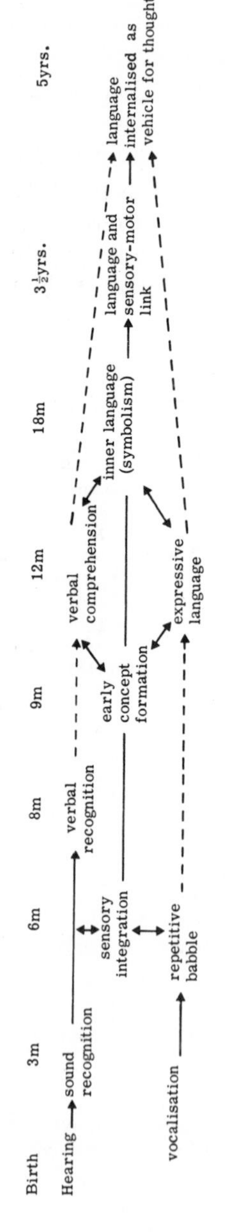

USE OF LANGUAGE

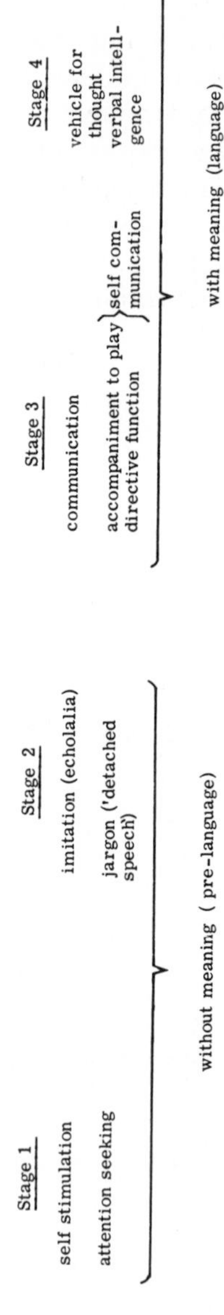

FIG. 5

progress of language development and four stages in the use of speech. Reynell suggests that each aspect of language must be seen in relation to the total language development, so that the interplay of all facets may be understood. This, she thinks, is particularly important in therapy with very young children when the developmental pattern is incomplete, so that there is then no emphasis upon one aspect of verbal language without reference to the whole.

The Incidence of Speech Disorders

In 1945, in a County Borough with a total school population of 12,200 we found that the incidence of defective speech was 3 per cent. Two per cent had defects of articulation, 0·7 per cent stammered, 0·2 per cent had defective use of speech associated with mental retardation and 0·1 per cent had sundry defects of speech. These included nine children with cleft palate speech, four who were partially deaf, two with dysphonia and one who had a developmental aphasia.

In addition, 92 children were referred by the teachers to the speech therapist but were found to have poor diction and no true disorder of speech. The proportion of these children was 0·8 per cent. Most of this poor speech was the result of environment with inadequate speech patterns in the home and poor use of tongue and lip movements when speaking. Such children require speech training, as carried out regularly in many schools, rather than speech therapy.

The mentally retarded children were being educated in the normal school at that time. Use of language was limited, and in some there was also defective articulation.

Thirty-four of the 87 stammerers were considered to have only a slight disability, but the remaining 53 were in need of immediate treatment.

One hundred and eight of the 273 children with defective articulation had such a severe disability that progress in school was being hindered.

Wohl (1951) in a similar investigation in the County of Dunbarton in 1951 found among 20,000 schoolchildren that 12 per cent suffered from some form of speech defect. Of these,

1·3 per cent were stammerers, 2·4 per cent were aphonic or dysphonic, 0·7 per cent had cleft palate and 7·7 per cent had other speech defects mainly of a dyslalic nature. These figures are considerably higher than those already mentioned and may have included many minimal defects of articulation.

The Study and Treatment of Disorders of Speech

In treating a disorder of speech we must, perforce, endeavour to treat something which as yet we do not fully understand. Through gradual increase of knowledge of the neurological processes involved, from careful personal observation and clinical experience our understanding of the problems and uncertainties will grow and widen. Knowledge has no finality. What we accept as true to-day is tentative, and may be proved false or incomplete to-morrow. The student of speech disorders, as of other sciences, must always be ready to consider and test the truth of such existing knowledge and beware of generalisations which do not agree with experience. He must be ready to change his opinion and continually discard ideas which are no longer valid in the light of further experience.

It is human nature to desire and seek for generalisations, and we tend therefore to see only what will give support to our theories and to neglect what does not. By so doing we distort our observations and hinder our search for reality. Accurate clinical evidence must be founded on careful observations of the facts and assessed with an ever-open and critical mind which is always willing to discard what is found to be false. But the facts as we observe them are personal to ourselves and are determined by our own experience and capacity to observe accurately and draw logical conclusions. They do not depend only on the object of our observations and the conditions under which we observe. The late Sir James Spence (1953) described clinical observation as 'the craftsman's skill in seeing quickly what he knows to be significant . . . It is the product not of guessing but of a sifted experience by which the significant is recognised with such rapidity that the steps of reasoning are not discernible to the uninitiated.' The student may learn much and better appreciate the nature of learning if he reads some of the history of medical science and of how information has been won through careful laborious and honest study based on accurate observation. Much that has been said has been forgotten, but the essential truths, however simple, persist and are substantiated through experience. Theories and generalisations, therefore, are not put forward here as finality but as hypotheses for criticism and for the opinion of others. They are not stated as essential truths but to be subjected to constant testing and examination in the light of continuing clinical experience, as we aim to approach as far as we are able towards reality.

Spence (1953) described 'clinical science' firstly as the planned study of disease, and its aim as 'to know disease in such a way as to enable us to infer its cause and to predict its course'. This involves the planned study of the disease, or speech disorder, in a number of persons, its cause, duration and final outcome, leading to a basis of knowledge and ability to advise or plan a course of therapy.

'The second kind of clinical science ... studies the phenomena of disease or disordered function and its aim is to explain their mechanism and their clinical significance.' This may be applied to the detailed study of a particular type of disorder of speech, and such knowledge will increase our understanding of the condition and may lead to further knowledge and discovery.

The objects of clinical research he defined as the discovery or decisive clarification of knowledge which involves 'clinical observation planned to answer a carefully prepared question. The plan is controlled by well-known criteria: (*a*) that the question is worth answering, (*b*) that it has not already been answered by someone else, (*c*) that a plan of observation can be designed which is likely to provide an answer to the question, and (*d*) that the observer is the sort of man who will carry out the plan.'

Although some of our time must be occupied with the clarification of thought and growth of knowledge, as therapists we are concerned primarily with the *patient* who has a speech disorder, and not only with the disorder itself. Because of the universal need and use of speech, the patient who has difficulty in communicating with others through spoken language will also experience some disability in his personal and social relationships. Speech therapy does not consist merely in the correction of speech, in the substitution of one phonetic element for another, but in treating the patient as a whole. An understanding of his own reactions and those of others to his speech disorder, the nature of his occupation, his age, his environment and his personality are all factors to be considered. The speech disorder will always be considered in so far as it interferes with the mental well-being and adjustment of the individual to his environment. Speech therapy is not concerned with dialectal variations unless they present a problem which the individual is unable to solve himself. Neither is it concerned necessarily with exact phonetic articulation. The need of the individual is to be able to communicate with others through intelligible speech, and under certain conditions a minor defect of which the patient is unaware may be allowed to persist. For anatomical or other reasons, accurate articulation of the true phonetic sound may not be easy and a defective consonant sound difficult to eradicate in an adult with long-established patterns of articulation. If intelligibility is not hindered, and it does not attract undue attention from others, it may be wise under certain conditions to allow it to persist.

In the young child, time and opportunity must always be allowed for any material and spontaneous improvement which may occur, therapy being required only under conditions where the child's speech is inadequate for his personal and social needs, where he is aware of, and concerned about his speech disorder, or when the child's difficulty fails to be understood and accepted by those in his environment.

The findings in this book are put forward as the outcome of over 30 years' experience and practice in the treatment of disorders of speech. A certain number of statistics are inevitable to substantiate the statements which are made, although it is appreciated that too many figures may lead to a precise assessment of human beings which is unreal and at times remote from true clinical findings in individual children, and may even distort rather than clarify the truth.

Walshe (1948) has said,

> For too many amongst us, also, the inadequate conception that science is measurement and concerns itself with nothing but the metrical has become a thought-cramping obsession, and the more a scientific paper approximates to a long and bloodless caravan of equations plodding across the desert pages of some journal between

small and infrequent oases of words, the more quintessentially scientific it is supposed to be, though not seldom no one can tell—and few are interested to ask—whither in the kingdom of ordered knowledge the caravan is bound. Whatever may be true of the physical sciences, the day is not arrived when all the truths of medicine and biology can be reduced to this bleak residue.

The figures in this book are to be considered as a guide to what may be expected under conditions similar to those under which they were obtained and do not express finality. It is hoped that what is here described may arouse a desire in others to evaluate the findings, disprove what may not be true, and form a basis on which others may continue to build in the light of further knowledge.

REFERENCES

Berko, J. (1958). The Child's Learning of English Morphology. *Word*, **14**, 50.

Brain, R. (1961). Neurology of Language. *Speech Path. and Therapy*, **4**, No. 2.

Bühler, C., and Hetzer, H. (1928). Das erste Verständnis für Ausdruck im ersten Lebensjahr. *Psychol.* **97**, as summarised by Lewis, M. M. (1936) in *Infant Speech*. London, Kegan Paul.

Cherry, C. (1957). *On Human Communication.* Cambridge, Mass., M.I.T. Press.

Chomsky, N. (1957). *Syntactic Structures.* Mouton, The Hague.

Chomsky, N. (1959). Review of *Verbal Behaviour* by B. F. Skinner, *Language*, **35**, 26.

Chomsky, N., and Katz, J. (1964). *The Structure of Language.* Ed. J. A. Foder. Englewood Cliffs, New Jersey, Prentice Hall.

Corder, P. S. (1966). Linguistics and Speech Therapy. *Brit. J. Dis. Commun. I*, **2**, 119.

Cruttendon, A. (1970). A Phonetic Study of Babbling. *Brit. J. Dis. Commun. V*, **2**, 110.

Fraser, C., Bellugi, U., and Brown, R. (1963). Control of grammar in imitation, comprehension and production. *J. Verb. Learn. Verb. Behav.*, **2**, 121.

Fry, D. B. (1957). *Jour. Laryng. Otol. LXXI*, **7**, 434.

Fry, D. B. (1966). The Development of the Phonological System in the Normal and the Deaf Child. In Smith, F., and Miller, G. A., *The Genesis of Language*, 187–206. M.I.T. Press.

Fry, D. B. (1968). The Phonemic System in Children's Speech. *Brit. J. Dis. Commun. III*, **1**, 13.

Gleason, H. A. (1955). *Introduction to Descriptive Linguistics.* New York, Henry Holt.

Haas, W. (1968). Functional Phonetics and Speech Therapy. *Brit. J. Dis. Commun. III*, **1,** 20.

Lenneberg, E. H. (1967). *The Biological Foundation of Language.* New York, Wiley.

Liebermann, A. M., Delattre, P., and Cooper, F. S. (1952). *Amer. J. Psychol.*, **65,** 497.

Luria, A. R., and Vinograd, O. S. (1959).

Luria, A. R., and Yudovich, F. (1959). *Speech and the Development of Mental Processes in the Child.* Ed. J. Simon. London, Staples Press.

McNeill, D. (1966). The Creation of Language. *Discovery*, **27,** 7, 34.

Mecham, —. *et al.* (1951). *Developmental Psycholinguistics in the Genesis of Language.* Eds. F. Smith, and G. A. Miller. Camb., Mass., M.I.T. Press.

Miller, G. A. (1951). *Language and Communication.* New York, McGraw Hill.

Morley, M., Court, D., Miller, H., and Garside, R. (1955). Delayed Speech and Developmental Aphasia. *Brit. Med. Jour.*, **2,** 463.

Morley, M. E. (1959). Defects of Articulation. *Folia Phoniatrica XI*, 1–3.

Morley, M. E., and Fox, J. (1969). Disorders of Articulation: Theory and Therapy. *Brit. J. Dis. Commun. IV*, **2,** 151.

Mowrer, O. H. (1950). Learning Theory and Personality Dynamics. *Selected Papers.* New York, Ronald Press.

Myklebust, H. M. (1957). Babbling and Echolalia in Language Theory. *J. Speech and Hear. Dis.*, **22,** 3, 356.

Mysak, E. E. (1966). *Speech Pathology and Feedback Theory.* Illinois, C. C. Thomas.

Reynell, J. (1969). A Developmental Approach to Language Disorders. *Brit. J. Dis. Commun. IV*, **1,** 33.

Sheridan, M. D. (1959). The Development of Speech and Hearing in Young Children. *Med. Press.*, Aug. 19th, 147.

Sherrington, C. S. (1947). *Integrative Action of the Nervous System.* Camb. Univ. Press.

Spence, J. C. (1953). Methodology of Clinical Science. *Lancet*, **2,** 629.

Teuber, H. L. (1960). Perception. In J. Field, H. W. Magoun and V. R. Hall (eds.), *Handbook of Physiology, Sect. I Neurophysiology, Vol. III.* Washington, D.C., American Physiological Society.

Vygotsky, L. S. (1934, trs. 1962). *Thought and Language.* Ed. and Trs. E. Haufmann and G. Vakar. Cambridge, Mass., M.I.T. Press.

Watts, A. F. (1944). *Language and Mental Development of Children.* London, Harrap.

Walshe, F. M. R. (1948). *Critical Studies in Neurology.* Edinburgh, Livingstone.

Wingfield, A. (1969). Methodology in Psycholinguistics Research. *Brit. J. Dis. Commun. IV*, **2,** 117.

Wohl, M. T. (1951). The Incidence of Speech Defects in the Population. *Speech*, **15,** 1, 13.

PART I

THE DEVELOPMENT OF SPEECH IN THE COMMUNITY

A Study of the Speech Development of the Children in 1000 Families in Newcastle-upon-Tyne

II. The Method of Investigation

THE speech therapist, spending much time working with children and adults who have defective speech, may lose a sense of proportion as to the relative importance of disorders of speech in the whole community; one's view may become somewhat distorted and one may even come to regard as a disorder what may well be within the range of normal. We were fortunate, therefore, that during the years 1950 to 1956 we were invited to study the speech development in a group of children representative of all social classes with young families in the city of Newcastle-upon-Tyne. The Child Health Department of the University of Durham and the Health Services of the city combined in an investigation to gain information and experience concerning the diseases and disorders of early childhood by means of a family survey. This survey was based on all children born within the city in May and June 1947 and is still continuing in 1956. The original number of children was 1142, but through deaths and removals the number in 1950 was 944, and in 1952, 847. Information concerning the first year of life has already been published (Spence *et al.*, 1954).

The speech of these children was investigated when they were between three and a half years and three years ten months, in 1951, and again at the ages of four years nine months, six and a half years and nine and a half years, in 1952, 1954 and 1956, the assessment being carried out by speech therapists in the children's homes.

The factors in speech development which were specially noted were the age at which speech developed, the standard of language ability, defects of articulation based on a phonetic analysis, the range and type of tongue movements, and the presence of stammering. The information gained was later analysed in relation to sex, position in family, social status and environmental and emotional factors.

Procedure

In carrying out this investigation it was not practicable to visit every child, and a sample of the whole was obtained by taking every tenth child of the original group of 1142 children, in order of registration. This provided a sample group of 114 children who at that time were aged three and a half years.

In addition, a preliminary survey of all the children was undertaken by the team of health visitors who were making frequent routine visits to the homes of the children. They were asked to report on three simple questions: (1) Does the child speak? (2) Is he or she intelligible to strangers? and (3) Does the mother think the child's speech is normal? The health visitors' observations on the speech of the child were also recorded.

When the speech investigation commenced, 944 of the original 1142 children remained in the survey. Excluding 114 of these who formed the sample group, the remaining 830 were classified on the reports of the health visitors as follows:

Normal speech development . . .	625
Defective speech development . . .	193
Stammering	12
	830
Sample Group	114
	944

The 625 children who were reported to have satisfactory speech development were not visited, and of the 193 whose speech was regarded as defective, 29 had defective articulation of the consonants [th] and/or [r] only. At three and a half years of age such a defect in isolation was considered to be within the range of normal development, and these children were excluded from the group with defective speech who were visited, leaving 164.

The speech of 278 children was therefore assessed by the speech therapists when visiting the homes of the children; 114 of these were in the sample group, and 164 were considered by the parents or the health visitors to have defective development of speech.

In addition, twelve children were reported initially to have some lack of fluency during the development and stabilisation of speech. The children whose speech was to be assessed could therefore be grouped as follows:

Sample Group	114
Delayed development of speech or defective articulation	164
Stammering	12
	290

At what age do children begin to speak?

In assessing the age at which a child began to use speech we were largely dependent on the mother's memory and the routine reports of the health visitors, as most of the children were already using speech to some extent at the time of the first visit when they were aged three years nine months. The mother's observations and memory are often unreliable and may be unduly optimistic, and it was unfortunate that an earlier survey had not been possible. There is here a possible source of error, but in the majority the mother's story correlated closely with the health visitors' reports, and the findings are also substantiated by general clinical experience.

We chose as stages in the development of speech the ages when (1) words were first used with meaning, (2) the child first used two or three words in sequence in simple phrases or sentences and (3) the child's speech was intelligible.

The first words used by the child with meaning are often remembered by the mother as a landmark in development, and she was frequently able to fix the time of this occurrence by its association with some family event such as a summer holiday, or a visit to a relative. The first words used by a child are often 'mum', 'up', 'bye bye' and so forth, and such simple words may be used for several weeks or even months before there is a period of more rapid growth of vocabulary.

The age at which the child ceased to use single words and made use of two- or three-word phrases was also noted. Although providing a less definite landmark, the mother could usually fix the time within one or two months. In some children this stage had not been reached at the time of our first visit, and we were able to assess it personally.

We also wished to know at what age the child's speech became intelligible to others. This could only be assessed when the child had developed the use of word sequences, as simple, single words are usually clear, or at least intelligible to the mother. Many children are intelligible from the inception of speech, and remain so, but it is known that others pass through a period when articulation is defective and often unintelligible, especially to strangers. It may be that language development has outstripped the accurate use of articulation, but constant substitutions and omissions are common and are the cause of varying degrees of unintelligible speech. In most cases another child or the mother can interpret such speech, the father is less likely to be able to do so, and to strangers the speech is unintelligible. This was our basis for the definition of 'unintelligible speech'. We wished to know (1) what proportion of children pass through such a stage and (2) how long it usually persists. Although an analysis of the articulation was based on the use of consonants in single words, intelligibility was assessed on the use of longer sequences of sounds in phrases and sentences.

The standard of language development

At the time of the first visit we also attempted to ascertain the standard of the language as used in conversational speech and when saying nursery rhymes. We wished to know what proportion of children used fluent speech and well-constructed sentences, and in how many there was a poverty of expressive language although the stage had been reached at which simple word sequences were being used.

Articulation

During the development of speech a number of children passed through a period when speech was not fully intelligible. This was usually the result of inaccurate use of consonants rather than of vowels, and a phonetic analysis of each child's speech was carried out at the time of the three visits at three years nine months, four years nine months and at six and a half years.

Tongue movements

Clinical observations indicate that in many children movements of the tongue are difficult or limited in extent. Some are unable to elevate the tip towards the nose and have difficulty in pointing it when protruded. Lateral movements may be slow or difficult, and the child may move the whole head when attempting to waggle the tongue from side to side, or assist elevation of the tip with the fingers, or by pushing upwards with the lower lip. We were interested to know if there was any significant relationship between defective articulation and such movements of the tongue.

Stammering

During the development of speech many children pass through a period when there is some interference with the fluent utterance of speech. We attempted to trace the parents' attitude to this difficulty and to ascertain the time of onset, the duration of the speech disability and the eventual outcome as related to the use of speech in these children.

CLASSIFICATION OF FINDINGS

The findings were ascertained and will be described for two main groups of children.

1. *The sample group.* In this group of 114 children each child was seen for detailed assessment whether speech was normal or defective. From these findings we gained a picture of the normal range of speech development in a representative sample of children.

2. *A group of* 181 *children with some disorder of speech development.* In the whole group of 944 children, 181 were found to have some disorder in the development of speech persisting at least until the age of three years nine months. These included delayed development of speech, defective articulation and stammering. No child had a severe degree of dysarthria and one child who was born with a cleft palate had developed speech normally following surgical repair. This group includes all children with defective development of speech whether found in the sample group or among the remainder of the 944 children, and includes 162 children who had varying degrees of defective articulation at three years nine months. Twelve children had been reported as having hesitant speech or stammering, but during the period of investigation 25 other

children were found who had some degree of stammering, that is a total of 37 children. Eighteen of these children also had defects of articulation and are therefore included among the children who had defective development of speech apart from, or in addition to, stammering.

From this group of children two smaller groups emerged. Firstly, we found 44 children with such severe defects of articulation that unintelligible speech persisted until the time of entry into school at five years of age. We have considered various factors in relation to their development of speech, as it was thought possible that such a severe speech disorder might differ in its underlying aetiology from that of children with a more transient disorder of articulation.

Secondly, in this group of 181 children we found 37 already mentioned who had a temporary or more persistent episode of stammering during the development of speech. Eighteen of these children also had defects of articulation. The speech of these 37 children who experienced some interference with its fluent utterance will also be described and its relationship to other factors.

Defects of speech at three years nine months could therefore be classified as follows:

Delayed development of speech		5	
Resolving defects of articulation		95	
Severe, persistent defects of articulation		44	162
Defective articulation and stammering	37	18	
Stammering only		19	19
			181

Our findings will be described for the following four groups of children:

114 children in the sample group.
162 in the whole group of 944 children who had varying degrees of defective articulation.
44 children who had severe and persistent defects of articulation, and
37 who encountered a period of hesitant speech or stammering.

In an investigation such as this many human factors are involved whose influence cannot be assessed. They affect both the response of the child and the judgment of the investigator. We have found, however, that this survey has given us a wider view of speech development and a fuller appreciation as to what we may expect to be within the range of normality.

REFERENCE

Spence, J. C., Walton, W. S., Miller, F. J. W., and Court, S. D. M. (1954). *A Thousand Families in Newcastle upon Tyne.* Durham Univ. Press.

III. The Development of Normal Speech

OUR findings concerning the development of speech will be described for those 114 children who form the sample group, giving a picture of what one could expect to find in a representative group of children, including the age range for the first use of speech and defects occurring during its development. The information obtained at the time of the first visit when the children were aged three years nine months has already been described by Ann Tattersfield, who assisted me in this investigation in 1951 and 1952 (Tattersfield, 1952).

THE AGE OF SPEECH DEVELOPMENT

Single words used with meaning

As described, we used as our first landmark in the development of speech the age at which the child first used one or two simple words with meaning. We found that the peak period was from 9 to 12 months when 66 per cent of these children are said to have first used single words as distinct from the usual babble utterances of infancy. The average age for the first use of words in this group of children was 12 months, but the age range extended from 6 to 30 months. By the time of their first birthday 73 per cent were using at least a few words to express their wants. A few children (seven per cent) were said to have done so before the age of eight months, and two per cent were late in beginning to speak and did not attempt to use words until they were over two years of age (Fig. 6). (Appendix, Table I).

The use of word sequences, phrases and sentences

The child passes from the use of one word with expressive gesture to the use of sequences of consonant and vowel sounds of varying length, and to the introduction into his speech of other words than nouns and proper names. These appeared mainly in the second half of the second year, 40 per cent of the children in the sample group reaching this stage at or around the age of 18 months, or 67 per cent between the ages of 17 and 24 months. By two years of age 89 per cent were using at least simple word sequences, and all but one child had achieved this level of speech development by three years of age. Nine per cent of the children were reported to have used phrases before they were 12 months old, but at this early age it is possible that such phrases were only the echo-like reproduction of sequences of sound often heard. In one child the words spoken were

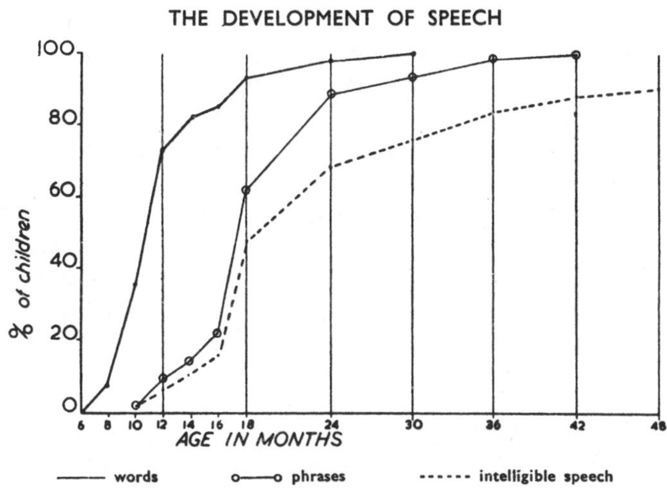

Fig. 6
Showing the growth in the use of words, phrases and intelligible speech in the 114 children in the sample group.

'Get down, Bobby' to the dog, and in another 'Up with your pants!' The average age at which these children first used word sequences was 18 months, and the age range was from 10 to 44 months (Fig. 6) (Appendix, Table I). All the children in this group were thought to have intelligence within the normal range, and we found no child with a severe delay in the development of speech beyond four years of age, or developmental aphasia.

Intelligibility

Although aware that many children encountered difficulties in the use of normal articulation, we found that a larger proportion of children passed through a period when speech was more unintelligible than we had expected. In the sample group two-thirds of the children were easily intelligible from the inception of speech, but the remaining one-third passed through a period when the speech they used was not intelligible (Fig. 6). It is also probable that in those said to be intelligible there may have been a transient use of unintelligible words or phrases, but this was not remembered by the mother and is therefore of little importance in the general picture of speech development. Most children have a few words of their own, or temporarily mispronounce words, but in many children the development of accurate articulation keeps pace with the growth of language.

In this group of children 69 per cent were intelligible to strangers by two years of age and 84 per cent at three years of age. Four children were still using unintelligible speech on entry into school at five years of age, and one was still unintelligible to his teacher and to strangers at six and a half years. These figures do not include children with lesser degrees of defective articulation where speech was intelligible. The average age for the acquisition of intelligible speech was two years (Fig. 6) (Appendix, Table I).

Relapsing articulation

During the gradual improvement of intelligibility, whilst newly developed patterns of articulation were still unstable, it was found that many children with apparently normal speech relapsed into their former patterns of defective articulation at times of excitement, emotional stress, or when self-conscious. Three children with normal use of articulation at six and a half years of age still had periods of such relapsing articulation, and this was also found among other children who had passed through a period of defective articulation. It persisted for varying lengths of time, and general experience suggests that this is a stage through which all such children may pass in their progress towards normal articulation.

Our findings therefore confirm the usually accepted age for the development of speech, that single words are first used at or about one year and sentences between the ages of 18 months and two years. Three per cent of the children were unable to use intelligible speech just before the age for entering school in addition to others with less severe defects of articulation. Such speech can be a source of difficulty and embarrassment to the five-year-old child, and if it persists to six or seven years it can be a serious handicap to educational progress in school.

Although these findings describe the general progress of speech development, they should not be taken to imply that language development proceeded at a steady and measurable rate. Words were used and lost again; and there were silent periods when little progress occurred. In some children words appeared and were quickly followed by the use of phrases and sentences, whilst in others there were long intervals of delay, in some children from 10 to 24 months after the use of single words before word sequences appeared, the average time being around six months. Two children used no words before two years of age, but phrases and sentences followed quickly, and both were using adequate speech at three and a half years of age.

There was a wide range of normality in the use of speech in this random sample of children. All but one were using intelligible speech at six and a half years, yet the age for the onset of the use of single words ranged from eight months to two and a half years, and for word sequences from ten months to three and a half years.

The Standard of Language Ability at the end of the Fourth Year

An attempt was made at the time of the first visit to ascertain the standard of language development as used in conversational speech and when saying nursery rhymes. Many children are too shy to speak freely before a stranger at this age, but we found that if attention was directed away from the child, as during conversation with the mother, he or she might be overheard speaking naturally. For others a picture book provided the requisite stimulus, and the speech of some was assessed whilst they were playing with other children in the road or garden. At this age also many children enjoy repeating nursery rhymes, and such repetition provided a useful opportunity for an assessment of the fluency with which words can be used in sequences under such conditions.

The child's use of language was graded as follows:

Sentences

A. Fluent and well-constructed sentences.

B. Minor defects of language, e.g. 'me' for 'I', as in 'Me did it', and so forth.

C. Sentences incomplete, with inversions or transposition of words, but adequate for meaning.

D. Limited and poor use of language. No complete sentences, but single words or short phrases used, often accompanied by gesture.

E. Not heard or uncertain, and not classified.

Rhymes

The use of rhymes was assessed as follows:

A. Says several rhymes without prompting.
B. Requires some prompting.
C. Repeats rhymes line by line or finishes each line only.
D. Can say no rhymes.
E. Uncertain or not heard.

Use of sentences

At three years nine months. As described, 89 per cent of the children in this group had begun to put two or three words together by two years of age, and at the time of the first visit at three years nine months all were using at least a few words in sequence. Sixty-three per cent of the children were using adequate sentences, 31 per cent had only minor errors in construction irrespective of the articulation used, five per cent were using incomplete sentences and one per cent only occasionally used one or two words in sequence. Six per cent therefore had a definite retardation in the use of language at this age (Fig. 7) (Appendix, Table VI).

At four years nine months. At the time of the second visit all but one of the children in the group were expressing themselves in useful sentences. Eighty-eight per cent were using fluent speech, 11 per cent had minor defects in the use of sentences, and only one child was using incomplete sentences (Appendix, Table VI).

Repetition of rhymes

The fluency in the use of words when repeating nursery rhymes is shown in Figure 8. At three years nine months 53 per cent of the children heard could repeat such rhymes fluently, whilst at four years nine months 77 per cent were able to do so (Appendix, Table VI).

LANGUAGE ABILITY

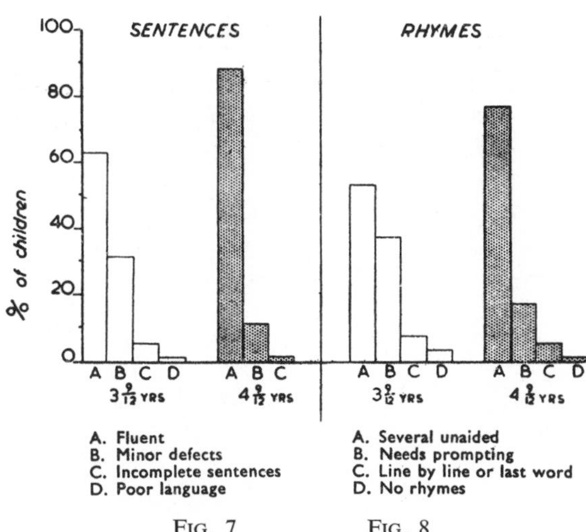

FIG. 7 FIG. 8

Showing the standard of language ability as assessed by the use of sentences, and the fluency in the use of words when repeating nursery rhymes, in 114 children in the sample group at two age levels.

DEFECTS OF ARTICULATION

A phonetic analysis of each child's speech was carried out at the time of the three visits at the ages of three years nine months, four years nine months and six and a half years. The assessment was based on (1) the use of consonants in words when naming pictures of common objects, and (2) the use of consonants in conversation and when repeating nursery rhymes. As the use of consonants often deteriorates in sentences, the phonetic analysis of articulation was finally made on the use of consonant and vowel sounds in single words only.

The children's articulation was classified as follows:

Group I Articulation normal, except for the defective use of [th] and or [r] only.

Group II Intelligible speech, but with some consonant substitutions other than, or in addition to, [th] and or [r].

Group III 'Unintelligible speech', that is intelligible possibly to other children or to those in close contact with the child, but not to strangers.

Group IV Delayed development of language, where there was insufficient use of language for the assessment of articulation.

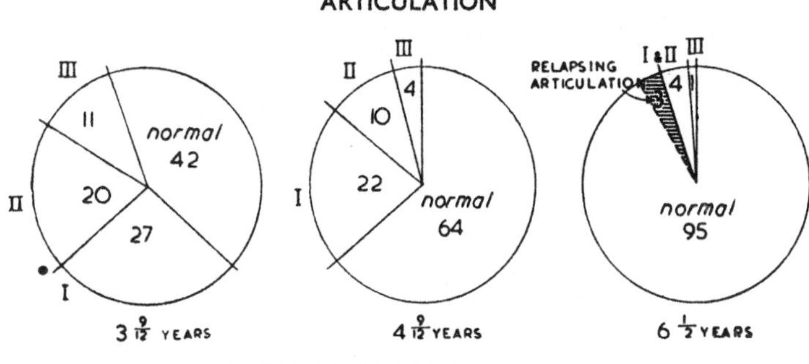

FIG. 9

Showing the classification of articulation in the 114 children in the sample group at three age levels and their progress towards normal articulation.

Dialectal use of vowel sounds was ignored throughout.

The articulation of the 114 children in the sample group is shown in Figure 9 at three age levels. It shows that 31 per cent of these children had defective articulation at the time of the first visit, 11 per cent being unintelligible, and that of the children aged four years nine months, about to enter school, 14 per cent had defective articulation, including four per cent who were unintelligible. Five per cent had obvious defects of articulation at six and a half years, although only one child in this group still had unintelligible speech. In addition, at this age, three per cent had articulation which was still unstable, and whilst usually normal deteriorated to varying degrees of defective articulation during moments of emotional stress (Appendix, Table IX).

Tongue Movements

It was considered advisable to carry out observations on tongue movements, and each child was encouraged to put out the tongue, raise the tip towards the nose and move it from side to side. Many children refused to co-operate due to shyness and inhibition as the result of parental correction in the past, and of 13 children in the sample group the tongue movements could not be assessed. In some children it was felt that awkward or clumsy movements might well be the result of shyness rather than of poor neuromuscular control. Other children, however, made valiant efforts to raise the tongue tip with the help of the fingers or the lower lip. Some children also assisted tongue movements with their fingers when attempting to move the tongue from side to side. No child in this group had a severe degree of tongue-tie.

The tongue movements of the children were classed as follows:

Normal movements of the tongue . . .	88	children
Tip of tongue could not be raised over the upper lip	9	,,
Poor control of the tongue for side-to-side movements	4	,,
Tongue movements not seen and not assessed .	13	,,

We did not find any significant correlation between these figures and defective articulation. Four of the children with apparently poor movements of the tongue had normal speech. This does not imply, however, a positive exclusion of such a possibility, and in certain children poor movements of the muscles of articulation are specifically associated with defective articulation. This question will be discussed further in connection with more obvious difficulty in the movements of the tongue in children with severe defects of articulation and with cerebral palsy. It is probable that some children are able to compensate for neuromuscular or anatomical difficulties. Children have been known to us who developed articulation which was acceptable and normal apart from the use of consonant [r] in association with a severe degree of tongue-tie when the fraenum was short and attached near the tip of the tongue. In two children the tongue tip could not be protruded beyond the lower incisor teeth, yet there was no obvious defect of articulation, and a useful and recognisable sound had been achieved for the consonant [r].

Further clinical observations have also demonstrated that many children who have good movements of the tongue, as described above, may have great difficulty in acquiring adequate control and direction of such movements for the accurate imitation and use of the consonant sounds of speech.

Summary

We found, therefore, that in a representative cross-section of young children of the city of Newcastle-upon-Tyne speech development commenced with the use of single words from the age of eight months, and that the majority had reached this stage by the end of the first year, the age range for the first use of words being from 8 to 30 months.

Most of the children began to use simple phrases around the age of 18 months although they were reported as early as ten months, and all were using phrases by three and a half years.

The majority were using intelligible speech by the age of two years, although approximately one-third passed through a period when articulation was defective and speech not always intelligible. In ten per cent speech was not intelligible at four years of age and in one child unintelligible speech persisted to six and a half years.

At nearly four years of age over 90 per cent of these children were using sentences appropriate to their age, although in one-third some errors of sentence construction were present. At nearly five years of age only one child was still using incomplete sentences and had therefore some retardation of language development.

REFERENCE

Tattersfield, A. C. (1952). The Speech and Language of the Pre-school Child. *Speech*, **16,** No. 1, p. 8.

IV. The Pattern of Speech Disorders in the First Seven Years of Life

In the whole group of 944 children at three and a half years of age, 181 (19 per cent) were found to have some form of disordered development of speech. Thirty-five of these were found in the sample group and 146 in the remainder of the 944 children. In addition, at this age 59 children were unable to use the consonants [th] and/or [r]. At the age of three years nine months, when these children were first seen, this was not considered to be abnormal, and they were therefore excluded from those children who were visited in their own homes. Where such a defect persisted to six and a half years of age, however, it was regarded as constituting a defect of articulation.

Of the 181 children, 37 had a transient period of hesitant speech. Eighteen of these 37 also had defects of articulation. We have, therefore, a group of 162 children with defects of articulation with or without delay in the development of speech. Four of these at the age of three years nine months had developed so little use of speech that articulation could not be fully assessed, whilst at four years nine months three children still had insufficient speech for assessment of articulation. The number of these children with delayed speech development was too small to constitute a separate group, and they will be described, therefore, among those with defective articulation.

Defects of articulation were therefore assessed in 162 children, the number varying slightly according to the age of assessment and the stage reached in the development of language. Ninety-three children (10 per cent of the whole group of 944) were not intelligible at three years nine months, and before this age a further 35 children were reported to have passed through a period when speech was not intelligible. One hundred and twenty-eight of these children (13·5 per cent) therefore had a period during which they had inadequate means of communication due to defects of articulation. This may be an underestimate, as in the sample group, where all children were visited, one-third were found to have had such a period of unintelligible speech. It may be, therefore, that in some of the children in the whole group such a period was short, considered by the mother to be of no consequence, and not reported. In those observed by us it varied in extent. In some it lasted for two or three months, but in 44 children (5 per cent) it persisted until four years nine months, and in six children (0·7 per cent) until the age of six and a half years (Fig. 10) (Appendix, Table X).

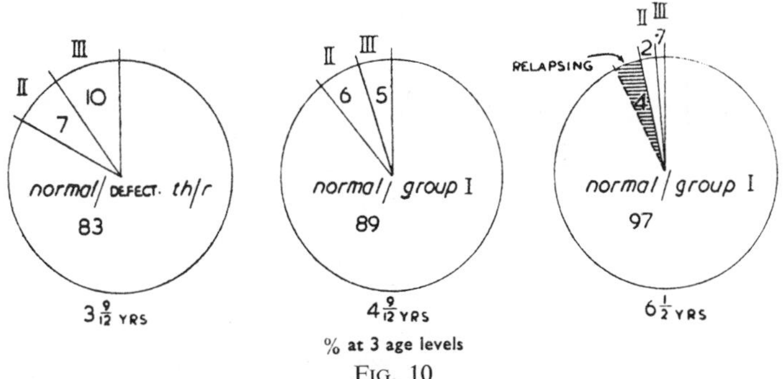

FIG. 10

Showing the classification of articulation in the whole group of 944 children at three age levels, again showing a gradual and spontaneous improvement. (Group classification as in Fig. 9.)

THE AGE OF SPEECH DEVELOPMENT

In 162 *children with defective articulation or delayed development of speech*

Comparing the age of development of speech in this group of children with that of children in the sample group representing a cross-section of the normal childhood population, we found that there was a general delay in the onset of speech (Appendix, Table II).

First words. Almost half of the children with defective speech development (44 per cent) were using first words at one year as compared with nearly three-quarters (73 per cent) of the children in the sample group. All these children were, however, using single words by the age of three years three months. The average age for the first use of words was nearly 15 months, that is almost four months later than in the sample group (Fig. 11).

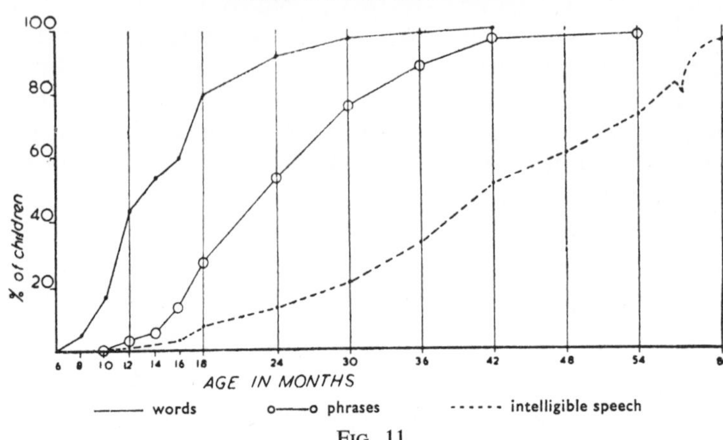

FIG. 11

Showing the growth in the use of words, phrases and intelligible speech in 162 children with defects of articulation.

Phrases. Apart from three children who were mentally defective and in whom speech was limited to the use of a few single words at five years of age, all but one of the children in this group were using at least two- to three-word phrases by three and a half years, as compared with three and a half years in the sample group, but at two years only half (54 per cent) were using phrases, whilst 89 per cent were doing so in that group of children representing a normal cross-section of the childhood population of the city of Newcastle-upon-Tyne (Fig. 11) (Appendix, Table II). The average age for the first use of phrases was 24 months as compared with 18 months in the sample group.

Intelligibility. Intelligible speech was used by only 13 per cent of these children at two years of age as compared with 69 per cent of those in the sample group, whilst 35 per cent were still unintelligible at four years. The mean age at which intelligible speech was used was 43 months, that is 19 months later than in those children who formed the sample group (Fig. 11) (Appendix, Table II).

In 44 *children with severe defects of articulation*

All the children in this group were thought to be within the normal range of intelligence, but later one child was transferred at the age of seven years to a school for backward children. The remaining 43 children were all educable in the normal school.

The age of speech development in this group corresponds closely to that of the whole group of 162 children with defective articulation (Appendix, Table III). The average age for the first use of words was 15 months and for phrases 25 months. Although the onset of speech was a little later in some of these children with severe defects of articulation, 18 (43 per cent) were using first words by the time of their first birthday.

Growth and development of language was rapid when it commenced, and at the age of two years 91 per cent were using words, whilst at three years the development in this respect had equalled that of the children in the sample group (Fig. 12).

There was similar development in the use of phrases. At two years the proportion of children in this group using phrases was 46 per cent, as compared with 89 per cent in the sample group and 54 per cent in the whole group of 162 children with defects of articulation. At three years 88 per cent were using phrases, as compared with 99 per cent in the sample group, and at three and a half years all these children were using phrases or sentences. At this age their development in this respect again equalled that of the children in the sample group (Figs. 13 and 14).

Severe defects of articulation, according to our findings, are not therefore associated with a delay in the use of language at three and a half years of age, but there was some initial delay in the onset of speech as compared with our findings for similar development in the children in our sample group.

In the group of 162 children with defective articulation the findings continued to be influenced by the fact that three of the children in this group were mentally defective and failed to develop adequate use of language at six and a half years.

In children who had a period of stammering

The age when words and phrases were first used was assessed in only 29 of the 37 children who passed through a period of hesitant speech or stammering (Appendix, Table IV).

There was some delay in the development of speech in these children compared with those in the sample group. In the

THE AGE OF SPEECH DEVELOPMENT

A comparison between four groups of children

A. sample group
B. 162 children with defective articulation
C. 44 children with unintelligible speech at 4 years 9 months
D. 29 children with stammer

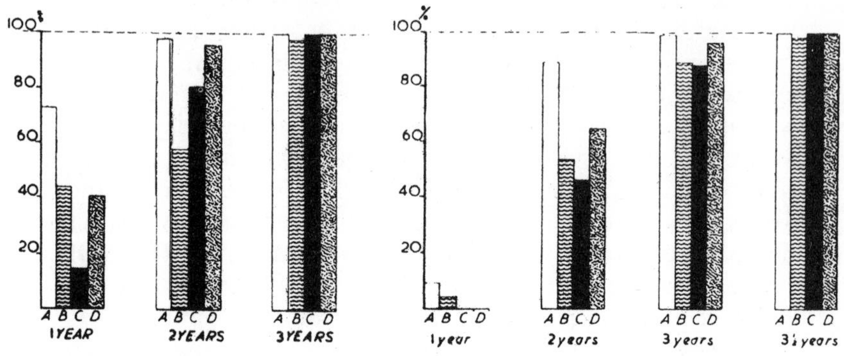

FIG. 12

First use of words.

FIG. 13

First use of phrases.

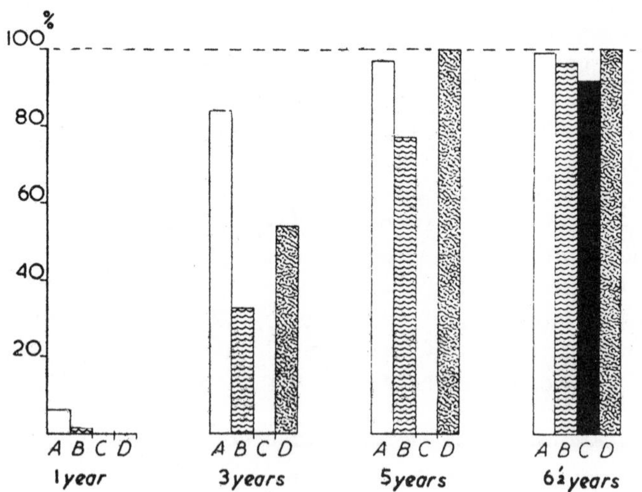

FIG. 14

Intelligible speech.

latter, 73 per cent of the children were using first words at 12 months as compared with 41 per cent in the group of children who stammered, the average age being 14 months, that is three months later than in the sample group. By two years of age only 65 per cent of these children were using phrases (89 per cent in the sample group), but all were doing so by the age of three and a half years (Figs. 12 to 14).

Many of these children also had varying periods when articulation was defective, but all were intelligible at four years nine months at the time of the second assessment. The average age for the use of intelligible speech was 35 months as compared with 24 months in the sample group (Appendix, Tables IV and V).

Our findings do not show that there was any marked delay in the age of development of speech in this small group of children who stammered, nor that the development varies considerably from that of the children in the sample group, and it tended to be slightly earlier than in the groups of children with defective articulation (Figs. 12 to 14). Although there was some retardation in the average age for the first use of words and phrases, all the 37 children developed adequate speech within the normal age range as assessed on the basis of speech development in the sample group (Appendix, Table V).

The age of development of speech and intelligibility for four groups of children is compared in Figs. 12 to 14. The onset of speech and the first use of words was considerably delayed at one year in all children with disorders of speech, and especially in those who later were found to have severe and persistent defects of articulation. At two years there was no delay in those who stammered, and marked progress had been made by those in the group with severe defects of articulation, whilst at three years there was little difference in this respect between the four groups of children (Fig. 12).

Delay in the use of phrases was most marked in children with defects of articulation, but again at three and a half years of age the difference had been eliminated (Fig. 13).

Although there was delay in developing intelligible speech in many of the children who stammered, at five years of age their ability in this respect exceeded that of the children in the sample group (Fig. 14).

The Standard of Language Ability

The standard of language ability as assessed by the use of conversational speech and the ability to repeat nursery rhymes has already been described for the sample group. A comparison of the level of language ability in this group with that of (*a*) 44 children with severe articulatory defects persisting to five years of age, and (*b*) 22 of the 37 children who had a period of stammering, is shown in Figure 15 (see also Appendix,

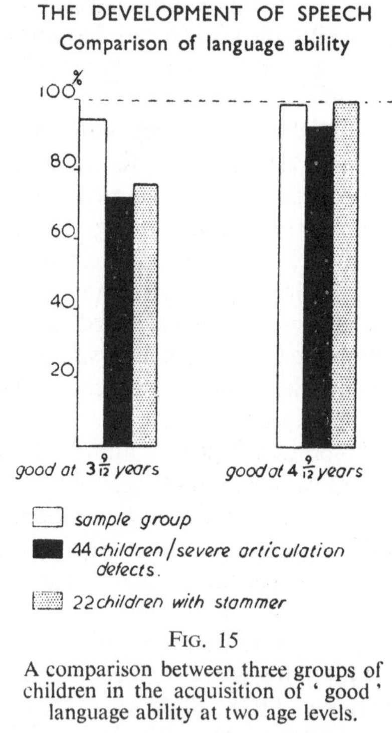

Fig. 15

A comparison between three groups of children in the acquisition of 'good' language ability at two age levels.

Tables VI, VII and VIII). The comparison is made at the age of three years nine months, and at four years nine months.

At three years nine months the children who stammered had better language development than those with severe defects of articulation, but in both these groups there was a less adequate use of language when compared with those children in the sample group. This difference was less marked at four years nine

	Plosives						Fricatives					
	Voiceless			Voiced			Voiceless				Voiced	
	[p]	[t]	[k]	[b]	[d]	[g]	[f]	[s]	[ʃ]	[tʃ]	[v]	[
Initial Position	4	12	67	3	3	35	42	58	68	53	11	5
Final Position	–	–	–	1	–	–	4	8	2	4	1	
Initial Position	4[t]	7[k] 3[s] 1[ʔ] 1[0]	61[t] 3[s] 1[ʔ] 1[0] 1[h]	3[d]	3[g]	34[d] 1[ʔ]	13[t] 10[p] 6[h] 6[s] 4[θ] 2[w] 1[ʃ]	33[t] 6[ʃ] 6[l] 3[˚θ] 3[0] 2[h] 1[w] 1[k] 1[ʔ] 1[n.p] 1[f]	30[s] 20[t] 5[t] 2[l̥] 2[k] 3[h] 1[ʔ] 1[w] 1[n.p] 1[0] 1[ts] 1[j]	26[t] 14[ts] 4[ʃ] 3[s] 2[k] 2[i̥] 1b [tʃ] 1[n.p]	9[b] 1[w] 1[ð]	30[10[2[2[1[1[1[1[3[
Final Position	–	–	–	1[d]	–	–	3[t] 1[p]	5[0] 2[t] 1[d]	1[s] 1[l̥]	3[0] 1[ts]	1[d]	1[1[

0 indicates that the consonant was entirel
Defects shown under 'Final Position' we
Defects under 'Initial Position' were defe
n.p. indicates nasopharyngeal sound.

F

Defects of articulation occurring in 162 children

Lateral and Semi-vowels			Consonant Combinations						
]	[w]	[j]	[s]	[l]	[r]	[θ]	[ð]	[r]	Defective consonants
5	6	21	79	45	96	118	22	85	
·	–	–	–	2	–	6	4	–	
w] j] 0] ʔ]	1[j] 1[j] 4[0]	11[l] 6[0] 3[w] 1[k]	78[0] 1[s] only	6[w] 37[0] 2[l] only	54[w] 34[0] 8[j, m or l]	71[f] 17[t] 12[s] 5[h] 6[0] 3[p] 1[b] 1[w] 1[ʔ] 1[l̥]	10[d] 7[v] 2[b] 1[z] 1[l] 1[j]	53[w] 14[l] 10[j] 4[0] 2[d] 1[b] 1[k]	Substitutions used.
not assessed	–	–	–	2[0]	–	3[0] 3[f]	4[0]		

ed.
ive in that position in words only.
tially only, or initially and finally.

fective development of speech (3 not assessed).

months when all the children who stammered were using complete sentences whilst approximately one per cent of those in the sample group and seven per cent in the group with defective articulation were not. By the age of five years, therefore, adequate and useful language was being used by most of these children apart from those who were mentally defective, irrespective of their ability to use normal articulation or fluent speech.

Defects of Articulation

In many children it appeared that the defective articulation could be regarded as due mainly to a limitation of the number of articulatory movements which had been acquired during the process of speech development. Normally, in the English language, 23 consonant sounds are used, but the consonant vocabulary of two children was limited to [p] [b] [t] [d] [w] and [j (y)], the last two being semi-vowels. Vowel sounds may also be defective, but are frequently normal in children with such defective articulation, apart from dialectal variations. In another child the only consonant sounds used in speech were [t] [d] [θ (th)] [l] [w] and [j (y)], and in another [p] [b] [k] [g] [θ and ð (th)] [w] and [j (y)]. The child either omits the sounds he has not acquired or substitutes the limited consonant vocabulary at his disposal (Fig. 16).

Twenty-five children had failed to develop use of one or more of the plosive consonants [p] [b] [t] [d] [k] [g], and 61 could not use one or more of the fricative consonants [f] [v] [s], [ʃ (sh)] [tʃ (ch)] [dʒ (j)] in the initial position in single words. We found three children, however, who substituted [s] for [t] and [k]. In some children the plosive consonants were normal but fricative consonants were omitted, or plosives were substituted. Ten children used [p] for [f] and 13 used [t]. Thirty-three substituted [t] for [s], 20 used [t] for [ʃ] and 26 substituted [t] for [tʃ] (Fig. 16).

Initial consonants in words were used more accurately and more consistently than when they occurred in the final or medial positions. Ten per cent of the children had defective consonant articulation in the final position in words only, consonant sounds in the initial position being normal. Omission of or defective articulation of final consonants may be sufficient to render speech unintelligible.

Voiced consonants were less frequently defective than the voiceless consonants in both the sample group and in the 162 children with defective articulation at three years nine months. (Figs. 17 and 18).

AN ANALYSIS OF THE TYPES OF CONSONANT DEFECTS

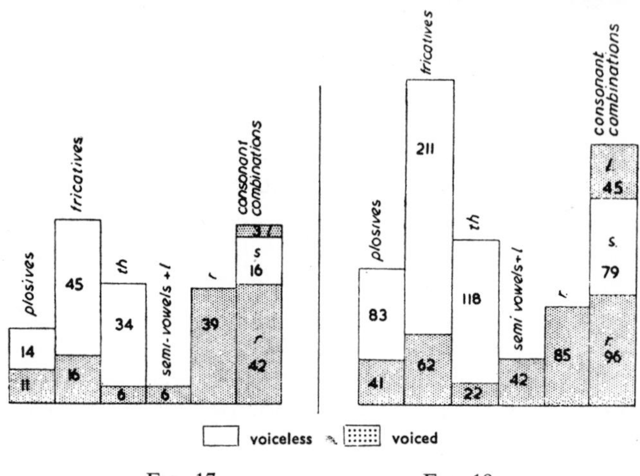

FIG. 17 FIG. 18

An analysis of the types of consonant defects in the sample group (Fig. 17), and in 162 children with defective articulation (Fig. 18).

In some children there was difficulty in co-ordinating the articulation of plosive and fricative consonants with phonation. Although the consonant could be imitated accurately in isolation, it was either omitted, or [h] or the glottal stop was substituted when the child attempted to combine such a consonant sound with a vowel sound, even in a simple syllable. Similarly, use of a combination of two or more consonant sounds, as [sp] in spoon, [sk] in school, [str] in street, presented greater difficulty and developed later than single consonants involving, as they do the combined use of fricative and plosive consonants with a vowel sound.

Commonly movements of the tongue for [k] and [g] were found to be acquired later than the bilabial and tongue-tip plosive consonants, but in a few children [k] and [g] were substituted for [t] and [d]. We found frequently that the articulation of consonants could be imitated normally in isolation but not used correctly in single words, or could be normal in single isolated words but defective when occurring in sequences of words and sentences.

Defective articulation of consonants in order of frequency

In the sample group the consonants most frequently defective were [r], 39 children; [θ and ð (th)], 34 children; [ʃ (sh)], 17 children; [tʃ (ch)], 15 children; [dʒ (j)], 14 children; [k], 13 children, and [g], 10 children. No child had defective use of [t] or [d]; and [p] [b] and [l] were each defective in one child (Fig. 19a).

In the group of children with defective articulation the order of frequency of defects of articulation was somewhat changed although [θ and ð (th)] and [r] and [ʃ (sh)] were again the most frequently defective. Five times as many children in the defective speech group had not acquired the consonant [k] as compared with those in the sample group, and whereas six [six per cent) of these had difficulty in using [s], 58 (37 per cent) of the children in the defective speech group were unable to do so (Fig. 19b).

Persistence of articulatory defects

At the age of six and a half years the chief residual articulatory defects as assessed by the articulation of single words were as follows (Fig. 19c):

[θ (th)]. At least 20 children still had difficulty in using this consonant sound. (The exact number was not assessed for the whole group.) All but one of those seen could use [ð (th)], this child substituted [n] at times.

Fourteen of the 31 children substituted [f] for [θ (th)], whilst other consonant sounds substituted were [t] [s] and [k].

[θr] as in three, tended to persist as [fr] when [θ] was being used normally.

[s]. Eighteen children still had difficulty in the use of this consonant. Ten children substituted [t], one omitted the sound entirely, one substituted [ts], one [k], one used a nasopharyngeal fricative sound, and one a lateral sound [l̥]. Three substituted [θ (th)].

(*a*) At three years nine months. In the sample group—112 children.																		Consonant Combinations with		
[r]	[θ (th)]	[ʃ (sh)]	[tʃ (ch)]	[dʒ (j)]	[k]	[g]	[f]	[ð (th)]	[s]	[j (y)]	[v]	[w]	[p]	[b]	[l]	[t]	[d]	[r]	[s]	[l]
39	34	17	15	14	13	10	7	6	6	3	2	2	1	1	1	0	0	42	16	3

(*b*) At three years nine months in 157 children with defective articulation.																				
[θ (th)]	[r]	[ʃ (sh)]	[k]	[tʃ (ch)]	[s]	[dʒ (j)]	[f]	[g]	[ð (th)]	[j (y)	[l]	[t]	[v]	[w]	[p]	[d]	[b]	[r]	[s]	[l]
118	85	68	67	66	58	51	42	35	22	21	15	12	11	6	4	3	3	96	79	45

FIG. 19a and b

Frequency of defects of articulation in order of incidence.

(*c*) Frequency of occurence in 31 children at 6½ years.																		Consonant Combinations with		
[θ (th)]	[s]	[r]	[ʃ (sh)]	[f]	[k]	[g]	[tʃ (ch)]	[b]	[t]	[d]	[ð (th)]	[dʒ (j)]	[v]	[p]	[l]	[j (y)]	[w]	[r]	[s]	[l]
20	18	14	7	4	4	4	2	1	1	1	1	1	1	0	0	0	0	16	19	4

FIG. 19c

Persistence of articulatory defects.

[r]. This sound was used defectively by 14 children. In seven it was weak, possibly a transitional stage in development, whilst other children substituted [w] [j] [v] and [l] in the proportion 3, 2, 1, 1 respectively. Four other children still used [tr] and [dr] for [kr] and [gr].

[ʃ (sh)]. Seven children were unable to articulate this sound in words and substituted [t]—2, [s]—2, [tʃ]—2, and [tʒ]—1.

[f] and [v]. Four children were still unable to use these consonants and substituted [p]—2, [t]—1 and [h]—1 for [f]. One used [pl] for [fl], but used [f] normally when alone in combination with a vowel. One child used [b] for [v].

[k] and [g]. [t] and [d] were still used by four children for [k] and [g].

[tʃ] and [dʒ]. Two children used [t] for [tʃ], and one child still used [ʒ] for [dʒ].

[t] and [d]. One child used [k] and [g] for [t] and [d].

[p] and [b]. [p] was used normally by every child, but one still used [d] for [b].

[l] and [w]. Normal in all children at the age of six and a half years.

It must be remembered, however, that many children still used consonant substitutions in conversational speech. They had reached the stage of development when they could articulate the consonant accurately in isolation, and perhaps in single words, on auditory stimulation alone and without conscious thought, but were unable to do so in long sequences of consonant and vowel sounds. It was also interesting to note that more difficult words acquired at a later stage of development were sometimes correct whilst defective articulation persisted in words in frequent use at an earlier stage of development.

Consonant substitutions used

The consonants used by the children in substitution for those they were unable to articulate varied considerably. For example, [f] [t] [s] [h] [p] [b] [w] [l̥] and [ʔ], the glottal stop, were all used by different children for the consonant sound [θ]. For [s], [t] [ʃ (sh)] [l̥] [θ] [h] [w] [k] [f], a nasopharyngeal fricative and [ʔ], the glottal stop, were used. In many children consonant substitutions were constant. In others there was erratic use of substitutions, although in general they were used consistently in the same words, or in a similar position, medial, initial or final, in words.

STAMMERING

Some form of interference with the fluency of speech, usually described as stammering or hesitating, was reported by the mother or the health visitor, or noticed by ourselves, in 37 of the children included in the survey between the ages of two and seven years, that is approximately four per cent of the 944 children.

This type of difficulty is also described by the mothers as 'can't get words out', 'becomes muddled when excited','hesitates when excited', 'repeats one word over and over again', 'becomes very excited and doesn't seem to get her words out'. For simplification we shall use the term stammering to describe this difficulty in using fluent and rhythmic speech. In only one of the children included in our investigation did this speech disorder persist in a serious degree until the present time.

Onset

In some of the children there were intermittent periods of stammering, but the initial onset, or the time when it was first noticed by the mother, health visitor, or ourselves in these 37 children was as follows:

Age in years	2–3	–3½	–4	–4½	–5	–6	–7
Number of children	1	6	14	6	6	2	2

In three children the onset appeared to be sudden. One child began to stammer following an attack of measles; another was reported to have stammered severely for two weeks following an accident when she hit her head against a door, cried for a long time and 'looked very white'. A third child was involved with her mother in an accident, and the stammer is reported to have been a sequel to this occurrence. In most of the children, however, the onset was gradual, beginning with a slight degree of occasional hesitant speech; and the age of onset, as reported to us, is probably the age at which the mother first became aware of the child's difficulty. The fact that it was reported by the mother again depends on her awareness and reaction towards the speech difficulty. Many more children than the 37 mentioned here may have passed through a period of hesitant speech, accepted by the mother as a normal and transient stage in speech development.

Degree of speech difficulty

In 12 of the children the stammer amounted to no more than a slight hesitation, which was sufficiently obvious to be noticed by the mother, health visitor or ourselves. In some instances the mother was in no way concerned, but on questioning answered that the child did have, or had had, a slight stammer. In 12 other children the difficulty occurred only occasionally when the child was in a hurry, excited or when anxious to tell a long story. It occurred perhaps once or twice a day, two or three days a week. In one child a slight hesitation at three and a half years cleared completely, but was followed by a more obvious but again temporary stammer at six and a half years.

We have attempted to classify the degree of stammering as follows:

1. Slight temporary hesitation occurring chiefly when excited, recognised as a stammer and sometimes corrected by the parents but clearing up within a few weeks or under six months			16
2. Lasting for a longer period of 6 to 12 months and of variable degree, with severe spasms occasionally, but not persisting in any severe form			
	for about six months	5	9
	6 to 12 months	4	
3. A more persistent stammer, not consistently severe, but lasting over a period of one to four years			4
4. An intermittent stammer, that is occurring or recurring at times of excitement or stress, lasting for a few days or weeks, with periods of normal speech between			7
5. Severe and persistent stammer			1
			37

In 16 of the 37 children who stammered the speech difficulty was temporary and did not last for more than a few months, or in some children for not more than a few weeks.

In 13 of the children the speech difficulty was more persistent, lasting from six months to four years. In at least eight of these there was an obvious stammer with tension and severe tonic spasms at times. In all these, however, speech eventually became normal and has remained so until the age of seven years, apart from two who still have very occasional short periods of hesitant speech at times of excitement.

In seven children the stammer occurred intermittently and was often severe, but not persistent. There were periods of obvious stammering, lasting a few days or weeks, followed by several months of normal speech and then a recurrence, sometimes associated with times of excitement such as Christmas, or a birthday party. In one of these children there were two marked periods of stammering, one in infancy at three and a half to four years, and another at six to six and a half years. In this group of 37 children two were considered to be backward, one being transferred at seven years from the normal to a special school for educationally subnormal children.

In five children at least there was a family history of stammering, and in the case of three more children there was a playmate who was reported to stammer.

The part that correction of the stammer plays in its persistence is important but difficult to ascertain without constant association with the family, and even with our frequent contacts it was not possible to assess entirely the part played by parental correction in the persistence of the stammer. In the children seen by us the mother was advised to ignore the hesitation in its early stages and to accept it as a phase through which many children pass during their progress towards stable speech. Again it is impossible to be certain how far this advice was actually carried out, and if so, what effect it had on the eventual achievement of fluent speech in all but one of the 37 children. In the case of some children, however, correction of the speech was certain. Brief notes concerning the speech of some of these children are included in Chapter XVIII.

In this survey we were able to see children with varying degrees of hesitant speech, only two of whom ever attended for treatment. The mother was reassured in each case, and it is possible that had the correction continued, some of these minor degrees of hesitant speech might have developed into a more persistent form of stammering.

Stammering and defective articulation in 37 children

Defective articulation is found to occur frequently in children who stammer. Whether there is a primary association between these two conditions, or whether the stammer develops as a result of parental correction, or the child's growing awareness of his speech inadequacy, it is not possible to say.

In this group of 37 children who had a period of stammering we found a high incidence of defective articulation. Half of these children passed through a period of defective articulation persisting at least until the time of the first assessment at three years nine months. In nine children, that is one-quarter, the speech at this time was not intelligible, and nine others had defects of articulation of less severe degree. Defects of articulation persisted in one-quarter of the 37 children until four years nine months, and in five to six and a half years, although all were intelligible by five years of age.

Although the proportion of children with defective articulation was somewhat higher in the group of children who had a period of stammering than in the sample group (50 per cent and 31 per cent respectively), this did not reach conventional levels of statistical significance. With *P* approximately 0·1, however, the difference could be accepted as suggestive, if not as firm independant evidence.

Summary

Articulation

Defects of articulation were present in varying degrees for varying periods and persisted in 157 children (17 per cent) to four years of age, 93 (10 per cent) being unintelligible to all but those who knew them well at that time.

At five years of age, when the children were about to enter school, 14 per cent of a random sample of the whole had serious defects of articulation, 4 per cent being unintelligible.

In the whole group at six and a half years, nearly 3 per cent had persisting defects of articulation, whilst six children (0·7 per cent) were still handicapped by the persistence of unintelligible speech. This figure might have been higher had not 13 children received speech therapy between four and six years of age. This was not offered when the children were visited, but was not refused if requested by the mother. In addition some children received treatment in the speech therapy department of the school health service after entering school and between the ages of five and six and a half years.

Many of these children had spontaneous improvement in articulation, and the defect was probably dyslalia, a functional disturbance where transient defective patterns of articulation arise and resolve spontaneously, or respond readily to treatment.

In a few where the defect was more severe and persistent there was probably an organic cerebral basis and the defects would be best described as isolated dysarthria or articulatory dyspraxia.

In considering the various articulatory defects we found a reduced number of learned articulatory movements with limitation of the number of consonants used. We also found that initial consonants were used more frequently and more accurately than final and medial consonants.

In some children it was thought that a difficulty in the use of certain groups of articulatory muscles such as tongue tip, blade or lips might be associated with, or the cause of the omission of, or substitution for, the relevant consonants. No significant correlation was found, however, between tongue movements and articulation in the sample group.

Voiced consonants tended to be more accurate than voiceless consonants, and plosives more so than the fricative consonants. There were difficulties in the co-ordinated use of articulation and phonation as when combining a consonant and vowel sound, or in the articulation of various combinations of consonant sounds.

As improvement in speech occurred, there were periods of relapse at times to the earlier defective patterns of articulation, and this still occurred when conversational speech was apparently normal.

Language

There was delay in the development and adequate use of language in some of the children with defective articulation, but three only, who were mentally defective, failed to develop useful language by six years of age. Some children with severe defects of articulation had no delay in the onset of speech.

Stammering

Stammering occurred in almost four per cent of the children. In general it was not severe or of short duration. One child had an obvious stammer which has persisted to the age of eight years, and two had a residual and very occasional minor degree of hesitation at times of stress. This would suggest that less than three children in a thousand will have a persistent stammer, and that of those who have a period of hesitant speech less than three per cent will develop a persisting disability.

V. Speech Development and its Relationship to Sex, Position in Family, Social Status and Environmental Conditions

THE relationship of sex, position in family, social status and environmental conditions was considered in connection with

1. The age of development of speech,
2. Defective articulation, and
3. Stammering, in four groups of children
   (*a*) The sample group.
   (*b*) 162 children with delayed speech development and defective articulation.
   (*c*) 44 children with unintelligible speech persisting until four years nine months.
   (*d*) 37 children who had a period of stammering.

SEX AND THE DEVELOPMENT OF SPEECH

In 1947, at the commencement of the investigation, there were 1142 children of whom 583 were boys and 559 were girls. At the time of the first assessment of speech, when the children were three years nine months, of the 944 children remaining in the survey, 490 were boys and 454 girls.

Sex and age of development of speech

(*a*) *In the sample group.* In the sample group of 114 children there were 55 boys and 59 girls. Forty (75 per cent) of the boys and 41 (70 per cent) of the girls were using first words by the age of one year, and 45 (82 per cent) of the boys and 55 (95 per cent) of the girls were using phrases by the age of two years. Words were first used by boys around 12 months and by girls nearly a month earlier, the average ages being 12 months and 11 months respectively. The average ages when phrases were first used was 19 months for boys and 18 months for girls

(Appendix, Table XIV). According to our findings there is no significant correlation between the age of development of speech and sex at the age of two years in the children of the sample group.

(*b*) *In 162 children with defective development of speech.* This finding is also supported by that in the group of 162 children with delayed development of speech or defective articulation. Here there were 103 boys and 59 girls of whom three, one boy and two girls, had so little language at the time of even the final assessment that the age when speech became intelligible could not be ascertained. Forty-five (44 per cent) of the boys were using single words at one year compared with 25 (42 per cent) of the girls. At three years of age, phrases were being used by 93 (91 per cent) of the boys and by 52 (88 per cent) of the girls. We were unable, therefore, to find any significant difference between boys and girls in the age at which speech develops, whether articulation was defective or normal (Appendix, Table XV).

There is, however, a highly significant difference between boys and girls in respect of the development of intelligible speech at the age of two years, and a less significant but suggestive difference at three years. In the sample group 30 (55 per cent) of the boys and 48 (82 per cent) of the girls were intelligible at two years of age, while a year later the proportions were 42 (77 per cent) of the boys and 53 (91 per cent) of the girls. This is again confirmed by the findings in the group of 162 children with defective speech which shows a highly significant difference between boys and girls for the age at which intelligible speech was used when compared at two years and at three years of age (Appendix, Table XV).

Sex and defective articulation

(*a*) *In the sample group.* At the time of the first detailed assessment of articulation at three years nine months we were unable to find any significant difference between boys and girls in their use of articulation. As described, the girls developed normal articulation more quickly than the boys and there was a significant difference in the age at which intelligible speech was used when compared at two and at three years of age, but this difference was gradually eliminated, and when the children were nearly four years of age the difference was only suggestive (Appendix, Table XVI).

(*b*) *In* 944 *children of whom* 162 *had defective development of speech.* Omitting five with delayed development of language, in whom articulation could not be adequately assessed, 157 had defective articulation at three years nine months, of whom 100 (11 per cent) were boys and 57 (6 per cent) were girls. At four years nine months defective articulation persisted in 64 (7 per cent) of the boys and in 33 (3 per cent) of the girls, and was still present at six and a half years in 17 (1·6 per cent) of the boys and 11 (1 per cent) of the girls (Appendix, Table XVII). These findings for this group of children show a highly significant difference between boys and girls for the age at which normal articulation is acquired.

(*c*) *In* 44 *children with severe defects of articulation.* Of the 44 children in whom unintelligible speech persisted until nearly five years of age, 34 were boys and ten were girls (Appendix, Table XVIII). There is again a highly significant difference between boys and girls in this group of children with severe defects of articulation, indicating that such defects tend to persist longer in boys than in girls.

(*d*) *In* 37 *children who had a period of stammering.* Of the 37 children who passed through a period of speech difficulty we have described as stammering 25 were boys and 12 were girls. The percentage of boys who stammered was 5·7 and of girls 2·7, and this difference is significant.

At the age of six and a half years one boy had a persistent stammer and one boy and one girl had very short temporary periods when there was some slight degree of stammering.

Position in Family and Development of Speech

The position in family was calculated from the number of older surviving siblings at the time of birth and not from the number of pregnancies. At the time of enrolment the position of the children in the family was as follows:

First	2	3	4 or more	Not stated	
540	334	146	119	3	1142

At five years of age, owing to deaths and removals, the position of the 847 children remaining in the survey was:

First	2	3	4	5	6	7	8	9 or more	
365	251	118	44	26	18	7	9	9	847

In the sample group of those children included in the speech survey the position at the time of the first visit was:

First	2	3	4	5	6 or more	
44	37	18	10	2	3	114

At this time 24 of the 44 first children were only children, and 20 the first children in a family of two or more. Fifty-one of the remaining 70 were the youngest children in the family and 19 occupied intermediate positions.

Position in family and age of development of speech

(*a*) *In the sample group.* 114 *children.* The number of first children who developed the use of words before and after twelve months was compared with similar development in children occupying other positions in the family (Appendix, Table XIX). Our findings showed no significant difference. The average age for the first use of words by 43 first and only children was around 11 months, compared with nearly 12 months for those 70 children in other positions in the family.

Similarly, there was no significant difference according to our findings between the ages for the first use of phrases, the average age for first children being 16 months and for the remainder 17 months (Appendix, Table XIX).

Intelligible speech was being used at two and a half years by 37 first children, that is 86 per cent of the first children in this group, and by 50 (70 per cent) of children in other positions in the family. The average age for the use of intelligible speech in first children was 21 months, and for the remainder 25 months, and at this age the difference is suggestive but not significant (Appendix, Table XIX).

Position in family and articulation

(*a*) *In the sample group.* In this group at three years nine months, 21 per cent of first children had defective articulation and 38 per cent of those occupying other positions in the family.

Five per cent of first children in this group were not intelligible, as compared with 16 per cent of children in other positions in the family (Appendix, Table XX).

At four years nine months, at the time of the second visit, defective articulation persisted in seven per cent of first children and in 17 per cent of the remainder, seven per cent of these being unintelligible. There were no persistent defects of articulation in first children at six and a half years, but two of the

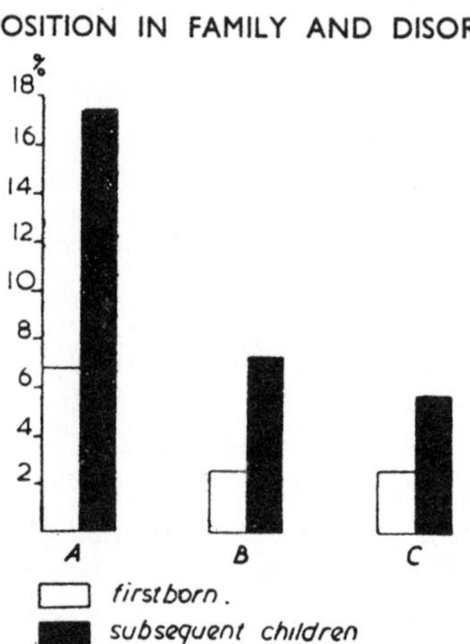

Fig. 20

Showing the relationship between defects of speech and position in family in

A. The sample groups at 4 years 9 months
B. 44 children with persisting defects of articulation at 4 years 9 months
C. 37 children who had a period of stammering.

children in remaining positions in the family had defective articulation, one being unintelligible.

In this small sample group these differences are not statistically significant in themselves, but the validity of the picture is confirmed by the next group.

(*b*) *In 44 children with unintelligible speech persisting until four years nine months.* In this group of children with severe defects of articulation there were nine first children (2·5 per cent all first children), whilst 35 (7 per cent.) of these children were in other positions in the family (Fig. 20). Defects of articulation were therefore less frequent in first children, and in this group the relative deficiency of severe defects of articulation in first children is highly significant (Appendix, Table XXI).

(*c*) *In* 37 *children who stammered.* The birth rank of these 37 children was as follows:

First	2	3	4	5	6	7	Birth rank
8	15	9	1	1	2	1	Number of children

Of the 944 children in the whole group at three and a half years of age, 423 were first children and 521 occupied other positions in the family. The incidence of stammering was eight (two per cent) among first children and 29 (six per cent) among the remainder, and as in the last group this difference is highly significant with a deficiency of stammering in first children (Fig. 20).

Social Status and Development of Speech

The social status of the children was determined by the father's work, and the occupational code of the Registrar General was used to group the families into five broad classes:

I. Employers, higher managerial groups, professions, etc.
II. Lesser employers, managers, etc.
III. Skilled workers—artisan.
IV. Semi-skilled workers.
V. Unskilled workers.
N.C. Not classed.

The following shows how the children in the sample group were classified:

I and II	III	IV and V and not classed	
12	63	39	114

Because of the small numbers in social groups I and II, and IV and V as compared with group III, groups I and II are taken together, as are also groups IV and V. The family survey excluded many of those families living outside the city boundary in the surrounding better residential districts, and this accounts for the small number in the groups I and II. Where the child was illegitimate, or the father unemployed, classification was not possible.

Social status and age of development of speech

The average age for the first use of words and phrases in these social groups was as follows (Appendix, Table XXII):

Social Group	*I and II*	*III*	*IV, V and N.C.*
First words . .	12	11·8	11·8 months
First phrases . .	19	18·4	18·8 months
Intelligible speech .	24	22·4	26·2 months

There was no significant correlation between the age of development of speech and social groups according to our findings. There was more difference in the age at which intelligible speech was established than for the first use of words and phrases, but again this difference was not, statistically significant.

Social status and articulation

Social status and defects of articulation in the sample group are shown in Appendix, Table XXIII, at three age levels. As in the findings for the development of intelligible speech, we were unable to show any significant correlation between social status and defective articulation at three years nine months, four years nine months nor at six and a half years in this group of children.

In 44 *children with severe defects of articulation.* In this group of children in whom unintelligible speech persisted until four years nine months there was, however, a highly significant correlation between social class and defective articulation (Appendix, Table XXIV).

Only four of these children were in social groups I and II, 14 in group III and 26 in groups IV, V and not classed. In view of the findings already described, it is possible that this may indicate a correlation with the persistence of severe defects to a later age rather than with their incidence, but this cannot be stated definitely. Better environmental conditions may contribute towards the more rapid improvement of articulation.

Social status and stammering

Only two of these 37 children were in social groups I and II, nine were in social group III, as were also two who were later transferred to group V. Fourteen of the children were in social groups IV and V. This distribution does not differ significantly from that of the children who did not stammer, and we could find no evidence that stammering was influenced by social status.

MISCELLANEOUS CONDITIONS

These have been considered only in relation to the 44 children with persisting unintelligible speech at four years nine months.

No significant correlation was found in this group between defective articulation and maternal capacity to manage the home and family, nor with the following conditions—fits, behaviour disorders, papular urticaria, tonsils and adenoids, squint, prematurity, nor attendance at a nursery. There was a possible suggestive correlation with enuresis and with acute otitis, however.

Deprivation. This included permanent or temporary loss of the father and/or the mother, absence of the mother whilst working, parental incapacity due to illness, and marital instability.

Social dependency, including neglect, unemployment and crime. In these two groups defective articulation was not found more frequently as the result of deprivation nor social dependency than in the normal cross-section of the childhood population (Appendix, Table XXV (*a*) to (*e*)).

OTHER DEFECTS

Cleft palate

No child in this speech survey had a cleft palate. With an incidence of 1 in 900 to 1000 births, one such child would have been expected. This was actually the case, but the child developed speech normally following surgical treatment at one year.

Dysarthria

Several children died in infancy following cerebral damage at birth, but no child survived to develop a severe dysarthria when speech was acquired.

Hearing defects

One child had a partial hearing loss, but speech was not seriously delayed. Intelligible speech was established at four and a half years and articulation was normal at six and a half years.

Intelligence

In the whole group there were four mongols. One died in infancy, and one later but before the time of the speech survey. Two are included in the figures already given. In both there was a serious retardation in language development. Single words were late in developing, and only limited phrases were being used at six and a half years.

One child had an intelligence quotient on the Merrill Palmer performance scale of 37 at seven years of age. There was a severe impairment in comprehension for speech, and he was at first thought to be deaf. He developed the use of a few words only, but at the age of seven could understand simple speech spoken in a normal voice. One other child, in whom speech development was slightly delayed and who also had a temporary period of stammering, was transferred at seven years of age, as already mentioned, from the normal school to one for educationally subnormal children, as also was one whose speech remained unintelligible at five years of age and who is included in the group of 44 children with severe defects of articulation.

One child who had no delay in speech development, and who had no apparent defect of articulation or disorder of the use of language, was later found to be ineducable in either a day or residential school for educationally subnormal children and was eventually transferred to a residential hospital for the mentally defective.

SUMMARY

We found no significant correlation between the age of speech development and sex, position in family nor social status.

In the development and use of normal articulation there was a significant difference in sex. Speech became intelligible earlier in girls than in boys. This difference was, however, gradually eliminated and did not persist at five years of age.

A relationship was also established between defects of articulation and position in family with a highly significant deficiency of defects in first children. The severe defects of articulation were especially more frequent in second and later children than in first children. The reason for this is not known.

Only in the group of 44 children with severe defects of articulation was there a significant correlation between social status and defects of articulation. Whether this is related to incidence or to the persistence of such defects to a later age we are unable to state, but there was no clear association between defective articulation in this group and unsatisfactory maternal care, deprivation, family dependency, nor neglect, so that the unfavourable domestic factor remains unknown.

PART II

THE DELAYED DEVELOPMENT OF SPEECH

VI. The Delayed Development of Speech

HERE we propose to describe abnormal delay in the acquisition of speech and the underlying causes associated with this delay in children referred to a speech therapy department.

As previously described, the child begins to have some understanding for speech from the age of perhaps six months or even earlier, and to use single words to express his needs usually between ten months and two and a half years of age. Two- or three-word phrases are introduced between 18 months and three and a half years, and an ever increasing vocabulary, with development in the use of sentences, follows, associated with the normal growth of the child. Although the period of speech development may normally extend from one to three and a half years, the period between one and two years of age is, in most children, that of maximum rate of speech development, and after three to four years use of speech is acquired with less facility.

CONDITIONS AFFECTING THE DEVELOPMENT OF SPEECH

Intelligence

It has always been recognised that defective or delayed general mental development is closely allied with delay in the use of and also the absence of or reduced need for speech. Mental defect also interferes with full comprehension for speech, although in the majority of such children with normal hearing understanding for simple speech associated with the basic needs of life may be adequate unless the mental defect is severe. There seems to be evidence, however, that delay in the adequate use of speech may be associated with development which in other respects is normal. One boy known to us, who used no expressive speech apart from a few isolated words until the age of five years, later became a brilliant student and medical specialist.

The development and use of speech results from the interaction of varying factors of which the general level of intelligence is only one. The neurological maturation of the perceptive and motor processes required for speech, the acuity of hearing, the personality and interests of the child and his environment may all influence the age at which he will begin to use speech and its subsequent development.

Developmental aphasia

The child with delayed neurological maturation for the central processes involved in the use of expressive speech may have adequate understanding for the speech of others. He may be friendly and co-operative and be making every effort to communicate with others and yet be unable to express himself adequately through speech. He appears to have little or no interest in the imitation of the sounds of speech, and often has been a silent child and made little attempt to use voice and articulate sounds in infancy. He may show signs of frustration when he cannot make known his meaning and will rely chiefly on gesture or well-developed mime to achieve his essential need for communication.

If development of speech is delayed beyond the range of what is normal, and the child's ability to formulate his thoughts into words and sentences is inadequate for his age, the condition may be described as developmental aphasia or dysphasia. Such a disorder may be associated with cerebral palsy, or exist in the absence of any obvious underlying neurological disorder and may possibly be the result of some cortical agenesis or dysfunction producing delay in the acquisition of the use of the audible symbols of speech.

Rarely there may be a lack of or limited appreciation for the meaning of spoken language which is not the result of nor proportional to any hearing defect or subnormal intelligence. These children may also use gesture to supplement their limited means of verbal expression. They show little interest in speech as a means of communication, usually fail to attend to the speech of others and make little or no attempt to use the visual sensory pathways, as in lip reading, for the understanding of speech. However, it is apparent that these children may have normal articulation for the words used in their limited or jargon speech, and therefore normal auditory perception. Developmental receptive aphasia is probably, therefore, a better term for this condition.

In children with varying types of obvious motor disability

arising as the result of non-progressive brain lesions, usually included in the term cerebral palsy, there may be such widespread damage that there is limited development of intelligence and of the mental processes required for speech in both its receptive and executive aspects. In others there is a more limited and specific defect affecting the development of expressive speech where intelligence and comprehension for speech are within the normal range. There is then a developmental expressive aphasia with delayed development and inadequate use of the verbal symbols of speech which may persist throughout life.

Before the diagnosis of developmental aphasia can be confirmed, however, it must be determined that hearing is adequate, intelligence, as assessed on performance tests and on general behaviour and development, is within the normal range, and that the child has good emotional relationships with those in his environment including a desire and need to communicate with others. He may use gesture and mime, and usually shows frustration when he cannot make his wants known.

Hearing

If hearing for speech is defective, the child may fail to respond to and to develop speech, or speech development may be retarded and articulation defective. The intelligent child may have an interest in speech which the child with developmental aphasia lacks, and may attempt to compensate for his disability through lip reading. In some children with partial hearing loss this may be so well developed that one is left in some doubt as to whether or not a partial hearing loss accounts for the delay in the development of speech unless care is taken to ensure that the child is unable to see the face of the speaker. If the hearing loss for speech is severe and yet the child is able to hear noises he may be certified as mentally defective. His response to sounds is regarded as an indication of normal hearing, and his failure to understand fully what is said, or to make suitable progress in school, as a sign of backwardness or mental deficiency. If the hearing loss is partial, speech may develop but articulation be defective. The child fails to hear normally the spoken sounds of speech, and can only imitate them as he hears them.

Emotional difficulties

A child may understand speech, but because of noncooperation, more serious behaviour disorders, or, rarely, actual psychosis, refuse or be unable to respond to the speech of others and have little interest in communicating with others through speech. In some such children development of speech may be adequate, but response to others and use of expressive speech is inhibited. Because speech is so useful to the child in obtaining what he needs, it is probable that he will use it if he can. His manner of speaking may be modified as a result of emotional disturbance, but this condition is more likely to occur at a later stage of his development, and not influence the early unconscious imitation of the speech he hears around him.

In the young of animals, in addition to inborn reflex reactions, there would seem to be an inherent and instinctive urge to imitate others of its kind. Walking in the upright position may only develop in a child who associates with other human beings. If there is absence of speech in the environment of the child, his speech will probably fail to develop, but the need to imitate others in the act of speaking is important to the child living in normal surroundings, and if at all possible he will attempt to do so. Laziness, the cause often suggested by the mother to account for the delay in the speech development of her child, is rarely, if ever, the cause, as most of these children are alert and active in other respects.

Many parents become anxious if their child is not speaking by the age of two and a half or three years of age, or even earlier if it is thought that the child does not understand speech. On the other hand, a mutual sign language of natural gesture may develop, the mother being in some cases unaware of the extent to which her child's understanding is dependent upon it. Again, a mother may maintain that her child is not speaking when she means rather that he is talking freely but she cannot understand what he is saying. He may be speaking in well-constructed sentences, intelligible to another brother or sister, but because articulation is defective the mother may insist that the child can say only a few simple words, these being the ones he can articulate normally and which she can understand.

CHILDREN REFERRED WITH DELAYED SPEECH DEVELOPMENT

In the past six years we have seen 280 children referred to the speech therapy department of the Royal Victoria Infirmary, Newcastle-upon-Tyne, with delayed development of speech.

The main conditions accounting for the delay have been mentioned. The number of children in each group are shown in Figure 21.

In 50 of the children with developmental dysphasia, normal speech developed late, between four and six years of age, but was eventually adequate. In 24 there was a more serious delay. The speech of these children will be described later.

In addition, children were seen with acquired temporary aphasia as the result of cerebral trauma or infective illness. These are excluded from this group of children with developmental delay in speaking.

	Boys	Girls	Total
Hearing defect	55	55	110
Developmental aphasia	56	18	74
Mental defect	41	30	71
Associated with cerebral palsy	15	7	22
Psychogenic retardation	2	1	3
	169	111	280

FIG. 21

The main conditions accounting for delayed speech development in 280 children

This table shows only the relative importance of the various underlying causes in a group of children referred with delayed development of speech. The incidence of delayed development of speech, as found in the study of 1000 children of all social classes in Newcastle-upon-Tyne, was described in Chapter III. At the age of four and a half years only four of these children were not using speech although sentences were necessarily not always complete. These were mentally defective and used only a few single words.

The age of referral of 258 of these 280 children is shown in Figure 22. The speech of 22 children with cerebral palsy will be described in a later chapter.

	Age in Years					Total
	1–2	–3	–4	–5	over 5	
Hearing defect	6	27	35	24	18	110
Developmental expressive aphasia	–	5	25	29	13	72
Mental defect	–	7	16	27	21	71
Psychogenic retardation . .	–	–	–	2	1	3
Developmental receptive aphasia	–	–	–	–	2	2
	6	39	76	82	55	258

FIG. 22

Delayed Speech and the age of referral in 258 children.

VII. The Delayed Development of Speech and Psychogenic and Mental Retardation

Speech and Psychogenic Retardation

In a few children we have thought that delayed or distorted development of speech was probably associated with emotional disturbance or psychogenic illness, and an account of the development of speech would be incomplete without some reference to the relationship between them, but no attempt will be made here to describe the emotional and behaviour disorders or psychogenic illnesses of childhood. They have been discussed at length by many more competent to understand and to treat them.

The social adaptation of the child involves his capacity to make contacts with other children and adults, and is closely associated with his emotional development, his capacity to feel and to express his feelings through speech and in other ways, and to develop the ability to control such feelings.

In some children emotional responses may be abnormal, exaggerated or diminished. The child may be solitary, and prefer to play alone, or for reasons which it is difficult to define, may be shunned by other children and excluded from their group and its activities. Fear of situations may be excessive, including fear of change of environment, with difficulty in adapting to changes even in the home. There may also be obsessive tendencies when the child persists in the same action or type of behaviour for a period and then changes and adopts another type of obsessive interest or behaviour. Development, either physical or intellectual, may be handicapped unless the child has a stable and satisfying environment in which he can grow and to which he can respond.

Interference with the development of speech may occur if emotional growth is not progressing harmoniously. There may be little need or desire for contact or communication with others, or speech, once acquired, may not be used freely or may be inhibited almost entirely. Extreme shyness or self-consciousness may hinder the gradual development and stabilisation of speech and prevent its free use as a means of self-expression.

Russell Davis (1954) defines psychogenic retardation as 'mental development slowed, distorted or arrested as the result of adverse psychological circumstances'. The result may be mental defect which renders the child incapable of education in school, or retardation of mental development. He divides the causes into (1) genetical or inherited and (2) environmental, which may be physical or psychological.

The single factor of 'intelligence', as assessed by the efficiency with which a child accomplishes certain standardised tests, cannot be isolated from the total personality of the child. The one with a strong desire to achieve all that is possible in spite of a lower intelligence quotient may yet go further and perhaps achieve more than the apparently more brilliant child with less urge for self-expression, or with inhibition of psychopathic origin, which makes it difficult for him to use his ability to the full. There may also be delay in emotional development and the attainment of maturity, again with resultant failure to make full use of intellectual capacity until later in life.

Some children, however, develop fully in spite of the most adverse conditions, which may even seem to assist rather than hinder the full development of personality. As Davis (1954) points out, 'There is as yet insufficient information on which to decide whether the apparent vulnerability of some children is due to inheritance by the few of a biological defect, or whether certain children develop psychoses only because of the particular combination of circumstances which they meet.'

If the arrested or defective development of speech is the result of, or associated with, psychogenic retardation, there will probably be signs of emotional difficulties and maladjustment in other respects. Such signs do not resolve with improvement in speech and with growth of more adequate means of communication with others through speech. This occurs frequently, however, where the emotional disturbance is secondary to the speech disorder and where much frustration has been experienced by the child with developmental aphasia or unintelligible articulation. Many children refuse to speak and take refuge in silence when they realise their inability to communicate effectively with others, or when they are subjected to repeated and misdirected correction of their speech at home.

It is probably true to say that a traumatic emotional experience occurring at the age when speech is developing may interfere with normal progress, but also that it may only produce a lasting adverse effect if the personality of the child is unable to meet the need. Delayed or disordered development of speech may then be part of the child's general emotional disorder. Normal speech may be used at times with intermittent periods of regression or inhibition of the use of speech. It is doubtful, however, if such disordered development can be regarded as a true disorder of speech, but rather as a symptom of a wider syndrome for the treatment of which speech therapy may or may not be indicated.

Such conditions are exaggerated in the autistic child.

Autism and Speech

Kanner (1943, 1944) was one of the first to recognise and describe childhood autism. Observation of the child's behaviour should be sufficient to indicate the need for further investigations. Such children, often highly intelligent, prefer things to people, may resent personal physical contact with others, and show little, if any, desire for affection from parents or other children. They play with toys alone, and resent any intrusion from others. As the desire to communicate with others, either physically or emotionally, is lacking, it is not surprising that these children have little use for speech. This does not necessarily mean that speech has not developed. The autistic child may have full understanding for speech but fail to respond in any way. Children who are successfully responding to treatment may unexpectedly begin to use speech, and while such speech may not, at first, be easy and fluent, it does perhaps indicate that it is rather an inability or refusal to respond to or to use speech, rather than lack of development of speech which is hindering communication through spoken language.

A report by Creak and others (1961) described the following symptoms as being diagnostic of the autistic child or 'schizophrenic syndrome in childhood': gross and sustained impairment of emotional relationships with children; apparent unawareness of his own personal identity; pathological preoccupation with particular objects; resistance to change in the environment; excessive, diminished or unpredictable response to sensory stimuli; acute excessive and apparently illogical anxiety (see G.M. p. 95); serious retardation in which islets of normal, near normal, or exceptional intellectual function or skill may appear. Furneaux (1966) has reported on the children she has studied and treated in a residential community. Through her daily contacts with these children she describes how they sometimes appear to gain information through touch and smell, sometimes of only one part of a person, or one item of wearing apparel. Sometimes these children close their eyes when they are under- or over-reacting to an auditory stimulus. She also describes what she calls 'gaze aversion' as being typical and completely different from the blank look of the seriously mentally subnormal, and thinks that these children are more aware of what is happening around them than is often immediately apparent.

From her observation and understanding of these children Furneaux thinks that although they do not use speech they undoubtedly understand a great deal of what is said to them. She observed that their speech development is highly complex. It may begin with a child of eight using infantile babbling, or a child of the same age suddenly repeating 'the whole of the television news he had heard the night before'. Echolalia is frequent, and a question may be repeated rather than answered. With improving personal relationships, increasing use of spoken language is frequently rapid.

Savage (1968) has summarised some of the literature on the subject of speech development in the autistic child. She states that of 63 children seen at the Maudsley Hospital 31 were mute at the initial interview, one child had normal speech development, and one quarter of the children had had a period of normal speech development before they regressed to the autistic state. Mittler (1963) saw 34 of these children at the Smith Hospital, mutism being apparent in 13; 17 children had grossly diminished vocabularies, comprising only a few words, and only 11 per cent had a normal-sized vocabulary.

It is important, therefore, to differentiate between the child with a true delay in the development of language, or developmental aphasia, and the autistic child. This can frequently be based on an assessment of behaviour. The child with a developmental aphasia makes normal contacts, physical and emotional. He is aware of his need to communicate with others and to express his ideas and wants. If unable to do this through spoken language he will frequently use expressive gesture, which leaves little doubt as to his meaning. At times he will be frustrated when the complexity of his ideas exceeds the means of communication at his disposal and when, therefore, others fail to understand his meaning. Temper tantrums, withdrawal or other signs may then be apparent, but these are the result of, and not the cause of the delayed speech development.

Many have thought that autistic children were partially deaf or have diagnosed them as having a receptive aphasia. However, Tubbs (1966), using the Illinois Test of Psycholinguistic Abilities, found that autistic children did not differ from her control group of normals or subnormals in the auditory vocal tests which required spontaneous output rather than the selection and utilisation of material. Frequently one detects a refusal to respond to sounds made to test hearing, rather than an inability to hear them.

However, the differentiation may not be as well defined as has been suggested. Some autistic children may have a true partial, or more severe delay in the development of speech. Other children with developmental aphasia may also have emotional problems which hinder their ability to develop other means of communication such as gesture, mime and even consistent vocal or phonic sound sequences to indicate certain objects, and thus become increasingly frustrated and unable to communicate, with signs indicative of a true psychogenic disorder.

In the group of 280 children referred with delayed development of speech, three only were considered to be the result of an emotional or psychogenic disturbance:

G. M. This boy was first seen at the age of five years. He was the second of two children, his sister being ten years of age at that time. The pregnancy and delivery were normal, but general development was slow and he did not walk until he was two years three months. He fed himself from two and a half years and sphincter control was established day and night by two and a half years.

Speech. He made no attempt to use even single words until four years nine months, but at five years he was able to imitate a few isolated words. Understanding for speech appeared to be adequate. He also imitated a variety of animal noises most realistically.

Hearing. He liked music and could sing in tune but without using words, and hearing was normal. He had a gramophone, and by some means not understood could identify the records and find the one he wanted, and which corresponded to the tune he was singing.

Intelligence. He was interested in books and would listen to a story for long periods, often asking questions. Play was constructive, his chief interests being jig-saw puzzles, which he did well, even difficult ones, and mini-cars. He did not respond well to intelligence tests and the first estimate at five years was an intelligence quotient of 50 to 60. However, on further testing at seven years of age he achieved a level of 100. On medical examination he was a well-developed boy with no signs of spasticity or other neurological abnormality. Blood tests of the mother and child showed no incompatibility nor antibodies.

Progress. Vocabulary continued to increase, but G. did not attempt to use phrases until nearly six years. At that time he was interested in numbers, could count to 100 and could appreciate numerical values up to ten. By the age of five years eight months he could read three or four little words, whilst at six years his reading age on the Burt scale was eight years. Three months later he was doing simple sums and could read a newspaper, whilst spelling ability was also up to the eight to nine years' level. At eight and a half years his reading age was eleven years. Tests for comprehension proved this was not purely a mechanical skill.

Personality. He was somewhat egocentric and introverted, although not lacking at times in affection nor awareness of others, particularly if they were absent from his environment, when he became unhappy until their return. His teacher reported that he showed little interest in games and did not enter into other children's play. He had obsessional fears and was at one time afraid of the speech recorder in the department. He fled panic stricken from the room when it was opened, and thereafter refused to enter the room during the next two years without first making sure as he opened the door that the recorder was not only closed but that the plastic cover was also in place. Consequently it was never possible to record his animal sounds, nor his accurate singing. All attempts to reassure him failed, and a fear of the gramophone at school persisted for several years although he was accustomed to and used one at home.

In spite of this child's ability in certain directions, he failed to make adequate progress in school. Speech was normal by the age of six and a half years and articulation was never defective. We have regarded this as a developmental dysphasia with distorted mental development associated with psychogenic retardation, perhaps autistic in type, his emotional and personal difficulties not permitting full growth and development up to the level of his intellectual capacity.

A. W., aged four years seven months, was the elder of two, having a younger brother aged three and a half years. Understanding for speech was adequate. The pregnancy and delivery were normal and she walked at 18 months. She was a quiet baby and made very few vocal noises or babbling sounds. She said 'Mummy' early, but use of words was limited until four years. Then she would use gesture rather than attempt to speak whenever possible. According to the mother, the child refused affection from the age of seven months, and pushed her mother away if she attempted to kiss her. On the other hand, she showed affection for her younger brother and for dolls. The mother felt that the child wanted affection but was too 'shy and reserved' to accept it, and therefore repelled any demonstration of affection by other people.

In addition there was a bilingual problem, the mother being Dutch and the father, who was frequently away at sea, being English. When the child was nearly twelve months old the mother returned to her parents in Holland for the birth of the second child, and they were resident there for eight months. A Dutch nurse returned to England with the family, and the mother conversed with the nurse at times in Dutch, although she stated that she always used English when speaking to the children. When A. was first seen the nurse had returned to Holland and the language of the home was entirely English except for the Dutch Radio to which the mother frequently listened.

Hearing. This was normal and A. had recognised the Dutch language on the radio as being like that of her grandfather and grandmother in Holland.

The younger brother was extremely voluble and spoke English well with no sign of defective articulation. A. spoke hardly at all, especially when her brother was present. At times she appeared to want to talk and made an abortive attempt, as though verbal expression were completely inhibited. So little speech was heard, even though she became friendly in a silent way, that it was not possible to ascertain whether or not articulation was normal or defective. Speech therapy, or other treatment, was not possible as she was abroad for long periods, but the mother reported slow but increasing self-confidence with progress in the use of speech at home. She made good progress in school, and intelligence was found to be within the normal range. She was, however, a silent member of her class.

In both these children use of speech was exceptionally delayed. They are described here not because they are representative of a type of speech disorder but rather to indicate the difficulties of assessment and the peculiarities of development which may occasionally be encountered. The developmental history is often normal, apart from behaviour difficulties, and the initial onset of speech may be at the normal age, but steady, progressive development may be lacking, with limited or intermittent growth in the use of language. Articulation may be normal or defective. Periods of relapsing articulation may be associated with gradual spontaneous improvement, until normal patterns of articulation become stabilised, or may indicate a true regression to a more infantile use of speech. In some, however, it is possible that this may indicate a resourceful attempt to regain attention which may have been unwisely and entirely directed to a younger child, and indicate mismanagement on the part of the parents rather than any serious defect in the child. Inhibition of and failure to use speech, however, is probably associated with a true psychogenic disability.

The Delayed Development of Speech and General Mental Retardation

Retarded mental development will affect the development of speech in both its receptive and expressive aspects, and is the most common cause of delayed development of speech when hearing is normal. The appreciation and interpretation of the meaning of word sequences is dependent on and in general varies according to the mental development of the child. Where there is poverty of thought there is little to communicate, and the need for speech is not urgent. In a few there may be an excessive flow of words, but the thought content is elementary, frequently irrelevant, and the vocabulary is limited.

Associated with retarded mental development there is usually delay in the onset of speech. The use of single words occurs at a later age, and this stage of speech development may persist with minimal growth in vocabulary for several years, with late onset of the use of phrases. These may be used in incomplete form for a long period, and in the majority are never used adequately.

Severe defects of articulation are not common, and the use of the sounds of speech is frequently normal apart from those who pass through a temporary period of defective articulation, or dyslalia, comparable to that through which many children pass at an earlier age. This may persist for a longer period than is usual, and in a few there may be an associated development, a dysarthria or articulatory dyspraxia, with more severe defects of articulation.

In 71 of the 280 children referred with delayed development of speech this condition was associated with general mental retardation.

First use of words

The age range for the first use of words was from one to six years, the mean age being three years, as compared with 11 months in the random sample of childhood (Chapter III). When words were used under two years of age, they were limited to one or two only.

First use of phrases

Phrases were not used before three years of age except in the case of one child. Twenty-two of these 71 children made no attempt to use word sequences until after five years, and nine children did not do so until they were between the ages of seven and nine years. The age range for the first use of phrases was from two to eight years, the mean age being four years, as compared with 18 months in the sample group (Chapter III). These figures do not indicate, however, the poverty of the language used and the limited vocabulary.

Comprehension for speech

Three children between four and six years of age had no apparent understanding for speech and no expressive speech. Two of them were at first thought to be severely deaf, but co-operation for audiometric assessment could not be obtained. Later it was found that these children responded to simple speech spoken in a quiet voice, and hearing was therefore adequate. Although the developmental milestones were not obviously delayed, two of these children were later found to have intelligence quotients of 37 and 45 respectively. The third, who also had had an operation for repair of cleft palate with a good physiological result, left the district and her further development is not known.

In these children it would seem that understanding for speech was more limited than would have been expected from their general motor development, and that some degree of developmental receptive aphasia possibly contributed towards their general mental retardation.

It is unusual in our department for the mentally defective child to be referred for speech therapy, but in these 71 children the diagnosis of mental defect was uncertain, or not at first suspected. In 32 of the 71 children the intelligence quotient was ascertained, the range being from 37 to 87, and the average 60. In only a few, therefore, was there a severe degree of mental retardation, and in some the delay in the development of speech was considered to be out of proportion to the level of intelligence as indicated by intelligence tests or by the development of motor skills and the milestones of childhood.

In order to gain more information concerning the speech of those with a severe degree of mental retardation, advantage was taken of a request by the regional psychiatrist to undertake a survey in a residential hospital for such patients of all ages. This was in order to assess the need for speech therapy and its possible value. In all, 82 patients were seen between the ages of 3 and 65 years for an evaluation of their speech. This was investigated as follows:

1. *Vocabulary*

(*a*) *Names of objects.* Pictures of common everyday objects were shown and the patient was asked to name them. They were arranged in groups according to the usual experience level of a child. In the first group were such things as a spoon, cup, baby and man (daddy). Common objects in the home comprised the second group, for example a chair, table and clock. In the third group were objects seen outside the home such as a bus, car and aeroplane. The fourth group contained pictures associated with increasing experience and knowledge of everyday life.

(*b*) *Actions.* Pictures showing actions were used and the patient was asked 'What is he doing?'

In both sets of pictures the patient was also asked to point to the picture named, especially if he could not name it himself, and he was also asked to 'Show me who is running—digging—sleeping' and so forth.

2. *Interpretation of pictures*

The patient was shown a picture and he was asked to describe it. He was asked, 'What can you see in this picture?' and 'Tell me about the picture.' The use of words, phrases and sentences was assessed according to whether the speech consisted of:

(*a*) The mere naming of objects in the picture.
(*b*) A description of obvious activities.
(*c*) An explanation of the meaning content of the picture.

3. *Articulation*

A phonetic analysis of the articulation was noted whilst the patient was speaking. If the use of speech was very limited, he was asked to repeat single words.

In carrying out these observations wider experience and understanding was gained of the extent to which the development of speech is affected by retardation of general mental growth, as differentiated from those in whom abnormal development of speech occurs in association with intelligence which is within the normal range.

After assessment the patients were grouped into five categories according to their age at that time, and a description of the language ability and the articulation used will be described for each. The number of patients in each group was as follows:

1. Under 5 years . . .	11 patients
2. Aged 5 to 10 years . . .	24 patients
3. Aged 11 to 15 years . .	32 patients
4. Aged 16 to 25 years . .	5 patients
5. Over 25 years . . .	10 patients
	82 patients

Assessment of Speech in Five Groups of Patients

From the study of these patients it was hoped to gain further information as to the relationship between the development of speech and mental deficiency, and to become more familiar with the picture it presents in children with delayed development of speech. Where there is a severe degree of general mental retardation, the diagnosis is not difficult, but the basic cause of delayed speech development is not always so obvious in children with a lesser degree of general mental retardation.

The general findings concerning these patients will be presented therefore for the development of language and articulation in each of the five groups, as it was felt that this would be of more practical value than a series of detailed statistics.

1. *Eleven children under five years of age*

In this group of children there were four mongols. They were seen in a nursery, and although happy and free to play with toys and with each other, the outstanding feature was the absence of the normal vocal sounds usually associated with children's play. There was little vocalising and no babbling. A few children used gesture, and one child obviously knew what she wanted and used gestures to explain her needs to the nurses. There was little constructive play of any kind, and little or no interest in each other.

Response to speech was extremely limited even when the children were at ease. Only one child aged four and a half years, with an estimated mental age of one and a half to two years, was heard to use speech to communicate with others. He had a vocabulary of about 20 words, and could also point to the pictures of the few words he knew. Articulation for these words was normal for many consonant sounds including [s] [k] [g] and [ʃ (sh)], also [p] [b] [t] and [d]. Other consonant sounds were not heard.

2. *Twenty-four children aged five to ten years*

In this group of children an attempt had been made to assess the level of intelligence. Eight children were unable to co-operate in testing and had not been ascertained. In the remaining 16 children the average intelligence quotient was 49, and the range was from 26 to 81. These assessments had been made by one of the teachers of the school attached to the mental hospital.

Language. One child in this group with an intelligence quotient of 81 used full sentences and could repeat nursery rhymes, articulation being normal except for [θ (th)]=[f].

Although the intelligence quotient obtained here is apparently not below the level usually accepted in the normal school, or in a school for backward children, he was resident in this hospital for special reasons, and with his brother, who was less intelligent, was receiving education in the school attached to the hospital.

Ten children used phrases of two or three words, and one with an intelligence quotient of 50 used longer phrases, but rarely used a complete sentence.

Eight children used only single words, and five children, aged seven to nine years, attempted no expressive speech whatever. Three of these five children had intelligence quotients of 29, 30 and 41 respectively, and in the other two the intelligence quotient could not be ascertained. These five children appeared to have very limited understanding for speech. Their ages were between eight and ten years.

Articulation. Eleven of the 24 children in this group had no obvious defects of articulation except for use of the consonants [θ (th)] and [r]. The articulation of the child who repeated nursery rhymes deteriorated when he spoke quickly, and another child had poor articulatory movements, resulting in articulation which was at times indistinct but not incorrect.

Eight of the remaining 13 children also attempted to use

speech but had defects of articulation with substitutions and omissions of consonants. In two of these the defect was only slight and comparable to the dyslalia which occurs during the early development of speech in so many children with normal intelligence. Here it persisted to a much later age.

Five children used so little speech that their articulation could not be assessed.

Therefore, in 19 of these 24 children who used speech, 11 had normal or near normal articulation, whilst eight had a dyslalia persisting longer than what is within the normal range for the development of articulation.

3. *Thirty-two children aged* 11 *to* 15 *years*

Four of the children in this group were of such low-grade intelligence that its assessment had not been possible. The average intelligence quotient of the remaining 28 children was 43, the range being from 21 to 46.

Language. Thirteen of these children were using sentences or phrases of four to five words. In two of these, however, the content of speech was largely irrelevant, and there was frequent repetition of phrases, often with little meaning.

Nine children used short, simple phrases of two or three words, and nine used only single words.

One child used no expressive speech and attempted only a few vague vocal sounds. Comprehension for speech was also very limited.

Articulation. Sixteen, or half, of these children had normal articulation, and in addition three had minimal defects, two having no defect except for the use of [th] and [r]. One child was unable to use the consonant [s] in speech, although it was used normally in single words.

In five children articulation was normal for the repetition of single words on request, but there was deterioration of varying degrees, amounting to slurring of articulation, and the use of some consonant substitutions during the limited conversational speech heard.

In six children only there was a more obvious defect of articulation. One probably had a dyslalia, and one had a dysarthria in association with cerebral palsy. No actual consonant substitutions were used except for [tʃ (ch)] which she pronounced as [ʃ (sh)], but there was limited movement of the soft palate, resulting in nasalised vowels and weak consonant sounds. She also had some dysphonia. One other child had clumsy and limited movements of the tongue with dysarthria, but without consonant substitutions. One girl aged 11 years, with some loss of comprehension for speech but no apparent loss of hearing, had a severe defect of articulation, substituting [ŋ (ng)] for [p] [b] [t] [d] [k] and [g], and [h] for [s] [f] [ʃ (sh)]. [l] [w] and [r] were used normally.

Two children had insufficient speech for the assessment of articulation.

Therefore, only six children of the 30 whose articulation could be assessed in this group of 32 children, had what could be described as an obvious articulatory defect. Although this is a considerably higher proportion than is usually found in the childhood population at this age, it is apparent that, with a low level of intelligence and poverty of language, the ability to imitate and reproduce accurately the sounds of speech may be adequate for the language used.

The children in the two groups just described, aged 5 to 15 years, were attending a school connected with the mental hospital, where the chief emphasis was on sense training, handwork and general behaviour, developed through games, simple acting, muscial plays and rhythmic work.

In the following two groups, where the patients were aged 15 to 25 years, they were only referred for examination if it was thought that speech therapy might be of assistance. Their speech will be described, but it must be remembered that it does not represent the level of speech attainment at any specific age in this special community.

4. *The speech of five patients aged* 16 *to* 24 *years*

Even at this age speech continued to be limited or defective. One man, aged 21 years, had useful language. Tongue movements were normal, but there was a severe defect of articulation with many substitutions, the only consonant sounds used being [p] [b] [t] [d] [w] and [l].

Three had a limited vocabulary and used incomplete sentences, although articulation was normal.

One woman, aged 19 years, rarely spoke and had very limited

understanding for even simple speech and the names of common objects. She used only the initial syllables of words and very few consonant sounds.

5. *The speech of ten patients aged* 25 *and over*

The age range of these patients was from 25 to 65 years, the average age being 41 years.

Language. Five used speech for communication, although the language was simple and in one patient was limited to short phrases. Three used only single words and comprehension for speech was also very limited, one probably understanding a few routine phrases only. Two patients, aged 41 and 44 years, appeared to have no understanding for speech, one using no expressive speech whatever. The patient aged 65 years had a speech difficulty which was severe, and probably not proportional to her general intelligence, which was higher than in the majority of these patients. She had defective articulation with variable consonant substitutions associated with apparent difficulty in finding the words she needed to express her meaning, and may have had a developmental dysphasia with an articulatory dyspraxia which had persisted into adult life.

Articulation. One patient in this group had normal articulation, and two had insufficient speech for its assessment.

One, aged 37 years, had a persistent minimal dyslalia. [th] was used for [f], and [s] was omitted in combination with another sound as in 'spoon'. Five patients had some degree of dysarthria, articulation for single words spoken slowly being correct but involving effort, and with deterioration during conversational speech. One of these five patients, aged 44 years, had very limited use of consonant sounds. Only seven different consonants were used, and he omitted all medial and final consonants in words. The remaining patient was the woman aged 65 years who had a persisting articulatory dyspraxia associated with limited use of language.

Summary

The outstanding feature in these mentally defective patients was the absence of or poverty of speech, rather than defective use of articulation. The onset of speech was severely delayed, and where it developed there was extreme limitation in the use of expressive speech persisting throughout life. A few used words more fluently but frequently with lack of meaning. Such speech was largely irrelevant and did not always appear to arise in a desire to communicate thought so much as from a desire to attract attention or to make a noise.

In the majority, comprehension for speech was better than executive speech, and the patients could point to an object named, or a picture representing some action, when the corresponding words could not be elicited.

Many of the schoolchildren could repeat nursery rhymes or sing songs. Some required prompting, and in others the repetition resembled echolalia with little or no apparent interest in or understanding of the meaning of the words used.

Although articulation was defective in some of these patients, more than half had normal or near normal articulation. Twenty had insufficient development and use of language for accurate assessment of their articulation, and of the remaining 62, 39 (63 per cent) had no serious defect of articulation.

It was also noticed that many of those who were more intelligent and had better use of language had the more severe defects of articulation, especially in the older age groups.

The general impression was, therefore, that although some of these patients had defects of articulation which tended to persist, the essential speech disability was a delay in its onset, with limited comprehension and expressive use of speech continuing throughout life. Some children with intelligence levels in the lower normal range or below may have delay in speaking which is out of all proportion to their mental retardation. Had speech development been proportional to their general intelligence normal education would have been possible, but with the additional handicap of developmental dysphasia education in a school for children with subnormal intelligence may be required.

Speech and Mongolism

Use of language is frequently affected in mongols, even the high grade mongol may have a severe retardation in comprehension and use of language. Many remain at the one-word sentence level with a limited use of vocabulary throughout life whilst others develop sufficient language skills for useful communication. Engler (1949), studying speech development in mongols, reported that the onset of speech was usually delayed, and found that 49·4 per cent had begun to speak by three years, 61·7 per cent by four years of age, and 81·2 per cent by five years of age. Others have suggested that language development might be more closely related to motor development in general than to intelligence, that is, related to maturation. If so, language training may not be useful until certain levels of maturation have been reached. A delay in maturation could be associated with a delay in phonological development, but it is probable that limited thought due to subnormal intelligence would be the most likely cause for delay in the use of expressive language.

Evans and Hampson (1968) studied the acquisition of language in mongols and the rate and manner of such development as compared with non-mongols. Their findings indicated wide variability in terms of development, and of language patterns; that a hearing defect was more common in these children than in other subnormal populations; and that these children have greater difficulty in using the grammatical structures of language. Mein (1961) also studying language development, found that mongols used a higher percentage of nouns when describing a picture than did non-mongols.

REFERENCES

Creak, M. *et al.* (1961). Schizophrenic Syndrome in Children. *Cerebr. Palsy Bull.*, **3,** 501.

Davis, Russell D. (1954). *Nurture and Mental Development, in Recent Advances in Paediatrics.* Ed. D. M. T. Gairdner. London, Churchill.

Engler, M. (1949). *Mongolism.* Baltimore, Williams and Wilkins.

Evans, D., and Hampson, M. (1968). The Language of Mongols. *Brit. J. Dis. Commun. III*, **2,** 171.

Furneaux, B. (1966). The Autistic Child. *Brit. J. Dis. Commun. I*, **85.**

Kanner, L. (1943). Autistic Disturbances of affective contact. *New. Child.*, **2,** 217.

Kanner, L. (1944). Early Infantile Autism. *J. Pediat.*, **25,** 211.

Mein, R. (1961). A Study of the Oral Vocabulary of severely subnormal Patients (2). Grammatical Analysis of Speech Samples. *J. Ment. Def. Res.*, **5,** 1, 52.

Mittler, P. (1963). Language Development of the Withdrawn Child, in

Communication and the Withdrawn Child. Proceedings of the Conference of the Guild of Teachers of Backward Children, Leicester.

Savage, V. A. (1968). Childhood Autism: Review of the Literature with particular reference to the Speech and Language Structure of the Autistic Child. *Brit. J. Dis. Commun. III*, **1,** 75.

Tubbs, V. (1966). Types of Linguistic Disability in Psychotic Children. *J. Ment. Defic. Res.*, **10,** 230.

VIII. Delayed Development of Speech and Defects of Hearing in Children

One of the most important causes of the delayed development of speech is a defect of hearing. Normally, children hear noises and the sounds of speech. Discrimination and perception for the recognition and meaning of such sounds gradually develops, and the child begins to understand spoken language. Imitation of sounds heard also develops, and the sound sequences become meaningful, are reproduced and eventually used for purposes of communication with others.

In this chapter, in a section dealing with delayed development of speech, only an outline of the basic facts is described, and is concerned with defects of a sufficient degree as to prevent or seriously hinder the development and use of spoken language in both its receptive and expressive aspects. In a later section (p. 352) on defects of articulation, lesser degrees of hearing disorders are considered and the clinical effects described. Such partial hearing losses may not influence the development of language, and may not, at first, be suspected. The child may be referred because of a defect of articulation. He speaks as he hears. Or he may be retarded educationally in school.

Although there can be no absolute division between the two groups, the clinical signs relating to speech differ. Hence the conditions are described according to their effects on spoken language, that is relating to delayed language development, and to articulation.

Sound

Sound travels through air, which, being an elastic medium, is capable of compression and return to its original condition. The rapid alternating displacement of particles of air with successive increases and decreases of pressure at any one point in space produces the phenomena which we recognise as sound. These vibrations of air exert a small force on any surface which they strike, and when they reach the tympanum of the ear they set up corresponding vibrations which are transmitted through the middle ear by means of the ossicles to the cochlea and the auditory nerve. The sensation of hearing is then experienced.

The intensity of a sound is measured by the energy which is transferred through the air. An increase in intensity is recognised by the ear as an increase in the volume of the sound or *loudness* which may also vary according to the frequency with which the vibrations pass along the auditory nerve to the brain.

The speed at which the vibrating particles of air move varies, and the number of complete cycles executed by each particle each second is known as the *frequency* of the vibration. Varying frequencies produce different effects on the ear which are recognised as variations in *pitch*. A more rapidly vibrating particle produces a sensation of higher pitch than one vibrating more slowly. There have been various theories concerning hearing, but probably the effect on the basilar membrane varies according to the frequency of the vibration, 1000 c.p.s. affecting most intensely that part near the mid-point, the pitch of a note as we experience it being dependent on the position on the basilar membrane which receives maximum stimulation.

Every simple harmonic motion of a particle is perceived by the ear as a simple tone, all others are resolved by the ear into a series of simple tones of different periods. Such a *pure tone* will excite with maximum response a region of the basilar membrane where the membrane has a natural frequency of the same period.

Musical notes, whether instrumental or vocal, are complex, and the *quality* of the note is dependent on the number of components of other frequencies which the ear can detect. This varies according to the instrument, and the pitch of the complex tone is that of the pure tone which is recognised as having the same pitch. When these other tones 'are inharmonic and are scattered indiscriminately through the audible pitch range, we describe the impression as a noise'. (Richardson, 1953).

Hearing and Sound

Hearing is the physiological process by means of which we recognise certain air vibrations as sound. Such vibrations may be set in motion in many ways, by the explosion of a bomb or by the vibration of a violin string; as the result of modification of expiratory air in the larynx during phonation, and by the movement of the lips and tongue during the process of articulation.

By normal hearing we understand that hearing response which is adequate for the reception of the sounds of everyday life, and for speech. The normal ear can respond to frequencies of vibration from about 16 c.p.s. to 20,000 c.p.s. If the frequency of vibration is below 16 c.p.s., the alternate increases and decreases of pressure acting on the ear are experienced as sensation of pressure or pulses. As the rate of vibration increases, such isolated beats are blended together and produce the sensation of a gradual rise in pitch of the sound. The lower level of hearing varies according to the individual ear but is about 16 vibrations per second. As the frequency of vibration increases, a point is reached at about 20,000 c.p.s. when the human ear can no longer react, and no sensation of sound is experienced. This upper response varies in different individuals and with age. Response to very high frequencies of sound diminishes with increasing age, but, in general, is not noticed until hearing for frequencies below a level of about 4000 c.p.s. is no longer adequate.

Hearing and Speech

Voice

The frequency of the fundamental tone originating in the larynx is between 100 and 400 vibrations a second, and is usually around 128 c.p.s. for the male speaking voice and 256 c.p.s. (middle C) for the female voice. Vocal sounds in man are produced by air issuing from the lungs as a result of their contraction and expansion. Vibration of this air originates at the laryngeal level, and this vibration is amplified and modified by the cavities of the larynx, chest, throat, nose and sinuses which act as resonators. It has been thought that the membranes of the larynx execute a simple harmonic motion, therefore producing a pure tone, but that the note issuing from the mouth is complex with various harmonics produced by the resonance cavities, at least two of which, the mouth and the larynx, can be adjusted or tuned at will. Pressman and Kaleman (1955), however, state that 'The fundamental pitch as well as overtones originates in the vocal folds of the larynx'.

The vocal cords have been compared to a reed stretched across the larynx, but for the production of voice the action of both vocal cords is necessary, as the sound waves are not produced by the vibration of a single cord. Richardson (1953) considers it is probable that voice may be regarded as 'being engendered by a sort of jet tone in which, however, the membraneous sides of the slit themselves take part, like the lips of a player on a brass instrument'. A stream of air issuing as a jet from a narrow slit sets up movements or vortices in the non-moving air around the orifice. It has been found that the frequency of a tone rises proportionately with the velocity of the outgoing air. Changes in the vocal folds both in tension and width of aperture may, therefore, affect the rate of expulsion of air during vocalisation and so vary the frequency and pitch of the sound which is being produced.

Pressman and Kaleman (1955) describe the action necessary for sound production as follows:

> Laryngeal sounds take place when the vocal cords are approximated by the action of the arytenoid cartilages and placed under tension by the action of the intrinsic and extrinsic musculature of the larynx.
>
> 1. The cords are adducted to the mid-line and placed under tension by the action of the adductor muscles.
>
> 2. Then either the entire length of the cords or varying segments of their more anterior portions, depending on the tone to be produced, are forcibly pulled apart by the action of those internal fibres of the thyroarytenoidei which insert into and become part of the cords. This is accomplished without any movement whatever of the arytenoid cartilages which remain tightly approximated.
>
> 3. The hiatus thus produced allows air to escape under pressure which more or less everts the already separated free margins of the cords.
>
> 4. The everted cord edges by virtue of their elasticity spring back into position without in any way affecting the degree of opening established by the pull of the thyroarytenoidei which remains as before.
>
> 5. This cycle is rapidly repeated, which repetition represents the vibrations of the vocal cords.

The work of Portmann and others, as yet largely unpublished, would indicate that the act of phonation is initiated by the cerebral cortex, which sets up the desired *clonic* movement in the vocal cords as opposed to the traditional theory of tonic contractions at the glottis.

During quiet whispering the differentiation of speech sounds is dependent on the resonance tones produced in the resonating cavities, chiefly the mouth, and excited by the quietly issuing breath stream. During forced whispering a fundamental tone may be produced which approaches but differs from the normal vocal tone. During oesophageal speech such tones in the lower part of the pharynx or oesophagus may be produced by air issuing through a narrow opening, causing vibrations in the air above and around the orifice or constriction. Such sounds may be used as a substitute for voice and as a basis for articulation.

Vowel sounds

Differentiation of the vowel sounds of speech is produced by alterations in the resonance tones, affected largely by changes in the position of the tongue in the mouth, and of the lips. The shape of the mouth may be altered at will so that the human being is able to tune this resonating cavity to imitate and produce many different sounds. For some vowel sounds the mouth is divided into two resonance chambers and the resultant sound is dependent on the proportionate adjustment and balance of resonance tones in the pharynx, mouth and other resonating cavities. Lack of such balance may be the cause of persistence of excessive nasal tone as for example in post-operative cases of cleft palate (see Chapter XVII).

It is probable that there is a fixed simple tone characteristic of each vowel sound which contributes to the complex tone produced by singing the vowel at any pitch. True differentiation and imitation of vowel sounds probably involves, therefore, the appreciation of harmonic tones of higher frequency than the fundamental tone of the human speaking voice, but this may not be essential for the approximate recognition and imitation of such vowel sounds.

Consonants

The consonants used in speech require for their discrimination adequate hearing for frequencies of sound at least up to 2000 c.p.s., whilst some may not be fully appreciated if there is loss of hearing in the frequency range 2000 to 4000 c.p.s. The voiced consonants [b] [d] [g] [v] [z] [r] and [l] have a low-frequency fundamental tone originating in the larynx, their differentiation depending on tones of higher frequency superimposed on the laryngeal tone and dependent on the position and mode of articulation. The voiceless consonants [p] [t] [k] [f] [s] [ʃ (sh)] and [θ (th)] are the result of interruptions of, or modified interference with, the expiratory air stream, the process of articulation involving the selection of the vibration rates necessary for the phonetic sound required. In such sounds there is no low-frequency fundamental tone, although they are closely linked to adjacent vowel sounds, and their differentiation and reproduction depends on appreciation of the higher frequencies of sound in the range 1000 to 2000 c.p.s., with component tones extending possibly to 6000 c.p.s. Consonants such as [s] and [θ (th)] may therefore be heard only approximately if there is useful, although only partial, hearing up to 2000 c.p.s. and may be considerably distorted or not heard if hearing between 4000 and 6000 c.p.s. is inadequate.

Fletcher (1929) and Watson and Tolan (1949) have stated that cutting off all frequencies of sound above 3000 c.p.s. reduces the intelligibility of speech by ten per cent, and above 1500 c.p.s. by 70 per cent. Cawthorn and Harvey (1953) found that the cutting out of frequencies above 3200 c.p.s. had a negligible effect, above 2400 c.p.s. the accuracy of speech reception was reduced by ten per cent, and above 1600 c.p.s. by 40 per cent.

Hearing for speech, therefore, is dependent on the adequate reception of sounds of varying frequency by the inner ear.

Defects of Hearing and Speech

Perceptive or sensori-neural deafness

In perceptive deafness there is a defect, developmental or acquired, in the inner ear, which affects the individual's response to sound vibrations of varying frequency. There may be a partial failure of response which is similar for all frequencies of sound required for speech, or, more usually, there is greater loss for the higher than for the lower tones (Fig. 23).

In a few children the loss is greater for the lower tones (Fig.

24), and in others the greatest loss occurs in the mid range of the frequencies required for speech (Fig. 25). Again there may be a marked difference of hearing for the lower and higher frequencies with almost normal hearing for the lower tones, but hearing for frequencies above 500 c.p.s. or 1000 c.p.s. may be seriously reduced (Fig. 26).

EXAMPLES OF PERCEPTIVE DEAFNESS

(Figs. 23-26 inclusive)

Right = O Left = X Air = —— Bone = ----

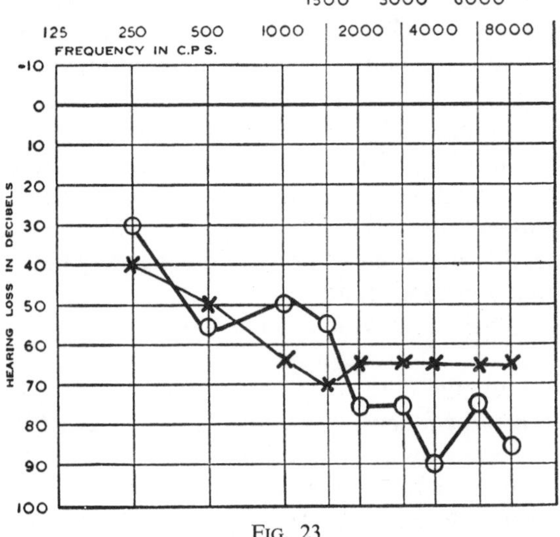

FIG. 23

J. B. Date of birth 15.9.49. Referred at four years two months. He tried to say single words at one year, but only the names of the family. He attempted sound sequences about two years, but speech was not intelligible. He used lip reading to assist his understanding for speech and used gesture freely to explain his meaning. His intelligence quotient on the Drever Collins performance scale was 135. The audiogram was obtained at four years nine months.

Very few people with a hearing loss are totally deaf and without some response to a few frequencies at maximum amplification, but there are many degrees and gradients of hearing loss, and the child's disability will vary according to the severity of the loss and the frequencies of sound most affected. The speech, as he hears it, will be distorted, and he will imitate it as it sounds to him. Even with amplification the sounds of speech, particularly the consonants, may not be received normally in perceptive deafness.

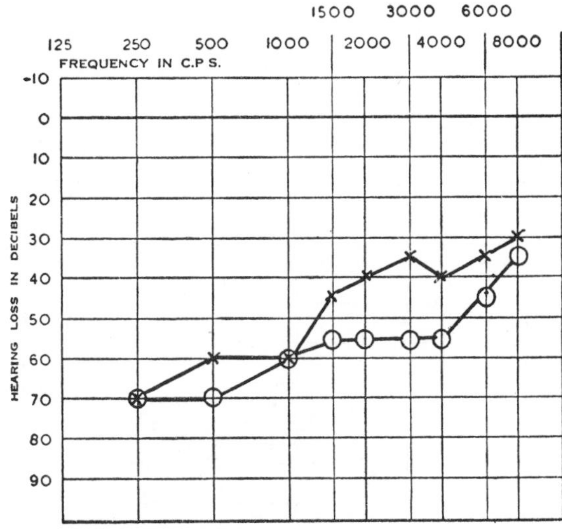

FIG. 24

B. P. Date of birth 27.7.37. Normal development and intelligence. He was referred at five years with no speech and no comprehension for speech except through lip reading. He used some inaccurate vowel sounds and excellent gesture. Special education was refused. At 11 years he drew well, and explained what he wanted by drawing it. He could copy writing. The audiogram was not obtained until he was 12 years of age. He was then using a few words with defective articulation.

Developmental receptive aphasia

In a few children there may be failure to comprehend speech fully when the hearing loss as assessed for various frequencies of sound would seem to be an inadequate cause and the ability to imitate and articulate accurately consonants requiring appreciation of the higher frequencies of sound is not affected. This defect may be associated with some failure of cortical development. Some of these children have normal hearing on audiometric assessment, whilst others show some degree of hearing loss insufficient to account for their marked failure to understand spoken language, and when articulation for the executive speech used is normal. Others show extremely variable responses to pure tone testing, even during the same session of testing. The reason for this is not understood. This condition of developmental receptive aphasia will be described more fully later (see page 138).

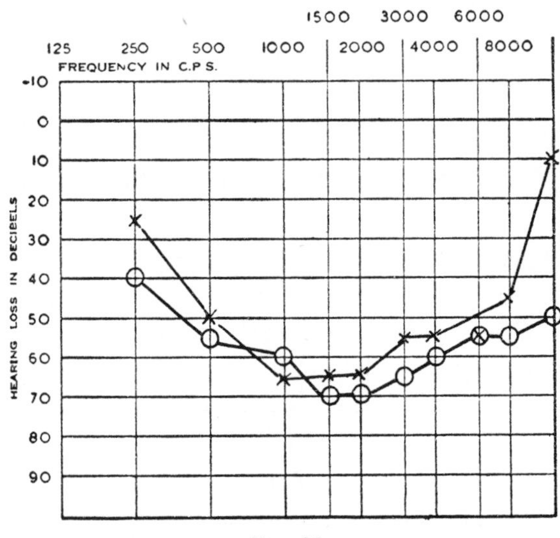

FIG. 25

E. L. Date of birth 8.3.41. He was referred at six and a half years. Normal milestones except speech. He had said 'Mummy' and 'Daddy' at two years, but there was no further speech development and very little understanding for speech. Subsequently there was slow development of speech with normal use of [s] and [f]. At 13 years speech was easily intelligible with good but not normal articulation. He had difficulty in imitating words he did not know. The audiogram was obtained at 13 years, intelligence quotient was then 100.

Central deafness

More recently, the description *central deafness* has been used for auditory impairment resulting from a supposed lack of normal function of the pathways leading from the inner ear to the subcortical, cortical receptive, and interpretative areas of the brain. Audiograms, as shown in Figs. 24 and 25, may represent some form of central deafness as compared with those in Figs. 23 and 26, which are typical of a cochlear hearing defect. Central deafness may therefore be distinguished from peripheral deafness, which includes defects in the outer, middle and inner ears, and in the auditory nerve and its nucleus in the brain stem.

Gordon (1966) uses the term auditory agnosia, and states that it is not surprising that sounds are ignored if they have no

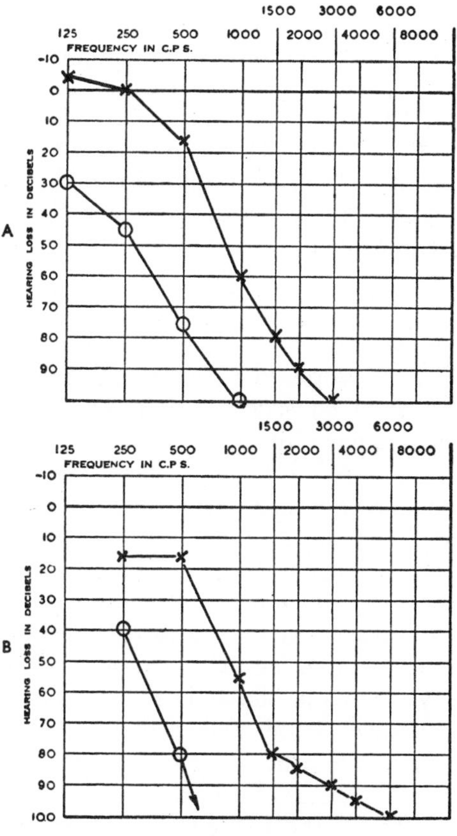

FIG. 26

A. L. This girl was first seen in a school for the deaf at 15½ years. Audiogram (*a*) showed normal hearing in the left ear at 250 c.p.s. but no useful hearing in either ear above 500 c.p.s. She was seen again at 21 years. Audiogram (*b*) showed some further deterioration in hearing. Comprehension for speech was good with lip reading, but was nil without. She had a limited vocabulary and use of speech, and this was generally intelligible.

meaning for the child. If the auditory impulse fails to reach the auditory cortex, or does not have meaning at the cortical level, the child so affected will be unable to develop language in the normal manner in its receptive aspects, and consequently also its expressive use.

This condition may be the cause of what we have described as developmental receptive aphasia, or be so similar in the clinical signs that absolute differential diagnosis may not be possible. In both, however, there is a failure to attach meaning to sounds heard, particularly the sequential sounds of speech, and to fully understand spoken language. At the same time the degree of the hearing defect, as indicated by pure tone hearing tests, is insufficient to account for the limited ability to develop adequate comprehension for speech nor consistent with the phonetic content in the speech used by the child.

Conductive hearing loss

Development and response of the inner ear for reception of sound may be normal, but such sounds may be unable to reach it adequately due to some obstruction or defect in the conductive mechanism of the middle or external ear. There may be wax, or even a foreign body in the external auditory meatus, or there may be inflammation in the inner ear with the possibility of temporary or permanent damage to the transmission mechanism. All sounds reaching the inner ear will then be reduced in strength, but raising the voice and increasing the intensity of the sounds may be sufficient to overcome the transmission defect, and may ensure that the sounds of speech are adequately received in the absence of any additional defect of the inner ear. In such cases sounds may be heard better if the tuning-fork or bone conduction apparatus of the audiometer is placed over the mastoid bone. The sound is then transmitted directly to the inner ear and the obstruction to sound transmission through the external and middle ear is avoided (Fig. 27).

Such conductive deafness rarely affects the development of speech, although, if persistent, it may prove a serious handicap to the child in school. Middle ear infections may not arise until adenoid growth or infected tonsils occur, well after the time at which speech has normally been acquired. Again such conditions are usually intermittent and hearing for speech is not affected continuously. Reception for speech is rarely defective for a raised voice, and in many cases of conductive deafness the higher frequencies required for the appreciation of consonant sounds are not affected, or to a less severe extent than the hearing for the fundamental tones of speech. The intensity of the vocal tones may be diminished, but there is then

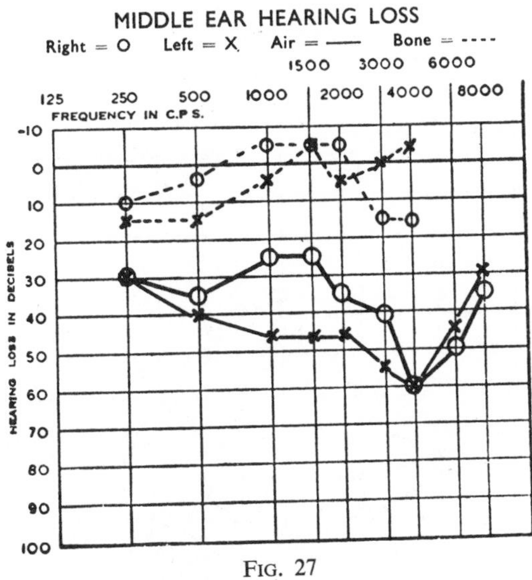

FIG. 27

R. McB. Audiogram showing conductive deafness. This boy had an 'abscess in his right ear' when aged six months, and had had chronic middle ear disease until the age of 11 years. Hearing is better for all frequencies by bone conduction than by air conduction.

little or no distortion of consonant sounds, and their discrimination may be unaffected.

Medical treatment is urgent in such children if advised by the otologist. Apart from the inconvenience and handicap such a child experiences in school, there is always the possibility that a temporary loss of this type may become a chronic ear disease with the possibility of a permanent impairment of hearing.

Mixed deafness

In some individuals there may be a combination of inner ear perceptive hearing loss and defective transmission of sound through the middle ear, and the defect may then be primarily one of transmission but with some reduced cochlear response. Such hearing loss will affect speech and speech reception according to the degree to which discrimination for the frequencies of sound in the consonant range are affected, but in addition there will be a reduction in the intensity of sound reaching the inner ear, with reduced hearing for the vowel sounds of speech (Fig. 28).

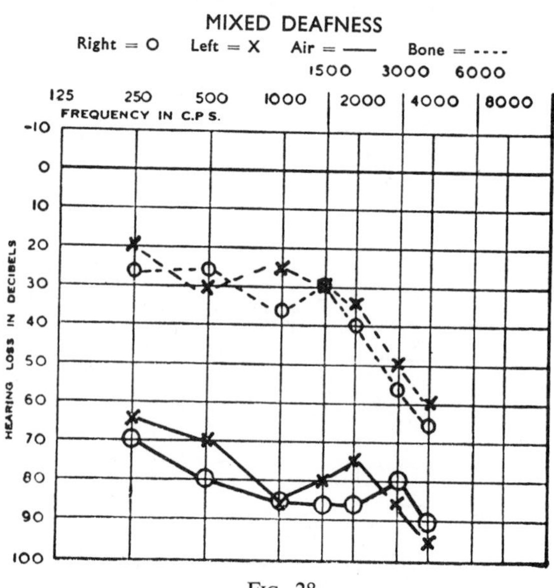

FIG. 28
Audiogram showing a hearing loss where there is a reduced cochlear response in addition to a transmission defect.

It follows, therefore, that with a severe congenital impairment of hearing of the perceptive type, resulting in failure of discrimination for the sounds of speech, there will be a serious delay in the development of understanding for speech with inability to imitate and use expressive speech.

The Delayed Development of Speech and Defects of Hearing

When a child is referred with delayed development of speech, it is important to consider the possibility of a severe hearing defect. This is almost always of perceptive or inner ear type, a conductive deafness rarely interfering with the development of speech.

If the hearing loss is very severe, there will be absence of and no comprehension for speech.

If there is a partial loss for all frequencies, there will be considerable delay in the onset of speech and articulation will be defective. Lip reading may have developed spontaneously to assist comprehension for speech.

Where the hearing loss is mainly for the higher frequencies, as in Fig. 26, with useful hearing for voice, there is usually little delay in the onset of speech. The child hears noises adequately, including voice, and there is therefore some appreciation of the use of speech, its rhythm and even intonation. Articulation is very defective, and again lip reading, spontaneously acquired, will assist understanding for speech.

We are concerned here with the severe hearing loss which is sufficient to prevent or seriously retard the development of speech. Partial hearing loss and its relation to defects of articulation will be described in Chapter XVI.

Hearing defects causing delayed development of speech in 110 *children*

In the group of 280 children referred with delayed development of speech to the speech therapy department of one hospital during the last six years, the cause in 110 children was found to be insufficient hearing. The hearing loss was of the perceptive, or inner ear type, and in 86 children was thought to be congenital, whilst in 24 an illness had occurred in infancy to which the hearing defect might have been attributed. Some of these children had in addition other associated conditions contributing to their disability such as cleft palate and general mental retardation (Fig. 29).

Congenital hearing defects

Of the 86 children with congenital hearing defects, eight were also mentally defective. Two children also had cleft palates, one of whom was, in addition, mentally defective.

Two children had a slight hearing loss of inner ear type, but failure to understand speech was considerable and out of proportion to the degree of hearing loss for pure tones as assessed by audiometry, and to the near normal articulation used in what expressive speech had developed. These two children were considered to be examples of developmental receptive dysphasia and are described in the chapter on developmental aphasia (Chapter IX).

In the remaining 74 children the underlying aetiology was not known, but in two cases the mother had had rubella early during the pregnancy (Fig. 30 and Fig. 31), and one child was known to have had kernicterus soon after birth.

Congenital . . .	86	Hearing loss only	74
		Hearing loss and mental defect .	8
		Hearing loss and cleft palate . .	2
		Slight hearing loss and auditory imperception	2
			86
Acquired . . .	24	. . . .	24
			110

FIG. 29

Perceptive hearing loss and associated conditions in 110 children, accounting for delayed development of speech.

Acquired hearing loss

Twenty-four children had had an illness in early life which might have resulted in defective hearing. These illnesses and the age when they occurred are shown in Fig. 32.

Tuberculous, meningococcal or influenzal meningitis probably accounted for hearing loss in 15 children occurring between the ages of three months and four years. Measles, which may have been complicated by other infections, was possibly the cause in three children between the ages of 3 and 12 months; whooping cough and pneumonia in two children at 5 and 12 months respectively, mumps in one who had already developed speech at three and a half years, but who subsequently lost the ability to speak, and an unspecified illness in three children at 13 and 15 months respectively, was thought to have been the cause of the hearing loss.

The problem of the deaf child has increased since the intro-

HEARING LOSS IN TWO CHILDREN WHERE THE MOTHER HAD RUBELLA IN PREGNANCY

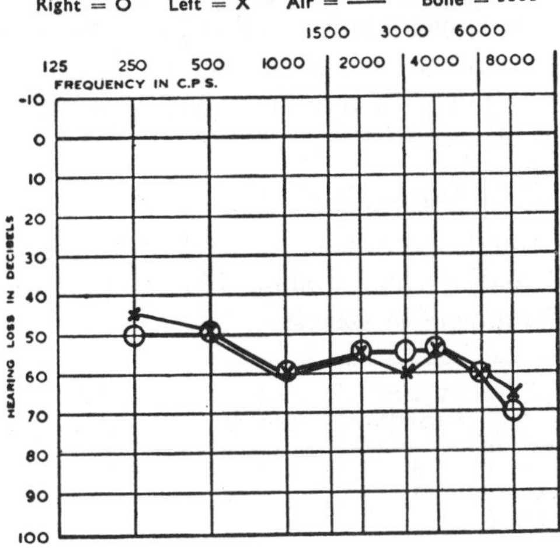

FIG. 30

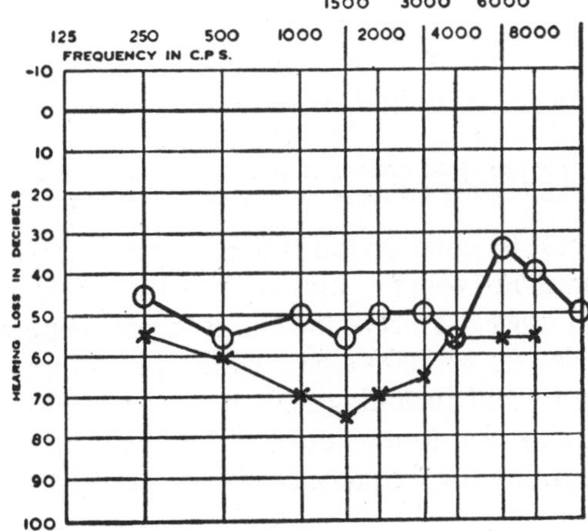

FIG. 31

The hearing loss in two children where the mother had had rubella early in the pregnancy. In both children the hearing loss was partial and similar for all frequencies.

Fig. 30. J. H. was aged six years nine months when **first seen. The mother had had rubella between the fourth and sixth weeks of pregnancy.**

Fig. 31. M. P. was first seen at three and a half years. **The above audiogram was obtained at nine years and confirmed previous ones. The mother had had rubella during the second month of pregnancy.**

duction of antibiotics. Children who now suffer from such severe illnesses as meningitis in infancy recover, and a minority are left with an impairment of hearing for which there is, as yet, no treatment, and with resultant absence of or delay in the development of speech.

The extent of the hearing loss

An approximate assessment of the hearing loss was obtained by pure tone audiometry for all but 19 of these 110 children with delayed development of speech.

Diagnosis	Under 6 months	6-12 months	12-24 months	2-4 yrs	Total
Meningitis	3	7	3	2	15
Severe measles	1	2	0	0	3
Severe whooping cough and pneumonia	1	1	0	0	2
Mumps	0	0	0	1	1
Unspecified	1	0	2	0	3
	6	10	5	3	24

FIG. 32

Table showing the age of occurrence of an illness possibly resulting in a loss of hearing which interfered with the development of speech in 24 children.

Nine of these 91 children failed to respond to any audiometric tone at maximum volume, and no hearing could be detected for any loud noise. Thirty-nine children had some response to all frequencies up to 8000 c.p.s., whilst 11 children had some response up to and including 2000 c.p.s. only. Four children had no hearing for tones above 500 c.p.s. and five had no detectable hearing for frequencies above 1000 c.p.s. (Fig. 33).

The age of onset of speech

Six of these 110 children had made no vocal or babbling sounds beyond crying and some pleasure sounds. Twenty-three children had not attempted to use single words although the mothers reported that they had made babbling sounds and other vocal noises. Thirteen children had first used words between one and two years, and the remainder had done so between the ages of two and eight years. The ages when these children first began to use single words is shown in Figure 34.

THE EXTENT OF THE RESIDUAL HEARING AND THE AGE OF SPEECH ONSET

No response at maximum volume above. . . .	Frequency in cycles per second							No response to any frequency	Total
	500	1000	1500	2000	3000	4000	8000		
Number of children . .	4	5	5	11	1	17	39	9	91

Not ascertained in 19 children.

FIG. 33

Table showing the extent of the residual hearing—in 110 children.

	Age in years							No words	No babbling	Total
	1–2	–3	–4	–5	–6	–7	–8			
Number of children	13	22	28	12	2	2	2	23	6	110

FIG. 34

Table showing the age of onset of single words in 110 children with a hearing loss.

In some instances the sounds thought to have been words may have been the result of optimism, and in the majority they were limited to the use of one or two words such as 'Mum' or 'Da', and speech failed to progress beyond this stage. In all these children speech was severely delayed as the result of a gross defect of hearing for speech.

We were also interested to know if speech continued to be limited throughout life, or to what extent it could be developed through special education.

In 1947 an investigation was carried out into the standard of speech development and degree of hearing loss in 112 children attending a residential school for the deaf. This assessment was made before the introduction of the Government hearing aid and none of the children assessed had used a hearing aid of any type.

Hearing Loss and Speech Development in 112 Children in a Residential School for the Deaf

Sixty-eight of these children probably had a congenital hearing loss, and in 44 there was the possibility of an acquired hearing loss in early life. Nine were known to have experienced an illness between 3 and 12 months of age which could have resulted in an impairment of hearing (Fig. 35).

Age in Years	Hearing Loss		Total
	Congenital	Acquired	
6	4	1	5
7	5	6	11
8	11	2	13
9	4	5	9
10	8	7	15
11	9	6	15
12	10	2	12
13	3	6	9
14	5	7	12
15	9	2	11
Total	68	44	112

Fig. 35

Age in years at the time of assessment of 112 children

When assessing the relationship between the standard of speech developed and the degree of hearing loss we could not exclude entirely the effect of other factors such as intelligence and the length of time the child had been in school receiving education and special speech training.

Thirty-six of the 112 children were either too young for reliable pure tone assessment of their hearing or were believed to have had some speech before the illness which caused the hearing loss.

In the remaining 76 children the hearing loss was congenital or occurred before the age of one year. They were between the ages of 6 and 15 years, and were able to give reliable responses to testing with a pure tone audiometer. Thirty-five were girls and 41 were boys. Our findings will therefore be described for this group of 76 children.

At the time this investigation was carried out in 1947 there were many partially deaf children attending the school, a number of whom had good or even near normal speech. With the increase in the number of severely deaf children, and the advent of hearing aids, many children with a partial hearing loss are now being educated in the normal school until adequate provision in a special class or school is available.

The majority of children who attend schools for the deaf develop understanding for written and printed language and are able to read and write. Spoken language may be largely understood through lip reading, and their ability to use intelligible articulation with normal intonation varies with their ability to hear or appreciate in other ways the sounds and movements of speech.

Assessment of hearing

In order to be able to compare the extent of the hearing loss with the type of speech developed, we took as a basis for comparison the average of the hearing loss in decibels in the better ear for three frequency ranges:

1. 256 to 1000 c.p.s.
2. 1000 to 4000 c.p.s.
3. 4000 to 12,000 c.p.s.

Fletcher [12] has more recently (1950) suggested that the hearing loss for speech might possibly be predicted by noting the loss in decibels for the frequencies 500, 1000 and 2000 c.p.s. An average is then taken of the two readings showing least hearing loss.

Assessment of speech

The speech of the children was assessed at three levels and the children were placed in one of three groups as follows:

A. Good or near normal speech.
B. Defects of articulation and limited use of language, but useful oral communication.
C. Very little, if any, intelligible speech.

This classification was based largely on the opinion of the school teachers who knew the children well. Because the standard of speech development was necessarily related to the age of the children and to the length of time they had been in school, these 76 children were subdivided into two groups according to age. The younger group included children aged six to ten years whilst the children in the older group were aged 11 to 15 years, as follows:

1. Aged 6-10 years . . 37 children
2. Aged 11-15 years . . 39 children

—

76 children

The level of speech development in these children is shown in Fig. 36. It will be noted that there are fewer children with good speech and more children with unintelligible speech in the

Speech	37 children aged 6-10 yrs.	39 children aged 11-15 yrs.	Total
A. Slight defects of articulation or normal speech .	2	11	13
B. Defective articulation with limited use of language, but useful oral communication	9	11	20
C. Very little or no intelligible speech . . .	26	17	43
	37	39	76

FIG. 36
The level of speech attainment in 76 children in two age groups.

younger age group than in those older children who had had the advantage of a longer period in school.

The average hearing loss in the better ear for three frequency ranges is shown in Figure 37 for each of the three levels of speech attainment.

Speech	No. of Children	Frequency in Cycles per Second		
		250-1000	1000-4000	4000-8000
(1) 37 Children aged 6-10 years				
A	2	45 db.	65 db.	70 db.
B	9	50 db.	63 db.	75 db. (2 nil)
C	26	70 db. (1 nil)	90 db. (9 nil)	95 db. (20 nil)
(2) 39 Children aged 11-15 years				
A	11	30 db.	50 db.	50 db.
B	11	50 db.	75 db.	90 db. (5 nil)
C	17	80 db. (2 nil)	90 db. (5 nil)	100 db. (17 nil)

FIG. 37

Average hearing loss for three frequency ranges in 76 children compared with their level of speech attainment,

Speech development in relation to the extent of the hearing defect

From the Table (Fig. 37) it will be seen that 44, or more than half, of these 76 children had no detectable hearing response for any frequencies of sound above 4000 c.p.s. Thirty-seven of these had no useful speech, and in the remaining seven it was severely defective. We cannot, however, conclude that these higher frequencies are essential for speech because all these children also had a more severe loss for the frequencies in the lower and middle range.

All the 13 children with good or normal speech, however, had some hearing for the frequency range 4000 to 12,000 c.p.s.

Their greatest average loss of hearing in the medium range was 65 db. and for the lower frequencies 45 db.

Twenty children had limited speech and defective articulation. Of these, seven had no hearing at maximum volume on the audiometer for any frequencies above 4000 c.p.s. The greatest average loss in the middle frequency range was 75 db. and 50 db. for the lower frequencies.

Forty-three children had very little, or no intelligible speech. Twenty-six of these were in the lower age group and had been in school for a shorter period than those in the older group where 17 of the 39 children had failed to develop useful speech.

Twenty-seven of these 43 children had no hearing response above 4000 c.p.s., 16 did not respond to frequencies above 1000 c.p.s., and in three there was no response to any pure tones on the audiometer even at maximum volume.

The approximate curves shown in Figure 38 indicate the extent of hearing loss for each level of speech development according to our findings in the older group of 39 children aged 11 to 15 years.

Markides (1970) has also analysed the speech of selected groups of deaf and partially hearing children with a view to identifying factors affecting the speech intelligibility of these children. Her findings showed that deaf children were 4–5 years, and partially hearing children 2–3 years, retarded in the use of vocabulary, also that retardation increased with age. The younger children in both these groups were less retarded than older children.

The most frequently misarticulated consonants were [s], [ʃ], [z] and [ʒ]. Final consonants were misarticulated more frequently than initial consonants, omission errors were more frequent among the deaf and substitutions among the partially hearing. As would be expected, linguistic development decreased and articulation errors increased in relation to the degree of hearing loss.

Assessment of Hearing

When a severe or partial hearing loss is suspected in a child referred with delayed development of speech or defective articulation it is of first importance that the extent and type of hearing loss should be assessed as early as possible. In the very young child with no speech this is not easy and may require much time and patience. It may usefully be carried out in the first instance by the speech therapist, who has been

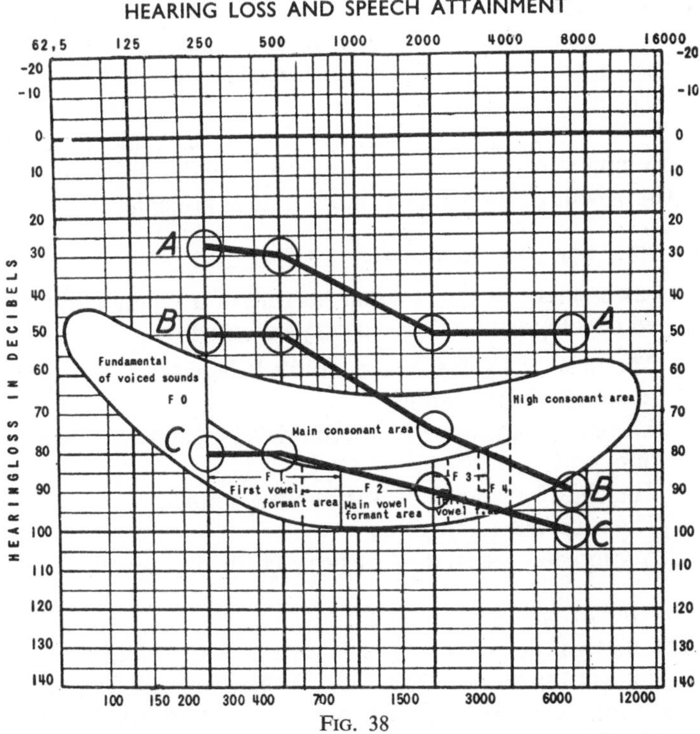

FIG. 38

Chart showing the formant areas for vowels and consonants. (Reproduced from *Acta Otolaryng.* 1953-54, 103-110, p. 12, Fig. 3. Supplement. Data from G. Fant (L.M.E.).) Superimposed are the approximate average hearing loss curves A, B and C, associated with three levels of speech attainment.

adequately trained in methods of testing the hearing of such young children. An audiometer should be available and considered an essential part of the equipment of a speech therapy department.

If the suspected hearing loss is confirmed, the child must be referred to the otologist for examination, diagnosis and medical treatment, if indicated. If the hearing loss is of the inner ear type and no treatment is possible, the mother must be advised, so that she understands the situation fully, and given guidance as to how she may help the child most usefully in the home.

Auditory training should be commenced under the guidance of the teachers in a school for the deaf, if possible, or by a speech therapist, using a hearing aid if it is found to be helpful. Arrangements must also be made, through the otologist or paediatrician, with the local education authority for the child's admission, when old enough, to a suitable school for education of the deaf.

All these arrangements depend in the first place on the ascertainment of the hearing loss, and secondly on as accurate an assessment of the residual hearing as is possible.

Methods for the Assessment of Hearing

An assessment of the residual hearing of a young child with delayed development of speech may be based on:

1. The mother's story of the child's behaviour and response to sounds in the home.
2. The extent and type of speech development and articulation.
3. The child's response to various test sounds.
4. The response to speech.
5. Audiometer assessment of hearing for pure tones.

1. *The mother's story*

The mother's observations are based on the child's natural behaviour in the home rather than in the unfamiliar conditions of the clinic, and are, in most cases, a useful guide. We have found the following questions most useful:

(*a*) Does the child come from another room when called, or when he is playing outside?

(*b*) Does he ever turn round when a door is opened or shut, or go to the door when there is a knock, or the bell rings?

(*c*) Does he listen to the radio, and turn it on or off (and not because he likes to see it light up)?

Does he ever turn round if it is suddenly switched off when he is not looking? If old enough, does he ever listen to speech in children's programmes or only to music?

(*d*) Does he listen to a story or nursery rhymes, and if so does he watch the speaker's face to assist his understanding for speech?

(*e*) Does the mother use gestures when she is explaining something to the child. She may be quite unaware of the extent to which she does this and may have to watch herself carefully to give a reliable answer to this question.

2. *Speech development*

The age of development of speech, if any, and the extent of the vocabulary and the type of articulation, as previously described, may be a guide to the degree of hearing loss. Perceptive deafness may be approximately divided into three types according to the effect it will have on speech development, always remembering, however, that there is no clear line of demarcation between them and that the level of speech attainment will be related to the extent and type of the residual hearing, other factors excluded.

(*a*) Very severe hearing loss for all frequencies.	No speech and no understanding for speech.
(*b*) Partial hearing loss for all frequencies.	Late development of speech—and defective articulation varying with the range of hearing loss, and with intelligence. Lip reading, spontaneously acquired, may be used to compensate for hearing loss.
(*c*) High tone hearing loss. Hearing for low tones and for voice may be normal, but hearing for consonants is distorted, with failure of discrimination.	Speech development probably at the normal age but may be limited in extent. Articulation severely defective, especially for the high frequency consonants [f] [s] and [θ] with inability to hear or imitate these accurately in isolation. Poor comprehension for speech apart from lip reading, with which it may approach normal in some children.

3. *Response to various noises*

In these tests it must always be remembered that although a positive response generally indicates that the child has heard the sound, failure to respond may result from lack of interest, refusal to co-operate, insufficient intelligence, or attention directed elsewhere to the exclusion of these test sounds.

If possible, the child's co-operation should first be gained through play. His attention should then be directed to some simple toy or game which does not demand his entire concentration. The sounds made should be interesting and varied. Ewing (1954) has described children who are apparently deaf when tested with loud sounds but who responded to instructions spoken in a moderately loud voice at six feet, and says, 'It is certain that other factors than pitch, loudness and duration of sound determine the child's response or failure to respond.' They also describe how, 'It is best to notice his reactions to quiet rather than to loud sounds, which occur regularly and naturally in his normal environment.' 'It is advisable to keep in mind that neither learned nor even reflex responses to sound are invariable and automatic, and that a form of sound that often or usually evokes a response from a child in a certain kind of situation may be ignored by him in other situations or circumstances.' The rustle of a sweet paper, the sound of a spoon in a cup, the ringing of a bell, the sound of a mouth organ, the squeak of a rubber mouse, a gramophone played with varying degrees of amplification, or pure tones from the audiometer delivered through a loud speaker may all be used in an attempt to obtain a reliable response.

The response may include eye movements alone, or a turning of the head towards the sound, or a questioning look round the room. It may also consist of momentary cessation of activity or even a look which indicates resistance to co-operation.

These tests may also be repeated when the child is using a hearing aid, but care must be taken to ensure that only a moderate degree of amplification is used at first. If there is no response it may be increased, but the child's co-operation may be entirely lost as the result of a bombardment of excessively loud noises.

McLaurin (1954) has described the development of response

to sounds and to speech in the very young child. He states that the child's first response to sound may occur soon after birth but becomes more definite by the end of the first month. It is usually a reflex response indicated by movement of the eyelids. During the first three months the child responds more readily to noises of varying kinds than to voice.

4-6 months	The response to noises and to voice is about equal, but a quiet voice is more effective than a loud one.
6-12 months	The child recognises meaningful sounds such as tapping the feeding-bottle or the noise of a spoon in a cup. He localises sounds and turns his head or eyes towards the source of the sound.
1-2 years	During this period the child responds to speech, again preferring a quiet voice, but not a whisper.
2-3 years	His capacity to localise sounds increases and speech and voice tests may now be used for testing hearing. Pure tones, as used for audiometer testing, usually do not interest the child at this age.
3-5 years	The child may now respond to audiometric testing. Speech and whispering may also be used for testing hearing response.

4. *Response to speech*

Response to speech should be tested if the child is over two years of age or is attempting to use speech. The speech stimulus must be interesting and suitable to the age of the child. One small boy who had failed to co-operate responded immediately when the mother said in a normal voice 'Get your coat, we're going home.' The following tests may be useful:

(*a*) Response to his or her name. This is probably the most familiar word to any child, and his response should be tested using a quiet voice, followed by the name spoken with increasing volume of sound.

(*b*) If the child is old enough he may be asked to pick out various toys from a box or bring them from the toy cupboard on request, to put the car in the garage, or put the dolly in the bed, and so forth. Response should be tested for single words, such as 'where is the *ball*' or 'give the *ball* to Mummy', the car, the chair (doll's size) and so forth. Again the child may be asked to pick out a picture of a common object from a row of pictures of objects such as a spoon, house, ball, baby, man and cat. Such tests should be carried out using at first a normal voice, or even a quiet voice if the child is near. A loud voice may be used if there is failure to respond, and again using increasing volume and at varying distances from the child.

(*c*) The child's ability to imitate certain consonant sounds or to respond to them may be tested. If the sounds [s] [f] [θ (th)] or [ʃ (sh)] are spoken close to the child, care must be taken that he does not turn because he feels the breath rather than hears the sound. Ability to respond or to imitate these sounds should be tested as an indication of response to the higher frequencies of sound.

(*d*) Response to speech using a hearing aid. In the very young child babble sounds such as 'bah, bah, bah' may produce some response from the child. He may show interest, move his lips, or even imitate the sound. If he is able to show that he can differentiate between two or three syllable babbles there is an indication of improved response to speech through amplification.

In the older partially deaf child with a conductive type of deafness there will probably be an immediate improvement in speech reception through use of a hearing aid, but the child with an acquired perceptive hearing loss subsequent to normal speech development will not necessarily understand speech more easily. Amplification of the low tones and surrounding noises may need to be increased to such an extent, in order that hearing may be improved for the higher frequencies of sound required for consonant discrimination, that the result may be compared with an attempt to listen to speech in a noisy factory for one with normal hearing.

The child with a congenital partial perceptive deafness, who has acquired some speech, may find that speech heard through a hearing aid resembles another language. Consonant sounds may now be heard which have never been appreciated before, whilst other sounds may seem to be distorted and unfamiliar. The hearing aid may need to be in constant use for six months or more before such a child learns to understand speech through a hearing aid.

In the child who has failed to develop speech a hearing aid will not make speech at once intelligible. Even if the aid is useful and suitable to the type of hearing loss, constant use of the aid and exposure to the sounds of speech for a year or two may be necessary before the child will develop understanding for speech.

5. *Audiometric assessment of hearing for pure tones*

The degree of hearing loss for pure tones of varying frequency can be tested using an audiometer. Pure tones of frequencies between 120 and 12,000 cycles per second are heard through ear-phones and a calibrated volume control enables the air conduction loss of hearing in decibels to be determined directly. If instead of the ear-phones a bone conduction apparatus is applied over the mastoid bone, it can be determined whether the loss by air conduction is the result of a conductive defect in the middle ear or of failure of response by the inner ear. In the former case the bone conduction test may show almost normal reception for sound by the inner ear when the air conduction tests indicate a partial loss of auditory acuity.

Audiometric tests usually present little difficulty in the older child and adult, or in young children who have sufficient hearing for speech to enable them to understand simple directions. It is much more difficult, however, in the young child who does not respond to speech and who may find the pure tones of the audiometer uninteresting and meaningless if not actually unpleasant. Many small children also dislike the pressure of the ear-phones and headband, even when they are detached and used singly.

Audiometric testing requires that the patient should indicate that he hears a pure tone when the volume is adjusted so that the sound can only just be detected. This is the threshold of hearing for that particular frequency and must be ascertained for each frequency in turn. The young child generally fails to respond to sounds of such minimal intensity, and allowance must always be made for the age of the child when considering the audiogram. This is also necessary in the case of a mentally backward child, many of whom may fail to respond until the intensity of the sound is 25 to 30 decibels above threshold, or even to very loud tones.

Various methods have been devised to assist the assessment of hearing in young children. In one the child is conditioned to respond to a given pure tone signal by carrying out some action. This requires the active co-operation of the child and the result obtained depends entirely on the child's response.

Another method, the psychogalvanic skin resistance test, is used in an attempt to obtain an assessment without the active co-operation of the child, and use is made of the physiological change in the electrical resistance of the skin to the passage of an electric current as the result of an external stimulus such as pin prick or mild electric shock. The emotional reaction to an unpleasant stimulus causes a physiological change. When this stimulus is associated with an audiometric tone, the child may be conditioned to respond in a similar way to this tone alone.

6. *The conditioned response*

Simple tests demand that the child should react when he hears the sound by performing some action which is interesting but not too absorbing.

1. A whistle is blown and the child picks up a marble and drops it into a box through a hole in the lid. It is helpful if the mother does this at first until the child wishes to try himself. The child also sees the tester blowing the whistle and perhaps responds to the action seen rather than to the sound heard if the hearing loss is severe.

2. When this reaction has been established, a large sheet of paper hides the whistle from the child. If the sound of the whistle has been important to the child in the conditioning, he continues to respond to the sound by putting the marbles in the box. The ringing of a bell and the squeak of a rubber mouse may also be used as test sounds. Whilst the child is listening

to the sounds it is useful if the audiometer ear-phone is held near his ear, although not in use.

3. The audiometric pure tone is next substituted for the whistle, either through the ear-phone or through a loud-speaker, and the test is continued. It is most important that the audiometer tone should be loud enough for the child to hear but not loud enough to be disagreeable or to frighten him. 500 c.p.s. is a more definite sound than 250 c.p.s. and should be used for conditioning.

In the very young child as few frequencies as possible should be tested as fatigue and failure to co-operate may occur at any moment. It is best therefore to test the frequencies in order of importance. This may vary somewhat for the individual, but probably 500, 2000, 250, 4000 and 1000 c.p.s. in that order will be found most useful in assessing approximately the usefulness of the child's hearing for speech. The length of the signal tone is also important. It should be of short enough duration to avoid fatigue but long enough for the child to be able to appreciate it, and an interrupted tone may give a better response than a long sustained one.

The time interval at which the signals are given must be varied or the child may accept a regular rhythm and react when he expects the sound rather than when he hears it. Reconditioning may be necessary at intervals, and the tester must continually ensure that the child is reacting only when the pure tone is sounding. The marble response is useful as the tester can hear the marble drop without turning to look at the child. One child became conditioned to the movement of the tester's head and dropped the marble when the tester turned to look at her.

The games should be varied to sustain interest. A small child may find it easier to place a large wooden cylinder into a hole in a block of wood, or coloured pegs may be fitted into a board. Many children invent games of their own, such as rolling the marble round the lid of the box before letting it drop in, or become more interested in sorting the colours of the marbles and pegs than in carrying out the response required. Such conditioning requires that the child learns to respond by the required action when he hears the sound, and, just as important, that he learns not to respond when he does not hear the sound.

The Hallpike Peepshow (1947). Here the child is conditioned to press a button switch when the pure tone is heard through the ear-phones, or through a loud-speaker placed at a known and constant distance from the child's head. The reward is a picture which is illuminated when the child presses the switch. The circuit is so connected that pressing the switch produces no result unless the pure tone is sounding.

Psychogalvanic skin resistance reaction in tests of hearing

Hardy and Bordley (1951) have carried out experiments since 1947 at Johns Hopkins University School of Medicine to develop suitable technique for an objective method of assessment of hearing capacity in young children.

The child is seated in a high chair or at a table and occupied with toys. Two electrodes are attached to the child's leg, usually the calf of the leg, about one inch apart. Stimulation of the sympathetic nervous system as the result of a slight electric shock in this circuit of which the child is a part increases the activity of the sweat glands, with resultant lowering of resistance of the skin. Two pick-up terminals are attached to the palm and back of the child's hand or foot, and changes in this circuit as a result of the alteration in the skin resistance are indicated by a galvanometer and recorded in wave form by a stylus attached to the moving needle of the galvanometer.

The audiometer ear-phones are placed in position and the child is then conditioned to react to a pure tone delivered through the ear-phones. A pure tone is given first, followed by a slight electric shock. A lowering of the skin resistance is then indicated by a change in the current strength. Eventually, the reaction takes place on production of the auditory stimulus alone, the child having been conditioned to recognise this as being associated with, and in anticipation of, the unpleasant sensation of the electric shock. Each pure tone can then be tested, movement of the galvanometer needle indicating when the child reacts to, and presumably hears, the tone given. Further reinforcement of the conditioning may be required at intervals during testing.

Hardy and Pauls (1952) claim that assessment of hearing by such means can be carried out on children from the age of four months with reasonable accuracy, but the interpretation of the result obtained is not always easy. Other extraneous stimuli are liable to produce emotional reactions with changes in skin resistance which may influence the readings. However, the observer is usually able to accustom himself to the reaction time of the individual child and can recognise those reactions which are probably the result of the auditory stimulus and those which are not. The assessment of hearing by this means requires skill, and is not precise nor infallible.

Measurement of Hearing Loss

In audiometry the degree of hearing loss is indicated by the number of decibels above zero, or the intensity level to which the volume of a pure tone must be raised to be just audible. This is the threshold of hearing for the particular frequency of sound, and requires the minimum energy of vibration which arouses auditory sensation. The standard unit of intensity of sound is that of a tone whose objective intensity is ten times that of the sound necessary to arouse minimal auditory sensation. This unit is the bel, but in practice one-tenth of this unit—the decibel—is used. The decibel scale is logarithmic, and expresses a ratio between two quantities.

The ratio of the loudest sound the ear can hear without pain to the weakest sound the ear can detect equals 12 bels or 120 decibels.

For a plane sound wave in air the volume or loudness of the sound depends on the intensity or energy of the sound wave, and the reference level of intensity has been measured as a pressure of 0·0002 dynes per sq. cm., which is approximately equivalent to the average threshold of hearing at 1000 c.p.s.

The audiometer is calibrated by reference to normal hearing at certain fixed frequencies of sound. The patient's loss of hearing can be read directly in decibels from the volume scale of the audiometer and the relationship of the patient's threshold of hearing for any frequency to normal intensity will determine the relative hearing loss at that frequency.

The approximate sound intensities of various familiar sounds in decibels above threshold are shown in Figure 39.

Although the audiometer is calibrated with reference to normal hearing, there are variations from time to time in the actual intensity of the tones and there is need for frequent checking and recalibration. There is also variation between different makes of audiometer. The Committee appointed by the Medical Research Council (1947) reported that 'It will be noted that the results show that large inconsistencies in the threshold readings, amounting to as much as 20 db., exist between individual commercial audiometers.' Allowance must therefore be made for the variations and differences of audiometer readings.

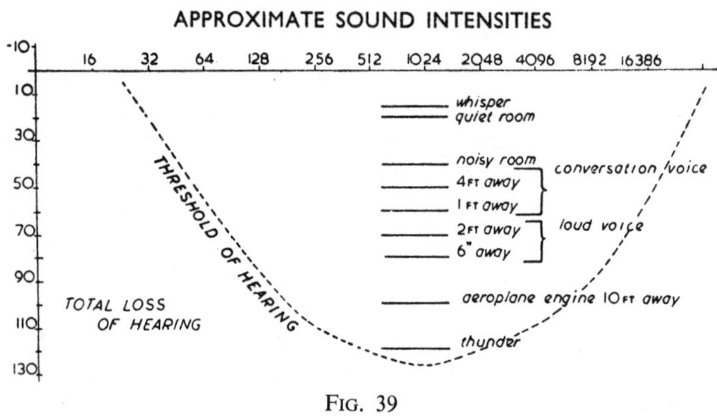

FIG. 39

The approximate sound intensities in decibels above threshold of a whisper, conversational and loud voice, and other sounds.

SPEECH AUDIOMETRY

Cawthorn and Harvey (1953) have pointed out that it would be a mistake to believe that it is always possible to estimate the ability to understand speech from the results of assessment of thresholds of hearing for pure tones. 'In conduction deafness there is a fairly constant relationship between loss of hearing for pure tones and speech. Perceptive deafness often behaves quite differently and it would be fair to say that an examination is not complete without a test of hearing capacity for speech.'

For this purpose the patient is asked to repeat the words on the Medical Research Council word list, and the test is therefore only of use in cases of acquired deafness and where hearing has been adequate for speech development. The threshold of detectability or zero level is defined as that 'maximum attenuation which enables a normal hearing person to detect the sound but not the meaning of about half the words'. The threshold of speech intelligibility is 'the level measured in decibels above the zero level at which the listener repeats 50 per cent of words correctly'. An increase of ten decibels or more raises the intelligibility to 90 per cent. The discrimination loss is defined as the difference between 100 per cent and the maximum intelligibility, which is equal to the highest percentage of words that the patient is able to repeat correctly.

They summarised their findings as follows:

1. In pure conduction deafness there is a close correlation between hearing for pure tones and for speech.
2. In mixed deafness there is a definite relationship but not so close as for conductive deafness.
3. In perceptive deafness the ability to understand speech may have little relationship with pure tone hearing.

It is important to realise, therefore, that even if an assessment of a child's hearing for pure tones is obtained it may give no accurate measurement of the difficulty the child will experience in hearing and imitating speech.

THE CHILD WITH A HEARING LOSS

The effect of a severe impairment of hearing on the development of speech has already been described. The child is unable to develop the normal means of communication through speech, but he may make use of natural gesture, which later may become a highly developed language of signs. He may also be taught to use the manual alphabet, or be trained by a special visual and kinaesthetic approach to make the best possible use of audible speech. He will also learn to understand the speech of others through lip reading, but his ability to express himself intelligibly through speech will be limited and determined largely by the extent of the hearing loss.

The child's difficulty is not limited, however, to his fundamental hearing loss, because his inability to make contacts with others through hearing and speech will cause interference with normal behaviour and development, and it is important that a real understanding of the cause of his difficulty should be ascertained as early in life as possible. Interference with this aspect of normal development at the peak period for the development of speech will cause frustration, resulting perhaps in temper tantrums and perhaps withdrawal from normal contacts with other children and may have a far-reaching effect on the future life of the individual. Such frustration is often felt more

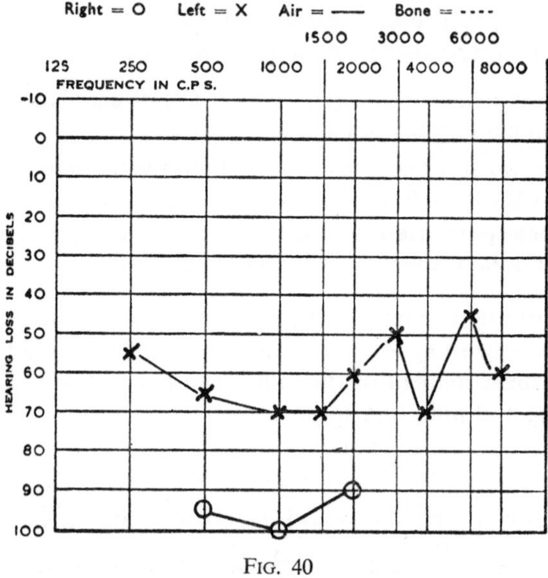

FIG. 40

F. A., aged six years two months. Audiogram showing a hearing loss which was not at first suspected.

keenly by the child with some residual hearing who can appreciate that speech is used by others and is yet aware of his own limitations.

F. A. was referred to the speech therapy department in 1948 at the age of five years. The paediatrician's report on the child when first seen at three and a half years was as follows:

This child exhibits a type of behaviour abnormality which has been termed autism, in that the child seems to be unaware of other people as personalities and to be content to enter into no human relationships. There is good understanding of concrete and mechanical objects, but none of abstraction. There is often a defect in talking and the child seems to feel little need for speech, as a result perhaps of her unawareness of, or lack of need for, other people; in this case the defect takes the form of almost complete absence of speech.

And again: 'Human voices mean nothing to her, but she listens intently to music. She hates loud noises.'

At three and a half years she had one word, 'Mummy', and a few words used indiscriminately. Between three and four years there was no further advance in speech. Music and dancing were her chief interests. She observed detail accurately and was very independent.

Between four and five years she began to play with other children, and led them without the use of speech.

Not until five years of age was a hearing loss suspected. It was noticed that she often failed to look up when spoken to, but when aware of speech she watched the face of the speaker. From this time speech developed more rapidly, and at five and a half years she could repeat rhymes and tell stories, though with some grammatical errors. She still used mime and gesture when trying to express herself. With development of speech she became more affectionate towards other people, and there was 'no further evidence of a gross behaviour disorder of the autistic type '.

Otological examination showed no abnormality, but audiometric assessment showed almost total loss of hearing in the right ear with a partial loss for all frequencies in the left ear (Fig. 40).

EDUCATION

The type of education most suitable for the child will depend on his ability to understand and use speech with or without a hearing aid. If he can learn through hearing, and understanding for speech is adequate, he should be educated in the normal school, but if the expressive use of speech is delayed beyond the age of four or five years it is probable that special education will be necessary.

Where there is some degree of delayed or defective development of speech but education is still possible through the auditory pathways, education should be in a school or class for the partially deaf where special methods are used to assist the child through understanding of his needs, and where the intelligent child can achieve a similar standard to that of the child with normal hearing.

If the hearing loss is more severe and the child is dependent to a greater extent on learning through the visual pathways, education should be in a school for the severely deaf.

The education of the severely deaf child requires special

understanding and knowledge and can best be undertaken by trained teachers of the deaf. The partially deaf child, being educated in the normal school, may be referred to the speech therapist for treatment of the defective articulation. The pre-school child may also be referred for an opinion as to the cause of the delayed speech development, and in the absence of suitable provision elsewhere may require help from the speech therapist.

The Pre-school Child

We have been fortunate in Newcastle-upon-Tyne in having a close association with the Northern Counties School for the Deaf. Until recently children had not been admitted to this residential school until the age of five, but a pre-school clinic was organised four years ago, and to this the mother and child could be referred when a hearing loss was confirmed. The mother and child attended for an hour at intervals ranging from once weekly to monthly attendances, and training and guidance were given by the teachers in the school. There was an additional advantage in that when the time of entry into school was reached the children were familiar with the staff and surroundings and were looking forward to their school life.

Where such facilities are not available, the speech therapist should be able to assist the mother and child. It is important that the mother should understand the situation. She is with the child constantly and can do more than anyone else in the early stages to encourage the appreciation of language.

Lip reading

The child can be helped towards realisation that lip movements have meaning. No attempt should be made to teach individual sounds, but simple words may be used in isolation, or in short phrases with repetition, always associating the lip movements with meaning. For example, whilst dressing the child the mother can pick up the shoes and, attracting the child's attention to them and then to her lips, say '*Shoe*, two *shoes*, here are your *shoes*.' 'Put on your *shoes*, one *shoe*, two *shoes*,' and so forth. Action words can be demonstrated such as 'jump', 'run', 'clap hands'. Toys may be put round the room and the child asked to bring one at a time. Nursery rhymes may be repeated, and associated with pictures, perhaps using only the first line of each, until the child can find the corresponding pictures in a nursery rhyme book. Pictures of objects may be collected in a scrap book, to be found by the child when named. The therapist will think of many other ways of interesting the child and giving him practice in watching and learning to interpret the lip movements for speech.

Daily repetition of words in this way will assist the development of lip reading, most of which will be spontaneous and without conscious effort. In the meantime the mother may use and accept gesture. Whilst aiming always at the substitution of understanding through lip movements, the mother must not increase the sense of frustration unnecessarily.

Sign language

Sir Richard Paget (1930) was of the opinion that speech was originally mouth gesture and believed that sign language should be encouraged in deaf children. He also believed that sign language should be used in addition to as much oral speech as is possible. Both lip reading and sign language are of limited use in that they are not possible in the dark. Sign language is also not universal and is limited to each community, each school of deaf children developing their own special sign language. Lip reading may be possible on television, but is of no assistance to the understanding of speech on the radio, and may be almost useless in a large group of people.

The deaf child's greatest difficulty is the acquisition of expressive language and verbal ability, and he lacks the mental stimulus of constant exposure to the sounds of speech in early life. When he has acquired the ability to associate printed verbal symbols with meaning and to read, his experience of language can develop more rapidly and fully, and he can subsequently use written speech as a means of expression.

Auditory training

Auditory training should be commenced as early in life as possible, either with or without a hearing aid if there is any response to sounds. Speech may then be helped to develop, so far as hearing permits, through the normal auditory pathways.

Fry and Whetnall (1954) have studied this problem and state that although methods of teaching deaf children to speak have existed since 1761, methods of auditory training have not yet been universally accepted. They believe that there are many children in schools for the deaf to-day who could have been in ordinary schools had they been given auditory training at the right age. They also state that 'It is now accepted that the cortical centres can learn to discriminate between auditory stimuli readily during the first three years of life, whereas after this period learning becomes increasingly difficult.' They define auditory training as 'the means by which the cortical areas are given additional practice in the discrimination of sounds—both the background sounds of everyday life and speech patterns', and believe that as far as is possible we should try to 'reproduce the conditions in which the normal child learns to listen during the first year of life'. 'There is no short-cut which will eliminate the need for repetition of sounds, if the auditory areas in the cortex are to learn, and the child trained at this age can develop speech during the normal physiological period.'

Ewing (1954) has pointed out that most deaf children use their voices for sequences of vowel sounds. In the hearing child such vocalising develops into babbling and speech; in the deaf child there is a tendency to become more silent. She finds that 28 out of 30 children were said to have used voice normally and believes that 'such use of voice must be continued so that the kinaesthetic sensations in the mouth may become established and serve as a basis for speech'.

Hearing aids

In the deaf child auditory stimulation and the encouragement of the use of voice may best be accomplished through use of a hearing aid, but only in those children where such amplification is useful and helps towards the appreciation of the sounds of speech and other environmental sounds.

Many small children, however, dislike a hearing aid and refuse to wear it for a sufficient length of time. A hearing child requires two years or more for the development of speech, and the partially deaf child requires a similar period of time for the development of appreciation and discrimination of the sounds of speech, and for the association of those sounds with meaning.

Hardy (1953) found that children with a hearing loss as great as 75 db. below normal could make use of residual hearing by means of a hearing aid, but considered that to learn to hear with amplification requires two years of constant exposure to the sounds of normal language and speech in order that the auditory pathways may develop. He believes that most children can learn to speak by means of amplification and that the best adjustment to the use of a hearing aid is made between two and three years of age.

The child may be helped to say words by feeling the breath on his hand, by feeling the vibration of the larynx or chest, in addition to watching the movements of his mother's tongue and lips. Words spoken clearly but without undue force close to the child's ear may also help him to an appreciation of the sounds of expressive speech. Such methods will supplement the use of a hearing aid, or be useful when a hearing aid is not tolerated.

An accurate assessment of a young child's residual hearing is difficult, as the majority of these children fail to respond to audiometric pure tones at threshold, and frequently only respond to such sounds when they are as much as 20 to 30 db. above threshold. Thus many may have more hearing than is indicated by their audiogram. Where there is any response to sounds, therefore, auditory training should be attempted, the child's response to such training being sometimes a better guide to the extent of his hearing than the standard hearing tests.

Where the hearing loss is less severe, the need for such auditory training may be even more necessary, associated with treatment for the defective articulation. The treatment of the partially deaf child will be described in Chapter XVI on defects of articulation associated with a partial hearing loss.

Author's Note. During the 15 years since this chapter was first written perhaps no subject in this field has developed more extensively than that of audiology. However, this section may still be useful to the speech therapist, who is not an audiologist, and provide an introduction to the subject.

Whilst some methods described may now be mainly of historical interest, other suggestions may still be useful.

REFERENCES

Cawthorn, T., and Harvey, R. M. (1953). A comparison between Hearing for Pure Tones and for Speech. *J. Laryng.*, **67,** 233.

Ewing, I. R., and A. W. G. (1954). *Speech and the Deaf Child.* Manchester Univ. Press.

Fant, G. (1948). Analys av de Svenska vokalljuden. *L.M.E. Report H/P*, 1035.

Fant, G. (1949). Analys av Svenska konsonantljuden. *L.M.E. Report H/P*, 1064.

Fletcher, H. (1929). *Speech and Hearing.* London, Macmillan.

Fletcher, H. (1950). *Speech, Hearing and Communication.* London, Macmillan.

Fry, D. B., and Kerridge, P. M. T. (1939). Tests for the Hearing of Speech by Deaf People. *Lancet*, **1,** 106.

Fry, D. B., and Whetnall, E. (1954). The Auditory Approach in the Training of Deaf Children. *Lancet*, **1,** 583.

Gordon, N. (1966). The child who does not talk. *Brit. J. Dis. Commun.* **2,** 78.

Hallpike, C. S., and Dix, M. R. (1947). The Peepshow. *Brit. med. J.*, **2,** 719.

Hardy, W. G., and Bordley, J. E. (1951). Special Techniques in Testing and Hearing of Children. *J. Speech Dis.*, **16,** 122.

Hardy, W. G., and Pauls, M. D. (1952). The Test Situation in P.G.S.R. Audiometry. *J. Speech Dis.*, **18.** 13.

Hardy, W. G., and Pauls, M. D. (1953). Hearing Disorders in Symposium on Hearing, Speech and Reading Difficulties. *Pediatrics*, **12,** 1, 62.

McLaurin, J. W. (1954). The Inarticulate Child. *Laryngoscope*, **64,** 454.

Markides, A. (1970). The speech of deaf and partially hearing children with special reference to factors affecting intelligibility. *Brit. J. Dis. Commun.*, **5,** 126.

Medical Research Council. *Special Report on Hearing Aids and Audiometers.* (1947). No. 261. London, H.M.S.O.

Paget, Sir Richard (1930). *Human Speech.* London, Paul.

Pressman, J. J., and Kaleman, G. (1955). The Physiology of the Larynx. *Physiol. Rev.*, **35,** 3, 507.

Richardson, E. G. (1953). *Sound*, 5th ed. London, Arnold.

Watson, L. A., and Tolan, T. (1949). *Hearing Tests and Hearing Instruments.* Baltimore, Williams and Wilkins.

Wedenberg, Erik (1952–1954). Auditory Training of Severely Hard of Hearing School Children. *Acta Otolaryng.*, Supplement **12,** 103.

IX. Developmental Aphasia

In contrast to the child whose delayed development of speech is the result of an impairment of hearing, and who may develop understanding for speech assisted by lip reading, and expressive speech proportional to the way in which he hears it, the child with developmental aphasia fails to develop the use of speech at the usual age, although general mental development and the sensory pathways for hearing are adequate.

Although a mechanistic analysis of such a finely integrated function cannot be pressed too far it is helpful to think of speech as a triple process, the reception of words by the ear or the eye, their interpretation and synthesis as language within the brain, and finally the expression of this language response in further spoken words. We regard *speech* as covering the whole of this receptive, formative and expressive activity.

Words are symbolic sounds which have a consistent range of meaning. In complete or embryonic form they are constructional units of thought and language, and in terms of the movement of speech are heard and understood, arranged and rearranged, and articulated and spoken.

Language is both the word library of speech and the sum of those meaningful association of words current in the life and literature of any society.

Speech may best be described as *spoken* language, as contrasted with *written* language. It involves both receptive and expressive aspects of speech, or the encoding and decoding processes, in the development and use of linguistic competence. However, communication with others through spoken language also requires normal appreciation of the phonemic system through hearing, just as appreciation of written language requires recognition of the accepted written or printed symbols through sight. When normal phonemic patterning is appreciated and used within a recognised linguistic system, speech becomes intelligible and available as a means of communication. It is necessary, however, that both the speaker and listener have full knowledge of the same linguistic system and phoneme usage.

Use of the word 'speech' should therefore not be equated with 'articulation'. Speech in the sense of articulation, without language, would be a sequence of sounds without meaning, whilst language without the use of a normal phonemic system would be unintelligible to others and useless for purposes of communication.

The meaningful content of speech is described by Brain (1952) as being 'based upon a constellation of associations built up by experience.'

At the physiological and anatomical levels the basis of such meanings is presumably a linkage of neurones. Visual impulses reach the cerebral cortex in the region of the calcarine fissure of the occipital lobes, auditory impulses in the posterior part of the post central convolution. It is to be expected, therefore, that the anatomical linkages of neurones upon which verbal meanings depend will join together these regions of the cerebral cortex, and these are found in the tracts of white matter known as association fibres which underly the grey matter of the cerebral cortex. In the majority of people who are right handed these association paths are situated in the left cerebral hemisphere but sensory impulses concerned in the reception of speech also reach the auditory and visual regions of the right cerebral cortex, which are linked to the left hemisphere by paths passing through the corpus callosum.

Goldstein (1942) describes the difficulty in deciding with certainty whether the left or right hemisphere is predominant in any one person and says that 'In many cases both hemispheres seem to be important for speech but that dominance is more definite for motor than for sensory speech.'

Stimulation of certain cortical areas has produced arrest of speech but so far has never produced speech. Penfield and Rasmussen (1960) have described how 'stimulation of two small areas on the pre-central gyrus has produced a well-sustained vowel cry—a cry without words'. 'It is complicated and includes innervation of the abdominal muscles, larynx, pharynx and tongue, lips and jaw, such as are necessary for word utterance.' He also states that 'vocalisation occurs with equal frequency from stimulation of the dominant, and the non-dominant hemispheres'.

At one time the physiological processes underlying the various aspects of speech were considered as being located in certain definite areas of the cortex, but it is now believed that the integrative processes required for speech involve a more general organisation of the entire cerebral system. Lashley (1938) states that 'In addition to their specific functions all parts of the cortex exercise a general facilitative effect upon the rest', and Goldstein (1942) describes localisation of a performance as 'not an excitation in a certain place but a dynamic process which occurs in the entire nervous system, even in the whole organism, and which has a definite configuration for each performance'. He also considers that 'The function of a specific region is characterised by the influence which the particular structure exerts on the total process.'

Aphasia is a breakdown in the comprehension and formulation of words giving rise to a disturbance of thought and a disorder of language. There is therefore both a receptive and an expressive component of aphasia. In some patients either the one or the other predominates, but in many there seems to be an impairment of more than one of the processes concerned, and this impairment may be either partial or severe.

Critchley (1952) recognises three types of faulty use of verbal symbols in adults:

1. Confusion in words, or paraphasia
   - (*a*) literal, where there is substitution of one sound for another,
   - (*b*) verbal, where there is substitution of one word for another—such speech may be gibberish, fragments of words being used, or one word may be substituted for another closely associated object as *chair* for *table*.'
2. Errors in the construction of sentences and word order, or paragrammatism.
3. Disturbed word finding.

Developmental Aphasia

Our present understanding of aphasia is chiefly derived from our experience of cerebral injury and disease as they affect adult patients, and in this context the phrase 'breakdown in the comprehension and formulation of speech' is a proper description of what has taken place. In the children with whom we are mainly concerned here, however, the process is a failure to develop the central processes of speech; a delay in building up the word library and creating a language. The condition resembles that seen in adult patients suffering from aphasia or dysphasia, involving literal or verbal paraphasia, paragrammatism, or word-finding difficulties. In spite of the essential difference, in that the child with developmental aphasia has not experienced the use of normal speech and subsequently lost that ability, we have used the word aphasia for this disorder of childhood. Since it becomes apparent during the time when speech is normally developed, we have qualified it with the word developmental, Morley *et al.* (1955).

In developmental aphasia the child is unable to appreciate and/or use speech on a symbolic or linguistic level, but is able to function adequately on a non-symbolic level.

A delay in the development and usage of a linguistic system for encoding, when decoding (understanding for language) is adequate, may be described as an expressive language disorder, or developmental expressive aphasia. It must be clear to the experienced therapist that the ability to understand spoken language must indicate that the child's phonemic system is fully developed, even when use of speech is absent or limited, when the phonemic patterning for the limited language used may be normal or defective.

Developmental Expressive Aphasia

Greene (1967) describes children at the age of three years who comprehend speech but do not speak. However, they show no evidence of such retardation in any other respect and are frustrated by their inability to express themselves. Masland and Case (1968) were impressed by the frequent occurrence of limitation of auditory memory in pre-school children with delayed development of language. Their vocabulary was limited to one- or two-syllable words at three to four years of age, and language usage was immature, even when it had passed the single word stage. They also found that, whilst the children comprehended short phrases, they appeared to have difficulty in appreciating longer sentences. They examined auditory memory under (1) temporal span, (2) temporal sequence, (3) temporal patterning of rhythm, stress and inflexion, and (4) patterning of phonetic detail. These four processes, they considered, were related to the process of serial order temporal integration, described by Lashley (1960) as basic to the language process.

Whilst the child attempts, during his development, to approximate to the language of his community, he has difficulty, states Byers Brown (1971) in mastering the rules which govern language. For some, maturation will ensure that competence is gained, others achieve partial mastery over the language process and may have a very restricted system for use in communication. She describes a *restricted* language system as inability to acquire the necessary sound differentiations simply by exposure to the environment, and a *fragmentary* system related to inability to organise the information extracted, and believes that short-term memory is probably a significant factor. The child is not abnormal in any other respect, but cannot acquire from his linguistic environment the information he needs.

Studies of aphasia in adults by Schuell (1966) showed that reduction of language may or may not be complicated by further disruption of auditory, visual, spatial or sensorimotor processes, and could be considered in terms of overall patterns of deficit produced by involvement of one or more of the functional cerebral systems tested. She suggests that this framework could be used to provide a systematic approach to the investigation of language disabilities in children.

Eisenson, writing in 1966, describes developmental aphasia as the cause of delayed speech development in only a small proportion of non-verbal children. The majority, with or without clearly determined central nervous system involvements, were found to be basically intellectually deficient. He regards aphasic children as those with central nervous system involvements that have resulted in perceptual dysfunctions for the processes that underlie the normal achievement of the comprehension and production of speech. He also suggests that the description oral, or verbal, *apraxia* might be used for those children who have good understanding for language but have a severe impairment for speech production, that is articulation.

Language and Thought

If the child is unable to use language is development thereby retarded? Kahn (1965) thinks that words enable us to build up thought processes, and that inability to use speech to express abstract ideas may hinder the development of abstract thought, also emphasised by Luria and Yudovich (1959) and Luria (1961). Vygotsky (1934) also believed that the use of words or signs to direct one's own mental processes is an integral part of the process of concept formation.

Hurst (1966) however, has conducted experiments with the deaf on thinking without language, both in its receptive and expressive aspects, and believes that the internal organisation of intelligence is independant of language systems. He believes that intelligent thinking does not necessarily need the support of a symbolic system, but that the comprehension and use of language is dependant upon the structure of intelligence. Greene, however, thinks that these experiments do not prove that abstract and logical thinking is possible without language. She advises therefore, once the diagnosis is established, that the therapist should institute useful training, particularly with the daily help of the mother in the home.

Developmental expressive aphasia involves a severe delay in the onset of speech. There may have been little or no vocal play and babbling; one or two isolated words may be used during the first two or three years of life, but vocabulary develops slowly. In some, a stage may be reached around four years of age or later when there is a sudden growth of vocabulary. This may be followed by rapid progress towards the uses of phrases and sentences with little or no sign of true developmental aphasia. Others may not develop adequate use of language until around six or seven years of age, after entry into school, when the condition may be described as transient aphasia. However, in others the difficulties persist with very slow progress in the use of words and phrases. Such a delay would probably indicate a more extensive dysfunction of the underlying neurological development for speech, with continuing limited use of spoken language.

Later in life there are obvious difficulties in the use of sentences. There may be confusion in the order in which words are used, or difficulty in word finding with omission of words, substitution of words not intended and inappropriate to the meaning, or the word for a closely associated object may be used, as 'hat' when 'coat' is meant.

The mispronunciation of words sometimes occurs when the consonants can be used normally in other words. The persistence of such defective pronunciation of words as 'aminal' for 'animal', of 'embelofe' for 'envelope', or 'heffalump' for 'elephant' occurs frequently in the speech of early childhood, but may be evidence of or closely allied to developmental aphasia when it persists to a later age. Such a persisting disability may be out of all proportion to the general intelligence of the child and to what is within the normal range of difficulty, as experienced by children in the development and use of speech.

In such children there may be no organic cortical lesion, but rather delay in or inadequate development of those neurological processes of maturation required for speech.

In 1897 Bastian wrote as follows: 'Speech has now become a truly automatic act for human beings, and that if children do not speak at birth this is in the main due to the circumstance that their nervous systems are still too immature.'

Failure of normal understanding for speech in the child with developmental expressive aphasia is rare, except when there is a partial hearing loss for some of the frequencies of sound required for speech, with which condition receptive aphasia may be confused. A failure to develop full appreciation of the meaningful content of words may, however, occur in association with some degree of general mental defect or slight hearing loss, but be more severe and out of proportion to the extent of either.

Associated defects of articulation

Dyslalia. Many children pass through a period when articulation is defective, but there is rapid and spontaneous improvement towards normal articulation. This frequently occurs in the early stages of speech development as previously described (Chapter III). The child with developmental dysphasia may also pass through such a phase in the early stages of the use of expressive speech, but at a later age than the normal child.

Dysarthria. This term implies slow clumsy articulation arising from dysfunction of the muscles used in speech. Such dysfunction is evident on physical examination. It does not necessarily involve any interference with the comprehension and formulation of words, although in some children with developmental aphasia there may be an associated dysarthria.

Articulatory apraxia. In this condition a difficulty is encountered in association with, or in the absence of any general muscular clumsiness, evident on examination. However, in some children muscular control may be adequate for general purposes other than the highly skilled integrated movements for articulation, with difficulty in controlling and co-ordinating purposive movements of the lips, tongue or palatopharyngeeal sphincter, when muscle tone and control does not appear to be otherwise abnormal. In children with developmental dysphasia associated with articulatory apraxia this articulatory apraxia may persist well into school or even adult life and is evident as speech develops. These conditions of defective articulation will be described more fully in Part III.

Developmental Aphasia in 74 Children

As already described, we have seen 280 children in the past six years with delayed development of speech of such a degree that the parents sought advice. Of these, 74 had a delay in the development of speech which was not the result of a hearing defect or of general mental retardation. We have considered that these 74 children had some degree of developmental aphasia.

The group of children with aphasia with whom we are mainly concerned here did not develop any recognisable words until two years or later, or phrases until four years or later. What is more, when words or phrases did begin they often developed slowly, and there was an obvious poverty of language. A few children had one or two words early in the third year, but the development of language was arrested at that point for some

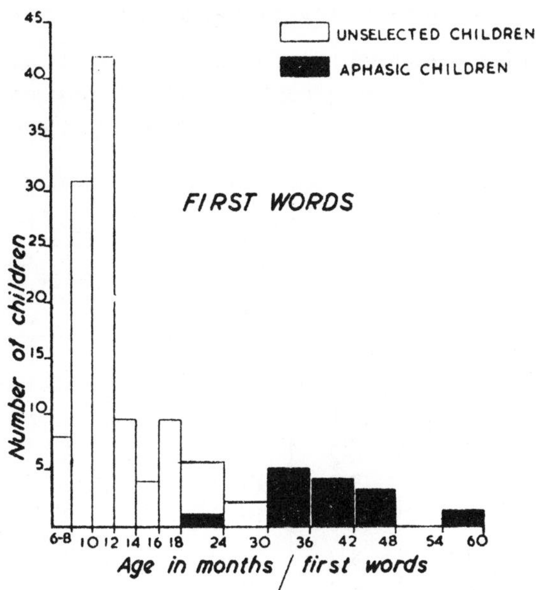

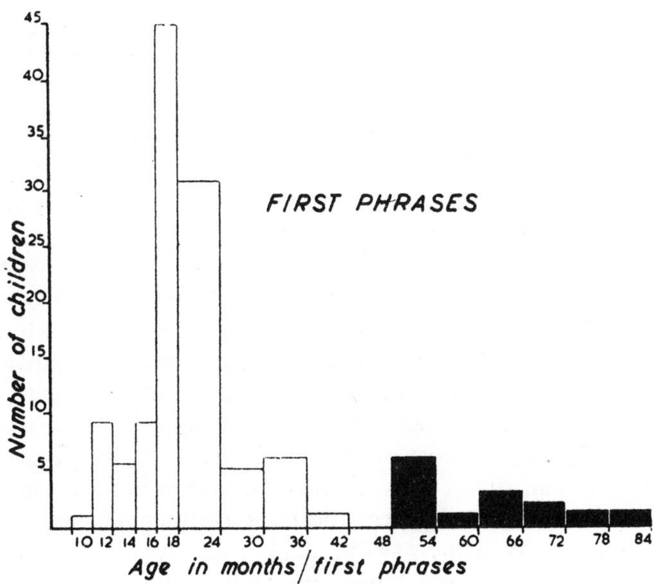

FIG. 41

Age of development of speech in 114 unselected children and in 15 children with developmental aphasia. Reprinted from *Brit. med. J.* (1955), **2**, 463.

time, with a further halting advance at four or five years or later. Our definition of developmental aphasia of considerable degree is of course an arbitrary one, but the delay in speech development

Case	Age (Years and Months)		Social Class of Father	Family Speech Disorders	Place in Family	Birth Weight	
	First Visit	Last Visit				lb. oz.	kg.
M.B.	8–3	16–2	V	–	5	7 0	3·18
G.D.	7–8	12–4	III	–	3	11 8	5·2
D.F.	6–2	10–11	III	–	3	6 0	2·7
A.H.	4–1	10–0	II	–	2	7 4	3·3
E.M.	3–6	9–4	III	–	2	9 3	4·17
D.P.	2–11	9–3	III	–	3	6 8	2·94
C.S. }	4–4	9–10	III	–	2	6 4	2·8
K.S. }						3 0	1·36
D.H. }	4–5	8–2	V	–	4	6 0	2·7
D.H. }						6 8	2·94
K.C.	4–3	8–4	III	+	3	10 4	4·65
D.W.	4–4	8–2	III	+	2	7 0	3·18
N.S.	6–2	6–5	III	–	3	5 1	2·3
A.W.	4–7	5–10	III	+	4	8 0	3·6
D.R.	2–11	5–3	V	–	3	Not recorded	

FIG. 42
Main features of 15 children with developmental aphasia.

in 14 children in this group in relation to a representative group of normal children is plainly shown in the chart (Fig. 41).

The 74 children, 72 of whom had mainly an executive and two a receptive aphasia, can be divided into three main groups. There were 50 in whom speech developed fairly quickly and successfully after the age of four and who could be regarded as the terminal gradient on the slope of normal development. We have called these transient developmental aphasia. The second and third groups consist of 16 children with a more prolonged delay and inadequacy who are the main concern of this chapter, and eight with intelligence quotients between 80 and 90 in whom the speech delay was out of all proportion to their mental retardation. We have called these prolonged developmental aphasia. None of the children in the first two groups was below normal intelligence. They appeared emotionally stable, had normal hearing and were free from other neurological abnormalities. The main features of 15 children in the second group are given in Fig. 42. One child with receptive aphasia (A.R.) is not included in these findings (see p. 169).

History of Birth Injury or Anoxia	Illness in First 3 Years	I.Q.	First (Years and Months)		Alexia	Defective Articulation
			Words	Phrases		
−	−	106	?	?	+	Apraxia
+	−	100	4–9	6	+	” Dysphonia
−	+	100	3–0	6–6	+	Apraxia
−	−	120	1–8	4–0	−	—
−	−	130	2–6	5–3	+	—
+	−	136	3–6	5–6	−	—
−	−	96	3	4+	+	—
+	−	93	3	4+	+	—
−	−	100	3–9	5–0	+	Apraxia
−	−	100	3–9	5–0	+	”
+	+	100	2+	5–6	+	”
−	+	106	3+	4+	+	Dyslalia
−	−	100	2+	4+	Not assessed	—
−	−	120	2+	4–6	” ”	Apraxia
−	−	99	2–6	4–1	” ”	Dyslalia

FIG. 42 (*continued*)
Reprinted from *Brit. Med. J.* (1955), 2, 463.

Social class, position in family and birth injury

The social class of these families was essentially similar to the normal range for our community. None of these children was a first child, and this is highly significant. Apart from two twins born at term but weighing only three and five pounds (1·4 and 2·3 Kg.) respectively, none was premature.

Birth injury

A mother's memory on this point is notably fallible and often ill-informed, so that reliable comment is difficult. In four children the possibility of perinatal anoxia or cerebral injury existed; G.D. was blue for several hours after birth: in D.P. normal breathing was not established for half an hour; K.S., the small second twin, was very ill for several days and was not expected to live; and K.C. had the cord tightly round his neck and was blue for the first two days.

Illness in the first three years of life

A similar factual difficulty is encountered when we try to assess the significance of illness arising during the normal period in which speech develops. Although this was specially asked for, illness was remembered in only three children. D.F. had measles at nine months; K.C. had severe measles on his first birthday, jaundice at 18 months, and chicken-pox at two; and D.W. had a doubtful rubella at one and measles at two years. None of these illnesses was associated with unconsciousness, prolonged drowsiness or convulsions, and there is nothing in the histories of these 15 children to incriminate early cerebral inflammation as a cause of aphasia. Infective and, especially, virus illness in the mother during pregnancy may be important, but we have no information on this point.

Intelligence

The results of the assessment of the intelligence of the 15 aphasic children are given in Figure 43. All the intelligence quotients were above 90, and therefore all the children may be regarded as not below normal so far as their intelligence is concerned. Non-verbal tests were, of course, used to measure the intelligence of these aphasic children.

Delayed reading

As the development of speech requires the association of memories for groups of sounds, and movements for articulation with visual impressions of objects and actions, so reading requires the development of associations between these sound patterns and visual impressions of the printed or written symbols which we recognise in reading. Reading involves the ability to discriminate between these isolated symbols or groups of symbols forming words and sentences, and to recall, in the early stages of reading the audible symbols of speech which they represent, with understanding of their meaning. In more rapid reading at a later stage the auditory memories are usually omitted in silent reading, and meaning is associated directly with the visual impressions of the written or printed symbols.

The absence of speech, with its delayed use of the audible

symbols of speech, can therefore interfere with the development of reading ability. Visual discrimination may be adequate, and the child may have no difficulty in picking out letters or words which are similar, but he is unable to recall the auditory symbols of speech which they represent. He may learn to read silently to some extent, depending chiefly on visual memory, and be able to understand something of the meaning of the printed words whilst still unable to read aloud. A few children may learn to associate auditory and visual symbols, such as plastic letters, before they are able to speak. They can pick out a letter when they hear the corresponding sound, or even a short word, whilst still unable to recall and use the sounds themselves.

Name	First Test	I.Q.	Second Test	I.Q.	Months between Testings
M.B.	A	106	—	—	—
G.D.	DC	100	WP	91	42
D.F.	DC	100	WP	98	39
A.H.	DC	114	A	120	31
E.M.	DC	129	WP	130	46
D.P.	MP	120	A	136	41
D.H.	RM	100	—	—	—
D.H.	RM	100	—	—	—
K.C.	DC	91	DC	100	30
D.W.	DC	106	RM	105	—
A.W.	DC	120	—	—	—
N.S.	WCP	100	—	—	—
C.S.	WCP	96	—	—	—
K.S.	WCP	93	—	—	—
D.R.	WCP	99	—	—	—

A=Alexander performance scale. DC=Drever Collins performance scale. WP=Performance tests of the Wechsler-Bellevue scale. MP=Performance tests of the Merrill-Palmer scale. RM=Raven's progressive matrices sets A, Ab, B. WCP=Performance tests of the Wechsler intelligence scale for children.

FIG. 43

Intelligence of 15 children with developmental aphasia.

Reprinted from *Brit. Med. J.* (1955) 2, 463.

The reading ages of ten of the children who were of sufficient age for testing were assessed on three scales, the Burt, Vernon or Durrell Reading scales. The reading ages obtained were approximately the same. Nine of the 12 children showed a severe delay sufficient to cause a serious handicap in school life.

The level of reading skills is shown in Figure 44.

Defective articulation

This was present in nine of the 15 aphasic children. In two it was a simple dyslalia which responded readily to treatment. The remaining seven, including the fraternal twins, had an articulatory apraxia. One boy had an associated dysphonia, one still stammers under stress, and the identical twins had a slight but persistent stammer from the age of six years.

Laterality

Eight of the 15 were right-sided, one left-sided and six showed crossed laterality.

Name	Chronological Age	Reading Age
M.B.	10-10	Nil
G.D.	12-4	9-3
D.F.	10-11	Nil
E.M.	9-4	5+
D.H.	8-2	6-8
D.H.	8-2	6-4
K.C.	8-4	Nil
D.W.	8-2	6-3
C.S.	9-10	6-5
K.S.	9-10	8-1

Assessment was made on the Burt scale. In addition, the Vernon and Durrell tests were also used in several children.

FIG. 44
The reading skills of 10 children with developmental aphasia and alexia (years and months)

Reprinted from *Brit. Med. J.* (1953) **2**, 463.

Delayed and defective speech in the family

Here again our information is almost certainly incomplete. The mother of D.W. stammered from four until nine years of age. A.W's brother, who is now ten, was also slow in developing speech, and a paternal cousin of K.C. did not begin to speak until the age of five. This is a very different family incidence from the children with developmental dysarthria (Morley, 1954), where speech disorders in other members of the family were present in more than half.

We have therefore found no evidence that social class,

position in family, birth injury, illness during the normal period of speech development, laterality, or family predisposition has any clear relationship to developmental aphasia, the aetiology of which remains unknown. In view, however, of the considerable delay in starting to speak, and the continuing difficulties with language which these 15 children experienced, we feel that they probably express a true cerebral disorder and not merely the extreme end of the normal range of speech development.

Expressive Aphasia

A. H., aged two, was the second child of intelligent professional parents. His birth was normal and general development satisfactory. Words began at 20 months, but phrases did not follow until after four years. At six he still avoided the use of verbs, and, though willing to tell a story with gusto, got it thoroughly muddled through omitting, transposing and mispronouncing his words. He had normal hearing and comprehension, and at eight years and ten months his intelligence quotient was 120.

He was, however, a tense, restless boy, and recovery may have been delayed by his personality and the parents' desire for rapid improvement and academic success. Though his speech continued to improve, his mother still considered him 'a proper Mrs. Malaprop'. His articulation was clear and his mispronunciations similar to those met with in acquired aphasia. Presumably this boy recalled sound sequences imperfectly. When he knew exactly what he wanted to say, his speech was sensible and clear; when he could not get the word or could not get the right one, distortions and word substitutions occurred and speech was jumbled and confused. In writing he expressed himself much more clearly. We considered this boy had an expressive aphasia, perhaps arising in part from a poor auditory memory for speech.

E. M., aged nine years four months, was the second child of three. His father was a skilled worker and there were no speech disorders in the family. His birth was normal and general development satisfactory. Three or four words came by the age of two and a half years, but there was little increase until after four. Phrases began at five years three months, and following this he developed a dyslalia which cleared within the next year. He seemed to understand speech from an early age and obeyed verbal requests very readily. He was always a very good-tempered boy and was happy and healthy, with normal hearing. His intelligence quotient at eight years three months was 130. From eight onwards his speech improved, though he was still a boy of few words. When excited or anxious, his speech might become halting and confused. We have regarded this not as a true stammer but as the disturbance under stress of a newly acquired and precariously balanced function with an underlying impairment of structural origin. At nine he still had a severe alexia. We regarded this boy as essentially an example of expressive or motor aphasia with associated alexia.

D. F., aged 10 years 11 months, was the third child in a family of five. Both parents were sensible folk and there was no history of speech disorder. He was born normally, but had severe whooping-cough at three months and measles at nine months. After his first year he developed satisfactorily apart from speech. Words began at three years, but phrases did not follow until six years six months. Although he understood some speech before he spoke, his comprehension of quite a number of common words was still uncertain when first seen in his seventh year.

He was lively and active, playing well but always talking much less than his brothers and sisters. On occasion his parents noticed that he whispered to himself as if to rehearse the word or phrase before using it. At nearly 11 he was a shy well-developed boy with normal hearing, and no abnormality in his nervous system. His intelligence quotient was 100. Even when you knew him he was taciturn, and had a marked economy of phrase. Articulation was still hampered by an associated slight apraxia, and he was still unable to read at all. This boy had a severe developmental aphasia, alexia and an associated articulatory apraxia.

Developmental Receptive Aphasia[1]

Developmental receptive aphasia describes a condition where there is inability to understand the linguistic system adequately with resulting failure to use expressive language normally. Phonemic patterning may be normal, but there is limited or abnormal use of syntax, resulting in what is often described as 'jargon' speech.

Gordon (1966) uses the term auditory agnosia for a condition where sounds in addition to those for language cannot be associated with meaning. At first these children may be thought to be peripherally deaf, but later found to have hearing but an inability to associate sounds with meaning which he describes

[1] First published in Speech Pathology and Therapy, Oct. 1960.

as central deafness. He suggests that a lack of sensory pathways to enable the auditory impulse to reach the appropriate areas of the cortex, and to be integrated at the cortical level, may be the result of selective damage from anoxia, pre- or peri-natal, or that such pathways have failed to develop. Assessment with E.E.G. audiometry has been found useful in excluding peripheral deafness, that is external, middle or inner ear deafness up to the auditory nucleus.

In 1956 I wrote that 'in over 20 years we have seen only two children who could be described as having a true receptive disability for speech. One was first seen recently, the other in 1942 at the age of six and a half years, and her development has been followed for 14 years.' Since then we have observed these and three others with a marked failure to develop normal comprehension for spoken language, and others with a less severe delay in understanding speech. In our experience this condition is still rare, but when it occurs it forms a severe handicap, preventing education in a normal environment. Although tending towards improvement with maturation and treatment, we have found the disability persisting in two of the five children to the ages of 22 years and 12 years respectively (1960) and now (1971) to the ages of 31 years and 18 years when last seen.

In this small group of children there were two girls and three boys, and there ages in 1960 were as follows:

TABLE I

	A. R.*	N. S.	M. F.	S. P.	S. C.
Sex	F	M	M	F	M
Age when seen	6·5 yrs.	6·5 yrs.	5·3 yrs.	4·1 yrs.	3·6 yrs.
Present age	23 yrs.	12 yrs.	8·5 yrs.	8 yrs.	6·5 yrs.

* A description of this child was first published in *Speech*, xi, 1, 16, 1947.

The general development of these five children is shown in Table II with details concerning pregnancy, birth weight and neo-natal condition. Sitting and walking were delayed in S.P., from the mother's description, possibly due to difficulties in balancing. Her intelligence quotient was finally assessed at 131. The estimated intelligence quotient of A.R. at the age of

TABLE II

General Development	A. R.	N. S.	M. F.	S. P.	S. C.
Position in family	Only	2nd—(twin)	3rd	2nd	2nd
Pregnancy	26 weeks	35 weeks	40 weeks	39 weeks	41 weeks
Birth weight	1 lb. 12 ozs.	5 lbs. 1 oz. (5 lbs. 4 ozs.) other twin	7 lbs.	6 lbs. 7 ozs.	8 lbs. 8 ozs.
Neo-natal condition	Blue. Not expected to live. In nursing home for 3 mths. weight then 4½ lbs.	Normal	Normal	Normal	Normal
Motor Development					
Sitting	18 months	7 months	8 months	16 months	9 months
Walking	2½—3 yrs.	13 months (twin 14 mths.)	18 months	2—2½ yrs.	18 months
Toilet control	2 years	18 months	16 months	18 months	Early
I.Q.	At 21 years, Ravens Progressive Matrices = 80	At 6 yrs. 2 mths. M. A. = 6½ yrs. At 6 yrs. 7 mths. = 100. W.B.S.C.	At 5 yrs. 4 mths. = 92 Merrill Palmer. At 5 yrs. 10 mths. = 90. W.B.S.C.	At 4 yrs. 5 mths. = 120. M.P. Performance. At 7 yrs. 6 mths. = 131	At 4 yrs. 7 mths. = 81. At 5 yrs. 1 mth. = 100. M.P. Performance

21 years was 80, but this does not correlate with her general behaviour, practical ability and appreciation of concrete facts. She has, however, difficulty when abstract thought is required and also little appreciation of number. The range of intelligence quotients in these five children is probably between 90 and 131, as assessed on performance tests.

The physical condition of the children is shown in Table III, including their hearing, ability to appreciate music, to sing in tune, rhythm response and general health. An E.E.G. was carried out for two of the children. At the age of seven and a half years N.S. had a series of three epileptic attacks. The findings were stated to be 'diagnostic of epilespy, acquired in nature', although there was no history, nor evidence of cerebral disease, neo-natal anxiety, nor illness. At ten years of age, when the E.E.G. was repeated the report was, 'still shows a considerable degree of abnormality. Well-marked independent spike foci are present in both temporal regions.' In spite of this report the condition was easily controlled with minimal dosage and there has been no recurrence of the fits. In the case of S.P. no abnormality was found.

At the time of examination by the neurologist there were no neurological nor clinical signs of associated general motor disability in any of these five children. Children with cerebral palsy, especially where the condition is predominantly that of spasticity, may have aphasia when intelligence is within the normal range, but it is more usual for this to be an expressive, rather than a receptive aphasia. Where there is athetosis there may also be a cochlear or more central hearing defect, particularly for sounds of high frequency, with or without associated difficulty for the use of language.

Others have described a language disability, not proportional to the hearing defect as estimated by pure tone audiometry, in children who had kernicterus due to the Rh factor. Goodhill (1956) describes damage to the normal auditory pathway, stating that it appears also that cerebral hypoxia and anoxia, with or without icterus, can produce lesions in this area simulating lesions of kernicterus which may involve cranial nuclear damage producing a special type of 'central deafness'. In the five children described here, however, the Rh factor was not involved.

TABLE III

Physical Condition	A. R.	N. S.	M. F.	S. P.	S. C.
Hearing	Slight loss at 7 years. Progressive loss	Slight loss	Normal	Low frequency Hearing aid	loss. Normal
Recognition of tunes	Normal	?	A little	Normal	Normal
Singing in tune	No	No attempt	Recognisable, not accurate	No	Yes
Rhythm	Normal	?	Normal	Normal	?
General Health	Measles and pneumonia at 6 years. Ts and As removed 6½ years. Whooping cough at 7 years	4 years ? fit. 7½ years—3 epileptic attacks. E.E.G.	Good	Good	Good

Hearing

An accurate estimate of the hearing is difficult to obtain, as these children present variable and unusual responses to normal testing methods and frequent assessment is essential. Psycho-galvanic skin resistance methods of testing are also unreliable. Rosen (1956) describes a case where it was felt that 'deafness' might be only slight although the child did not respond to tones of less intensity than 50 to 60 db. Cohen (1956) quotes Byers as saying that the estimated impression by parents and therapists of the degree of the child's hearing defect may also be at variance with the audiometric tests. Byers (1955) believes that this suggests a higher level of perceptual involvement than the cochlear nuclei, whilst Cohen describes these children as having a language disability showing many characteristics of the aphasic adult. Although the Rh factor was involved in these children, the disability in some, where it is essentially a language, rather than a hearing problem, may be similar to the condition we have seen in the five children described here. The child (S. C.) with a normal audiogram, had a severe associated articulatory defect at first. A. R. appeared to have normal hearing when first seen apart from some variations due to nasal infections which disappeared following adenoidectomy. An audiometer was not available until 1946 when she was eight years of age. The following four assessments (Table IV), obtained at 10, 17, 19 and 22 years of age, show a progressive deterioration with unknown cause. She has variable articulation in the speech she uses, but all consonants can be used normally at times. As hearing has deteriorated she has begun to use some lip reading.

The following audiograms show the responses of these children to pure tones, obtained after repeated testing (Table IV).

Hearing and Perception

Cawthorn and Harvey (1953) pointed out that in inner ear (perceptual) deafness there may be little relationship between the thresholds of hearing for pure tones and for speech. Fry and Whetnall (1954) stressed the need for early auditory stimulation and training to improve cortical perception for sounds in the child with a peripheral (cochlear) and perhaps also a more

Table IV

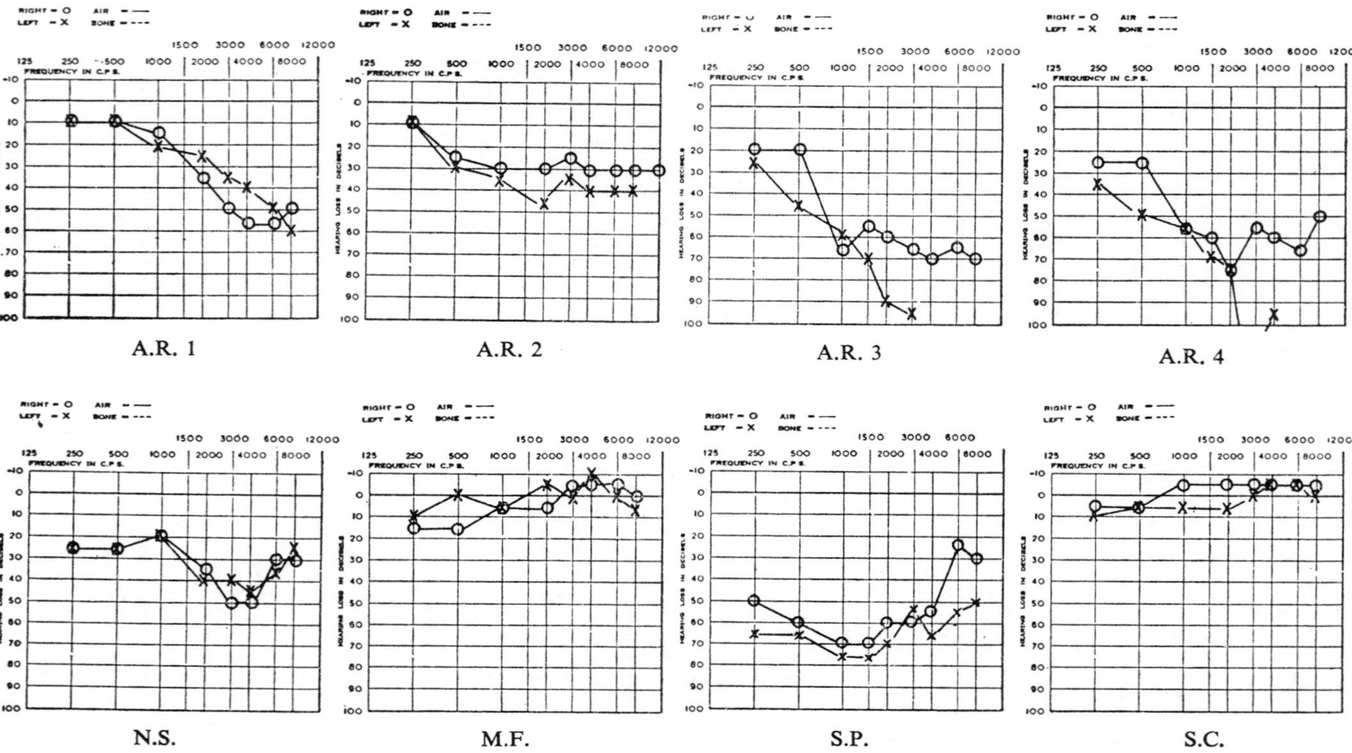
RIGHT = O AIR = —
LEFT = X BONE = - - -
FREQUENCY IN C.P.S.
125 250 500 1000 1500 2000 3000 4000 6000 8000 12000
HEARING LOSS IN DECIBELS
-10 0 10 20 30 40 50 60 70 80 90 100
A.R. 1
A.R. 2
A.R. 3
A.R. 4
N.S.
M.F.
S.P.
S.C.

central hearing defect involving perception. Resulting improvement for sound perception in such children, who probably have no associated receptive aphasia, has been reported by many. Myklebust (1956) points out, however, that in some children there may be a mixture of peripheral and central damage, or deafness and aphasia, particularly as seen in the Rh child. Eisenson (1966) also finds some degree of hearing loss in many of the children with developmental aphasia, but the degree of impairment in the use the children made of their hearing was invariably greater than would be implied from the hearing loss as indicated by a pure tone test of hearing.

Children with partial deafness use lip reading and may respond to the use of a hearing-aid. Where there is a receptive aphasia, as in the five children described with little or no hearing loss, lip reading is not used. This was also noticed by Hannigan (1956) in the Rh child. These children also fail to benefit significantly from the use of a hearing aid, even when the audiogram would indicate that it might be useful. (See S. P. audiogram).

It may be, therefore, that on the one hand a receptive aphasia may exist with little or no failure of peripheral hearing response, auditory discrimination, or perception for the sounds of speech, as in the five children described here, and that on the other hand an obvious hearing defect may be associated with some degree of central failure of perception, and perhaps also, in certain cases, of symbolisation, or receptive aphasia.

Table V shows the age of speech development, articulation, and related abilities such as reading, writing, spelling and number.

Reactions to Speech

Reactions to spoken language vary according to the severity of the condition. These children frequently present a general picture of inattention due to interest in their environment rather than in the conversational speech of others. They have little or no interest in stories and radio programmes apart from music, and even television may fail to hold their attention if the sound is incomprehensible. The abstract, unusual, or unfamiliar aspects of language present especial difficulties, and they tend to understand better the speech of someone who is familiar,

TABLE V

Language and Speech	A. R.	N. S.	M. F.	S. P.	S. C.
Language Expressive	Gesture—3 to 6 yrs. Words, 7 yrs.; phrases 9 yrs. some jargon, limited language	Gesture. Words, 2 yrs. (a few). Vocalising, 4 yrs., phrases, 7 yrs.; perseveration, jargon	Words, 3 yrs.; phrases, 6+	Words, $2\frac{1}{2}$ yrs.; phrases, $5\frac{1}{2}$ yrs. Jargon	Words, $3\frac{3}{4}$ yrs.; phrases, $5\frac{1}{4}$ yrs.
Articulation	Variable use of consonant sounds	All sounds used. Not always in correct order	Normal sounds by 8 yrs. Not always used correctly.	At 5 yrs.—Dyslalia. At 6 yrs.—Normal	Severe apraxia. No consonants at 5 yrs. Using a few at 6 yrs.
Reading	11 yrs. Poor comprehension. Can follow a recipe	Reading age at 9 yrs.—nil; at 10 yrs.—6 yrs. 1 mth.	8 yrs. R.A. = 6 yrs. Not full comprehension	Reading age at 6 yrs. 3 mths. = 7 yrs. 2 mths.	Nil
Spelling	Good	At 9 yrs.—nil; at 10 yrs. = 5 yrs. 5 mths.	Own name	Mostly normal	—
Writing	Incorrect construction	Copies well. Can write own name	Nil. Some copying	Construction faulty	—
Number	Poor	At 9 yrs. = 6 yrs. 2 mths. At 10 yrs. = 7 yrs. 5 mths.	7 yrs.—simple addition	Simple sums at 7 yrs.	—

rather than that of a stranger. There is commonly a delayed reaction to speech, also noted by Hannigan (1956) and also by the headmistress of the school which A. R. attended. Because they lack appreciation of environmental speech they tend to seek interest elsewhere, and may at first be considered over distractable, or even hyperactive, where this may result from situational factors rather than from a true neurological condition and hyperkinesis.

Expressive speech develops later than the normal and useful gesture is employed. There may be a period of jargon, ranging from complete unintelligibility to the use of recognisable words, with normal articulation but with misuse of words, for example, 'sit on' for chair, 'cut with' for scissors, 'up in air' for aeroplane, and transposition of syllables, perseveration, particularly of well-known simple phrases and paragrammatism. Alternatively, expressive speech may be limited to a few single words and simple phrases or sentences. Fluent use of jargon tends to decrease with the child's increasing awareness of his speech inadequacy in social situations.

Examples of Expressive Speech

A. R. at 11 *yrs.* I a Christmas tree, a bicycle, crackers pink, purple crackers, boys and girls party, Christmas tree, my house, pencil, Christmas present, book, Christmas present, all boys and girls, 21 people party, Holiday (meaning holly) on table, pink cake with Father Christmas.

At 21 *yrs.* We had a lovely time at the party. We have lots of presents. There are twenty-three 21st birthday cards. We have some beautiful presents. We have some iced cakes, birthday cake, beautiful cakes, four roses, great white key. We have some pearl necklace, gold watch, some silver silver. I have nice pink and white party frock. My mummy too, black dress colour with some lovely lily of valley spray. Daddy and me have beautiful photographs camera man, Mr. Nicholson, enjoyed the party. Thank you very much for lovely party. I came home 12 o'clock, late finish the party. New Year 12 o'clock. We help me at 7.30 change ready for the party. We had white fur cape—gold watch, necklace and flower on my head, hyacinths pale pink and lily of valley. My cousin pale blue frock and pale blue hyacinths. Mummy long glove, white, my silver gloves short one.

N. S. at 7 *yrs.* [Describing a picture.] Bus—wheel—two wheel—in that in that. Little bit—house—house side the bus, side the bus.

Bus run—hard—going little bit. At door there, a door there—a gate—a gate. Bus, bus, car, all down.

At 8 yrs. [Conversation with therapist whilst looking at picture. From a recording. Therapist's speech in brackets.] Look at that, the big one. Look at a big one. Look at a car, a car. Had a one. Look at this. Lolly, lolly, lolly. Look at that, all that. [Cherries, Neville, cherries.] Look at a gous,* a gous, a gous. [Yes, Father Christmas.] Look at that—he come down this, we go to sleep, we go to sleep. Got a gous, a gous, a gous, got a gous, got a gous. Come down this and this. [What's this,—what's this, Neville, a bath?] Look at that one, come down. Look at that one. Look at this one. Mummy had a one, Mummy had a one, had a one. [What is it?] Mummy had a one, Mummy had a one. Look at this big one, look at ding ding, roller, roller, [a steam roller, Neville], roller, roller. Had a one, had a one, had a one. [A Christmas tree, Neville?] He broke it, he broke it, bang. [Snowman,—snowman—what is it, Neville?] Look at that, he's coming down, down there. [Dolly in a bed?] Go to sleep, go to sleep. [There's Humpty Dumpty, Neville.] Look at that, look he's fall, fall down. Got his hat off. He fall, fall there. [What are those, Neville?] Look at that big one, big one. [Look at the little ones, how many are there? Count the the little ones.] A big one, a big one. [Big ones and little ones, count the little ones, Neville.] That's a big one, a big one, a big one.

M. F. at 3½ yrs. A very few phrases such as 'open the door', 'mind Mommy', 'get passed'.

At 8 yrs. [Describing a picture.] That's party—had orange juice—girl—boy—birthday cake. Having cake. Got a coat on. That one. Candles—cake birthday, cake—blow. Man [this was a postman] letters, hat on, give girl. Mix it up. Got penny on. Sit. [Buying a ticket on a bus.]

Articulation

Defects of articulation have not been an important feature in these children. However, (S. C.) had what may have been an associated articulatory apraxia. Hearing was normal for pure tones, and he could sing in tune. Muscle tone, and movements of the muscles for articulation, was also normal except for the learned movements necessary for accurate articulation. At first he used no consonant sounds whatever, and later had difficulty in co-ordinating consonant with vowel sounds. At 6 years of age, however, he began to make more rapid and spontaneous progress, simultaneously with improvement in com-

* Phonetic symbols for a word, the meaning of which was never clear.

prehension and use of spoken language. It was interesting to observe the change in his behaviour as he became increasingly interested in, and attentive to the speech of others. A. R. has had, and still has variable use of articulation. She can use all consonants normally, especially in single words and simple speech, but tends to relapse when she is hurried, or nervous. S. P. and N. S. each had a partial hearing defect, as shown by response to pure tones, yet each developed normal articulation spontaneously. S. P. could not use (k) and (g) when first seen, and M. F., with a normal audiogram, could not at first use (s) in combinations with other consonants. No therapy was given for articulation. In these children, however, variable use of articulate sounds is common.

Reactions to Music

Three of the five children could recognise tunes with which they were familiar, but only one (S. C.) with the severe articulatory defect, could reproduce tunes accurately. Appreciation of rhythm was normal in three, and doubtful in two. The two girls, A. R. and S. P., enjoy dancing and ballet, A. R. having taken part in public presentation of ballet whilst at school.

Visual Perception

Visual appreciation for the discrimination and perception of printed or written symbols may be normal, or even especially well developed. Words could be matched to pictures by A. R. before she could understand any spoken words. This has also been described by Hannigan (1956). She could read aloud at the age of eleven years, but had, and still has imperfect comprehension, depending on the level of the reading material. S. P. began to read at 5½ years and at 6 years 3 months had a reading age on standard tests of 7 years 2 months, but again there was limited comprehension. Her articulation was always normal when she was reading, and in simple, short sentences, although jargon speech was not intelligible. M. F. began to read a little at 8 years of age, but N. S. had a reading age of 6 years at 10 years of age, and may have an associated dyslexia.

Thursday 8.th 1952

Dear miss morley

I hope you are having very nice time at holiday. before Easter, I went to school last monday I am going to coming newcastle for next year. to see you next time. My mummy she get on well feeling better now. I am going to ballet. on Friday. tonigth. about half past six, we have lovely time in garden. with my mummy. and daddy. I went to Doncaster and Nottingham My cousin name Marlene. gone home,. about four week. no morn. holiday with mummy,. and Adèlè to coming to see you at newcastle next year.,..

Love from.

Adèlè.. Best wishes

Friend

All these children can copy, and A. R. and S. P. can write letters (see samples at 15 and 7 years respectively). Spelling is good but the paragrammatism persists in written as in spoken language. N. S. can write his own name; M. F. and S. C. do not attempt to write although both enjoy drawing.

Acalculia

A failure to appreciate number is common in these children. A. R. has little understanding of quantities greater than approximately 15 to 20, and cannot give accurate change for more than one shilling. At 8 years of age she could, however, count indefinitely. Simple mechanical arithmetical processes, such as addition, subtraction, and so forth, may be slowly developed, but abstract appreciation of number is very limited. How far this may be due to failure to understand the teaching of arithmetic it is difficult to say, but this does not appear to be the entire answer. M. F. and S. P. can add and subtract simple numbers, and at 10 years N. S. had a mental age for arithmetic of 7 years 5 months, rather higher than his reading age.

Dear sister
Thank you very
much. give me Stars of on
sums book I very Good. I
hope have lovely Christmas
tree. lots of presents and
xmas pudings its Jelly custard.
I lots Book give you kisses
and kisses two Girls two boys
I have been mine seven
days old. mine birthday party
invitation birthday cards

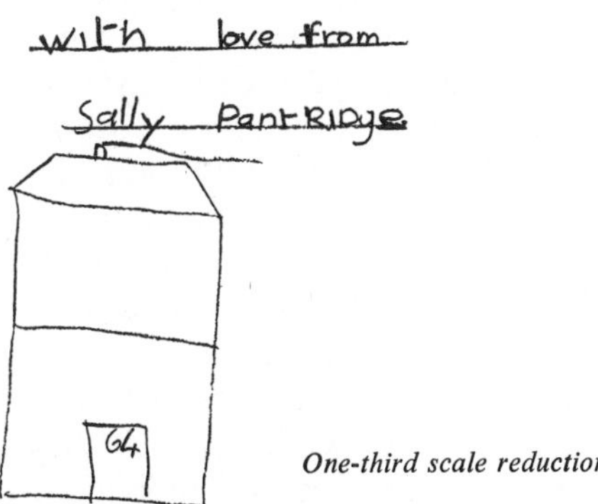

One-third scale reduction

Visual appreciation of figures, as for the number of a required bus or the number of a house, seems to be adequate for practical purposes.

Emotional Factors

The surprising fact is that clinically these five children present a reasonably normal picture of practical intelligence, independence and emotional relationships. But as they grow older they become increasingly aware of their social inadequacy where speech is concerned and also in the competitive aspects of school life. They find this difficult to understand and reactions to the situation vary, but their initial spontaneity tends to be damped. As she grew older A. R. appeared less sophisticated than was normal for her age, but she took part in school games and social activities such as tennis, cycling, horse riding, guide camps, and has always enjoyed and been particularly good at cooking. She is popular with her friends and even one of the leaders in her social group. She dresses well, choosing her own clothes and cosmetics, and maintains good social relationships within a limited environment in spite of her handicap. It is not possible yet to assess the outlook in the four younger children, but they all show adjustment appropriate to their intelligence level to what is a most severe social handicap.

Education

Each of these five children began his or her education in the normal school, but, as teaching became increasingly verbal, it was apparent that their failure to fully comprehend speech prevented adequate learning in the normal school situation. A. R. became increasingly unhappy at around eight years of age, but recovered when some individual teaching and encouragement was instituted. She later continued her education in a private school where she could compete successfully with others in games and other activities, if not in school work. In order that general education should progress within the limits of the child's potential it would seem best that they should be educated in a school where there can be individual teaching, where there is full understanding of their problem, and where there can be specialised help with language development. N. S. therefore attends such a school for children with severe speech handicaps,* and S. P. and M. F. may also attend this residential school. S. C. will at present continue to attend the normal school unless it becomes apparent, as in the others, that such education is not appropriate.

* Moor House School, Hurst Green, Surrey. The only special school in Britain for children with speech handicaps and normal intelligence.

Employment

Only one of these five children has left school and is in employment. A. R. is working in a florist's shop, making up bouquets, sprays and so forth, and also delivers flowers in a surrounding suburban district. It is probable that only essentially practical occupations will be possible for those with this severe, and within the limits of our experience, persisting disability.

Continuing follow-up, 1957–1971

A. R. continues to work in the florist's shop. At 35 years of age she is still handicapped by limited understanding for language, spoken and written, although there is some continuing improvement. Actual auditory perception (or hearing) shows some improvement, and reaction to spoken language within her comprehension is apparently normal.

N. S. continued at the school for children with severe speech handicaps until he was eighteen years of age. Since then he has been working steadily in the Post Office Engineering Service. He has always had good practical ability and can understand when shown. Although he still has limited understanding for speech there has been a continuing, slow gradual improvement in this respect over the years. He is now 24 years of age.

S. P. after three years in a local Convent day school, was transferred to the John Horniman School for three years, the preparatory school for Moor House School, where she went later when aged 11 years. Reports at that time were as follows:

Professor of Paediatrics. 'The thought behind her language is remarkably mature but the difficulty is still in constructing and understanding language. She speaks a lot, but the order of sentences, and of words in sentences still tend to be jumbled. Articulation is still clear, and reading and spelling good.'

The Psychologist's report was: 'A girl with superior intelligence who functions at the dull, normal level in verbal comprehension and expression. She gets more from the written than from the spoken word.'

Professor of Audiology. 'I cannot see how one can relate the phonetic content of this child's speech with the audiogram. She has no difficulty in producing any speech sound whether of high or low frequency, almost all her difficulties are syntactic.'

Summary of School report. Quick to learn and to retain new words. Ungrammatical sentence construction. Is discouraged easily because she is anxious to do well. Shows signs of strain and fatigue. She attempts to cover her difficulty by intelligent guess work. Good at games and practical subjects such as cookery.

However, shortly after entering Moor House School, regular audiometric testing began to show deterioration in hearing for pure tones, first in the right ear and then in the left. There was no apparent cause for this, but it continued until at 18 years of age a recent audiogram in March 1971 shows the extent of her hearing loss (Fig. 45). She now finds a hearing aid indispensable.

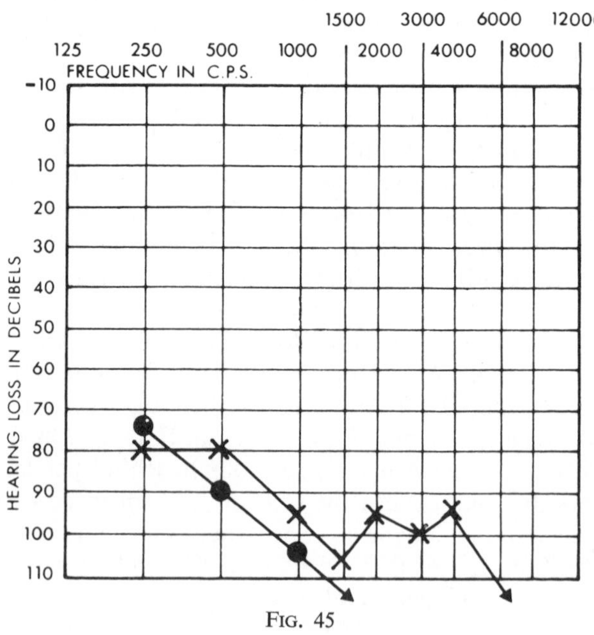

FIG. 45
S.P. Audiogram at 18 years

Because of the hearing loss she was once more transferred to the Mary Hare School for Deaf children in September 1964.

A few months later it was noticed that there had been a marked change in her intonation, and that articulation was becoming slurred and indistinct. Because the hearing aid compensated well for her increased hearing loss, it was thought that the change could only be the result of imitation of the speech of the deaf children amongst whom she was now living.

She continued to make good progress in domestic subjects, sports, riding, hockey, netball, badminton, dancing and cookery. She represented S. W. Berks. at the County athletic meeting in throwing the javelin.

She trained at school as a copy typist, and is now doing well in a Government Office, having passed the Civil Service test. She has many friends, in work and in the badminton club to which she belongs. She has an extremely good memory for facts and details in her work. At the age of 18 years she is happy and content. Expressive language is reasonably good, although probably inadequate for her intelligence level. Articulation and intonation still resemble the speech of the deaf child, and she does not always understand spoken language at first, and asks for repetition. She hears a voice of normal volume when using her hearing aid.

Summary

The condition described is that of an isolated developmental receptive aphasia where intelligence is within the normal range, there is no general motor disability, and cochlear hearing responses, and perception for consonant sounds, is adequate for the accurate reproduction of these sounds in speech. Some children, however, show a partial hearing defect for pure tones on audiometric assessment.

The onset of speech is delayed and comprehension for language, spoken and written or printed, is defective. Use of spoken language is attempted, and this may consist of jargon, or limited intelligible speech, and involve paraphasia, perseveration and paragrammatism.

Associated articulatory defects are not common, but dyspraxia occurred in one child with a normal audiogram on pure tone testing.

Visual perception may be well developed and permit reading without full comprehension. Spelling may be good, but written language shows errors of construction comparable to those in spoken language.

Acalculia, and difficulties with abstract thought are common in the children described.

It seems probable that children with a marked cochlear hearing defect may also have a more central defect affecting perception, whether resulting from limited stimulation or not, and that in a few there may also be an associated receptive aphasia.

When the major disability is a cochlear defect, or defect of perception, there may be appreciable improvement in comprehension following increased auditory stimulation and treatment, but where there is a true receptive aphasia, our experience so far indicates a very limited response to treatment, and a persisting disability which may prove a serious handicap throughout life.

There are many degrees of developmental aphasia or dysphasia in children, but if useful expressive speech is achieved by five or six years it will cause little hindrance to education in the normal school. Should the failure to develop speech persist beyond the age of six years, or use of speech be inadequate, there will be interference with normal education. This is especially so if there is failure to develop sufficient comprehension for speech, when education in a special school for children with speech disorders may be necessary.

THE TREATMENT OF DEVELOPMENTAL APHASIA

As has been described, children normally develop phonological and linguistic competence within a period of approximately two years, and between the ages of 6 months and 3 years. There would therefore appear to be a critical period for language acquisition, dependant on the requisite level of maturation for the functions involved. If there is a marked delay in the use of speech, as described in developmental aphasia, there may be a subsequent lack of adaptability and inability for reorganisation in respect of the neurophysiological processes. The greater the delay in the onset and use of language, and the more severe the underlying disability, the greater the probable effect on the ultimate use of language.

Therapy, in the form of language stimulation, should therefore begin as soon as possible, or when the interest and co-operation of the child can be obtained.

Because speech is acquired as the result of neurological maturation, attempts to teach a child to speak will produce little result. Treatment for receptive or executive developmental aphasia can only aim to stimulate and assist the normal processes of speech development and ensure that nothing is done which may hinder the progress of language development.

When a child is late in using speech the parents become anxious and fear that the child may be 'dumb' or mentally retarded. The child may be constantly worried by relatives who bombard him with requests to say this or say that. If he does use a word, so much notice may be taken, with requests to repeat it for the benefit of other members of the family, associated with unwise praise and remarks, that the child becomes self-conscious and withdraws once more into his shell of silence.

The inherent natural urge to imitate sounds and to speak is usually so strong, and such a useful means of obtaining one's needs, that most children will speak if they can, at least in early life. Appreciation of this need may, however, be encouraged through contact with other children and enhanced by the mother's attitude. She should not always respond immediately to gesture, but should so manage the situation that the child appreciates the usefulness of words rather than signs. She must, however, accept the child's temporary limitations and be careful not to induce excessive feelings of frustration or even temper tantrums. She may also take advantage of all occasions when the child takes her to show her what he wants, or uses gestures, to speak to him the words he has failed to use. She should repeat these two or three times and at the moment when the child's interest and attention is focused on what he wants.

Development of Understanding for Speech

Understanding for speech precedes its use, and the first emphasis should be on 'input'.

Whilst expressive speech is delayed, the parents should do all that is possible to build up the child's vocabulary and language in its receptive aspect. Whilst dressing, washing or feeding the child, the mother can almost continuously speak to the child, using simple language or isolated words, naming shoes, coat, spoon and so forth. She does not ask for, but accepts, any verbal response on the part of the child without unwise comment.

Games can be invented so that the child runs to any object in the room on request, carries out various actions, or brings his toys one at a time, as named. He may point to pictures of objects, or pick out objects named in a large picture. A scrap book with highly coloured pictures cut out of magazines may encourage interest in the names of objects or actions. Although he may not yet be expressing himself through words, he is doing so through action and movement in response to words.

Naming. Objects should be named, especially those of interest to the child. 'This is a . . .', and then to encourage response, 'Where is the —?', accepting an action response from the child. This can be followed by 'What is this?', hopefully, the child may reply if ready. But children rarely respond to 'Say —'!

Most of this work is best carried out by the mother in the home, whenever the child's co-operation can be gained. The therapist should also see the child at regular intervals and use her skill and knowledge to guide the mother in as many ways as possible to provide interest for the child and stimulate and sustain the mother.

Language training should continue through learning to read and write. In some cases the usual class teaching may need to be supplemented in clinical sessions, if the child's linguistic competence is still inadequate for his age.

When the receptive developmental aphasia is more severe and persists into school life, special education will probably be necessary, and a more definite approach may be required. A scheme has been devised by Lea (1965) for helping children with such a disability. He points out that these children differ from the normal in that to them the spoken word is meaningless, and that they have marked difficulty in acquiring the subtleties of grammar and syntax. The child also fails to generalise. A blue ball may be 'a ball' but he does not necessarily apply this word to a smaller red ball. There is also difficulty in associating verbal ideas.

Lea outlines the main requirements in teaching such children as the development of expressive language in the order in which the normal child proceeds, and to link language with concepts in day to day needs, aiming to give the child the means to express what he needs and wants to express. He places the greatest emphasis upon the visual stimulation and presentation of language. Words may be represented by lines of varying colours, built into a pattern such as

(red)	(yellow)	(red)	(green)	(red)
The boy	is running.	A	fast	car.

Words may be represented by coloured lines as: nouns red, articles red, verbs yellow, adjectives green, prepositions and conjunctions blue.

In stage 1 he uses a basic vocabulary of approximately 200 words and has designed a series of booklets, aiming to provide practice in the correct patterning of words in phrases and sentences. Continuing the work into stage 2 he expands and continues the work in stage 1, and introduces reading concurrently.*

Development of Expressive Speech

If the child has been unusually silent and there has been little or no vocal play or babbling, it may be possible to encourage this through the imitation of vowel and consonant sounds either in the form of animal noises (moo—baa baa, and so forth) or simple babble drills. The child is thereby building up the necessary normal patterns of articulation, and delay in doing this spontaneously may be responsible, in some, for the delay in the use of executive speech. The child should enjoy this vocal play so that he associates pleasure with the use of the sounds he makes.

When the stage of speech readiness is reached, the child will attempt to echo what he hears, and is then ready to imitate simple words. He may subsequently continue to develop speech rapidly with no more than the normal stimulus at home.

If not, he should now be encouraged to name the pictures in his scrap book. He can be encouraged to count (steps up to bed,

* See also *The Colour Pattern Scheme. A Method of Remedial Language Teaching*. By John Lea. From—The Secretary, Moor House School, Hurst Green, Oxted, Surrey, £0.80 including postage.

his fingers and toes, and so forth) and to imitate the words in children's songs and nursery rhymes, even if only the last word in each line is spoken by the child. Or he may enjoy singing or speaking in unison with his mother.

As he progresses he will enjoy listening to stories and can be asked to repeat phrases from the stories after his mother or the therapist, and eventually attempt to retell the story himself.

Luria (1961) describes how the focussing of the child's attention by means of descriptive speech on details of the form, properties and uses of objects and their significant relationships in the external world around them constitutes the most potent means of educating the child and developing intelligent understanding.

Greene (1967) believes that adequate assessment* is essential, of language development (comprehension, production, auditory memory and discrimination) and motor and visuomotor development. She also considers that such assessments can be more successful when made during observation of play, arranged so as to be diagnostic (rather than by the use of speech tests). In treatment, play is planned so that every activity is a language entity. Mime and visuomotor training are used, and language is developed through pictures, story telling, drawing, articulatory play as in babbling, and listening training.

Byers Brown (1971) also uses therapy through interesting activities, in the first step, play through activities accompanied by speech from the therapist. This input must be that to which the child will attend, progressing from sounds to words, and

* 1. The Illinois Test of Psycholinguistic Abilities (I.T.P.A.) was devised to assess language abilities in children aged two and a half to nine years of age. It is available for, and used by speech clinicians in the United States, but only by psychologists in Great Britain. This is unfortunate, as the speech therapist with knowledge and experience of language development and its disorders could learn much from observation of the child's method of approach and achievement, giving her a better understanding of the child's problem. Phillips (1968) described some of the modifications which may be necessary with children in this country, where there are certain vocabulary differences from United States usage. (See References.)

2. Reynell Developmental Language Scales. Obtainable from the National Federation for Educational Research, 2, Jennings Buildings, Thames Avenue, Windsor, Berks. SL 41 QS.

3. The English Picture Vocabulary Test by Byrne and Dunn. Pre-school Version (3 to 5 years); Test 1 (5 to 8–11 years); Test 2 (7 to 11 years 11 months). From Educational Evaluation Enterprises, 5, Marsh Street, Bristol 1.

to the development of syntactical structures. Therapy is designed to meet the needs of each individual as they arise, based on linguistic factors and a linguistic analysis of the child's speech.

Many speech therapists have devised methods for working with these children, each of whom presents an individual problem. Hence the difficulty in defining schemes and describing specific methods of treatment. The speech therapist is presented with one of the greatest challenges, requiring the best that he or she can give in appreciating the problems, ingenuity, and encouragement and support for the child and his parents.

Articulation

As speech develops, articulation may be normal or he may pass through a period of dyslalic speech. He may also have an associated developmental dysarthria or dyspraxia, when articulation will be more seriously defective. If this is so, there should be no correction of the pronunciation of words except in so far as this can be achieved by saying them clearly and repeatedly to the child. Any interference with the developing use of expressive speech in its early stages may hinder progress in language development and must be avoided.

The practice of simple babble exercises may continue for a few minutes each day at home with the mother, and very simple rhymes may also help towards improvement in the use of articulation.

Older children may be helped by associating the phonetic sounds of speech with plastic letters and simple words built with these letters. A few of these children are able to associate sounds with such visual symbols before they can recall and use words fluently in speaking.

Later more consistent speech therapy may be required to assist the development of intelligibility. Therapy may also be required if there is an associated dyslexia, or if language retardation has hindered the development of reading skill at the age when it was being taught in school.

If a child of five years has understanding for speech, as most of these children have, he can attend a normal school. If intelligence is adequate, he can learn if he cannot speak. Such children may suggest a general condition of mental retardation, and it is important that the teacher should understand the child's disability.

Brain (1952) has stated that 'internal verbal formulation is not necessary, at least for the simple forms of logical thought. It is probably required for abstract thinking and is necessary for the communication of the product of thought to others.'

It is probable, therefore, that in the child who cannot express himself through speech the processes of thought may yet be possible and that attention, memory, recollection and other processes required in learning may be possible in association with delayed development of the expressive use of speech. If this is considerably delayed until six or seven years, or later, there will be increasing interference with educational progress and resultant delay in other language fields such as reading and writing. Again, if there is lack of ability to clarify thought through the process of verbal expression, and contact with others through communication is hindered, there is likely to be some eventual hindrance of intellectual development and educational progress.

REFERENCES

Bastian, H. C. (1897). Some Problems in Connection with Aphasia and Other Speech Defects. *Lancet*, **1,** 933.

Brain, W. Russell (1952). *Diseases of the Nervous System.* London, Oxford Med. Publications.

Byers, R. K., Paine, R. S., and Crothers, B. (1955). Extrapyramidal Cerebral Palsy with Hearing Loss following Erythroblastosis. *Pediatrics*, **15,** 248–254.

Byers Brown, B. (1971). *Application of Linguistics.* Selected papers of the Second International Congress of Applied Linguistics. Eds. G. E. Perren and J. L. M. Trim. Cambridge Univ. Press.

Cawthorn, T., and Harvey, R. M. (1953). A comparison between Hearing for Pure Tones and for Speech. *J. Laryng.*, **67,** 233.

Cohen, P. (1956). Rh Child. Deaf or 'Aphasic'? 'Aphasia in Kernicterus'. *J. Speech and Hearing Dis.*, **21,** 411–412.

Critchley, J. Macdonald (1952). Articulatory Defects in Aphasia. *J. Laryng.*, **66,** 1.

Eisenson, J. (1966). Perceptual disturbances in children with central nervous system dysfunctions and implications for language development. *Brit. J. Dis. Commun. I*, **1,** 21.

Fry, D. B., and Whetnall, E. (1954). The Auditory Approach in the Training of Deaf Children. *Lancet*, **1,** 583.

Goldstein, K. (1942). *After Effects of Brain Injury in War.* London, Heinemann.

Goodhill, V. (1956). Rh Child. Deaf or 'Aphasic'? 'Clinical Pathologist Aspects of Kernicteric Nuclear "Deafness".' *J.S.H.D.*, **21,** 407–410.

Gordon, N. (1966). The child who does not talk. *Brit. J. Dis. Commun.*, **2,** 78.

Greene, M. C. L. (1967). Speechless and Backward at Three. *Brit. J. Dis. Commun. II*, **2,** 134.

Hannigan, H. (1956). Rh Child. Deaf or 'Aphasic'? 'Language and Behaviour Problems of the Rh "Aphasic Child" Child.' *J.S.H.D.*, **21,** 413–417.

Hurst, G. F. (1966). *Thinking without Language: Psychological Implications of Deafness.* New York, Free Press.

Kahn, J. H. (1965). *Human Growth and the Development of the Personality.* Oxford, Pergamon Press.

Lashley, K. S. (1938). Factors Limiting Recovery after Central Nervous System Lesions. *J. nerv. ment. Dis.*, **88,** 741.

Lashley, K. S. (1960). *The Neurophysiology of Lashley. Selected Papers.* New York, McGraw Hill.

Lea, John (1965). A language system for children suffering from receptive aphasia. *Speech Pathology and Therapy*, **8,** 2, 68.

Luria, A. R. (1961). The Role of Speech in the Regulation of Behaviour in the normal and oliogophrenic child. *Ed. Psych. in U.S.S.R.* Ed. B. Simon. London, Routledge and Kegan Paul.

Masland, M. W., and Case, L. W. (1968). Limitation of Auditory Memory as a factor in delayed language development. *Brit. J. Dis. Commun. III*, **2,** 139.

Morley, M., Court, D., and Miller, H. (1954). Developmental Dysarthria. *Brit. med. J.*, **1,** 8.

Morley, M., Court, D., Miller, H., and Garside, R. (1955). Delayed Speech and Developmental Aphasia. *Brit. med. J.*, **2,** 463.

Myklbust, H. R. (1956). Rh Child. Deaf or 'Aphasic'? 'Some Psychological Considerations of the Rh Child.' *J.S.H.D.*, **21**, 423–425.

Penfield, W., and Rasmussen, T. (1950). *The Cerebral Cortex of Man*, p. 91. New York, Macmillan.

Penfield, W., and Roberts, L. (1959). *Speech and Brain Mechanisms.* Princeton Univ. Press.

Phillips, C. J. (1968). The Illinois Test of Psycholinguistic Abilities: a report on its use with English children. *Brit. J. Dis. Commun.*, **3,** 143.

Rosen, J. (1956). Rh Child. Deaf or 'Aphasic'? 'Variations in the Auditory Disorders of the Rh Child.' *J.S.H.D.*, **21,** 418–422.

Schuell, H. (1966). Some dimensions of aphasic impairment in adults considered in relationship to investigation of language disturbance in children. *Brit. J. Dis. Commun. I*, **1,** 83.

Vygotsky, L. S. (1934, trs. 1962). *Thought and Language.* Cambridge, Mass., M.I.T. Press.

X. The Differential Diagnosis of Delayed Development of Speech

FACED with the child who has delayed speech, we have to decide whether this is due to mental deficiency, severe or partial hearing loss, to developmental aphasia or, in rare instances, to psychogenic retardation or arrest.

Mental deficiency is without doubt the commonest cause of delayed speech development, but information concerning the child's general development may be withheld by the parents, who have a natural reluctance to consider this explanation. Their answer to questions may therefore be consciously or unconsciously inaccurate. On the other hand the failure of the deaf or aphasic child to understand speech may lead all too easily to the false assumption that he is mentally defective. To complicate the situation further, the absence or limitation of speech in all three rules out the more satisfactory verbal methods of intelligence testing.

We have found the following simple questions and observations useful in the initial assessment: Does the child respond intelligently to everyday sounds? Does he respond to speech, especially when his back is turned, or from another room? Does he watch the speaker's lips? Does he grasp simple and more complicated requests, easily or with difficulty? How does he make his wants known? How do the family respond to him —by speech or by gesture? What kinds of play interest him most, and can he play for reasonable periods on his own? Does he take care of his toys or is he disturbingly destructive? What is the child's temperament—sensible, good humoured and interested, or restless and lacking in attention and concentration? If tantrums occur, are they capricious or only related to failure on the part of others to understand what he wants?

While this history is being taken from the parents, the therapist can usefully watch the child's behaviour with the toys in the consulting room. She can then begin the direct examination by showing the child a number of familiar pictures and asking him to point to the ones named. If speech is forthcoming, its extent and quality can be assessed. Suspicion of mental defect will be aroused by excessive restlessness, lack of concentration, inability to design and sustain individual play for any length of time, destructiveness and capricious emotional behaviour. However, the exact diagnosis of moderate mental retardation demands expert assessment before suspicion is allowed to harden into certainty.

A careful examination of the child by his own doctor or paediatrician may be advisable, especially of the ears and nervous system and with special reference to the presence of spasticity or athetosis.

With severe deafness for all frequencies the child fails to respond to some or all of the everyday noises as well as to speech. What is more, he may be so frustrated by his failure to understand and be understood that he has violent tantrums and may be first brought to the doctor as a behaviour problem. In the child with high-frequency deafness, on the other hand, the beginnings of speech are not greatly delayed and so the condition is frequently missed, sometimes well into school life. Such a child may be treated for defective articulation unless enquiry has recorded that the child responds well to sounds and music but hardly at all to speech and stories unless he can watch the speaker's face.

The most difficult children to distinguish from those with developmental aphasia are children with varying degrees of partial deafness, particularly with loss in the middle-frequency range. These children are not silent even though speech is delayed, and sensible parents have often failed to recognise the true state of affairs. In any child with delayed speech, especially where comprehension is defective, hearing must be thoroughly investigated by tests and audiometric methods suitable for children of different ages. Only in this way will these children with partial deafness be discovered and proper training instituted with the use of hearing aids where necessary. The distinction between partial deafness and receptive aphasia can be particularly difficult and may require further observation or even a period of residence in a special school. Moor House School is the only school in the country at present which caters for the more complex disorders of speech.

Where the delayed speech is due to a mainly expressive aphasia there is good understanding for speech, and if the child's intelligence is normal there should be little difficulty in its recognition. The psychotic child with delayed speech, though uncommon, may go unrecognised for a long time under the label of mental defect or behaviour difficulties. Gradually, however, a more bizarre pattern of behaviour becomes evident and psychiatric help is sought.

The Differential Diagnosis of Associated Conditions

The following is a summary of the chief signs associated with the various basic conditions which may cause a delay in the development of speech.

General mental retardation

General development. Delayed.

Behaviour. Lack of interest in toys with little or no constructional play.

Destructive tendencies not associated with the curiosity of the intelligent child. Poor concentration with short attention span.

Memory may not be well developed or there may be some well-developed memory which may be misleading.

He may be unable to take part fully in the games of other children or be excluded from the group.

The mother distrusts the child's ability to look after himself and is afraid to let him play outside the house because he wanders away and does not return.

Response to sounds. Immediate response at times, especially to those he associates with some satisfaction such as feeding, e.g. rattle of a spoon in a cup.

Speech. Understanding for simple language usually adequate. Little interest in stories.

Delay in the use of speech with failure to develop and use adequate expressive speech.

Psychogenic retardation

General development. Normal milestones.

Behaviour. Abnormal.

Defective emotional responses which may be lacking, excessive or variable.

There may be greater interest in things than in people.

Interests may be obsessive, limited to one, or a few.

Desire for maintenance of familiar conditions with failure to adapt easily to changes.

There may be excessive and unreasonable fears.

Response to sounds. Normal unless inhibited with obvious refusal or inability to co-operate.

Speech. Comprehension usually normal, but this is not always apparent.

Development may be normal followed by speech arrest, or normal but partially or wholly inhibited.

Articulation may be normal or there may be a persisting dyslalia with some regression at times to an earlier level of speech development.

Hearing loss—congenital or acquired before the development of speech.

(*a*) *Severe*

General development. Normal milestones except speech.

Behaviour. No response to speech or noises unless very loud.

No interest in radio apart from turning switch to produce a light.

May show keen interest in television and concentrate well.

Good use of gesture.

Interested in pictures but not in stories.

Frustration often apparent as child grows older, with temper tantrums.

Response to sounds. Nil or only when very loud.

Speech. No understanding for speech unless lip reading has been acquired. It may not develop in the child who fails to realise the existence of communication through speech.

There may be vocal sounds, babbling or even a few words

depending on the age of child and extent of residual hearing, or the child may be mostly silent.

Gesture is used freely.

(*b*) *Partial hearing loss for all frequencies of sound*

General development. Normal apart from speech.

Behaviour. Normal apart from frustration due to defective means of communication.

Response to sounds. May listen to radio when loud or to music, but not to radio stories or speech.

Speech. Failure to understand speech easily, unless using lip reading.

Development of speech delayed.

Defective articulation when speech has developed.

Frequent use of gesture for communication.

(*c*) *Hearing loss chiefly for high tones*

General development. Normal apart from speech.

Behaviour. May be normal, but appreciation of inability to make contacts through speech produces lack of confidence which becomes increasingly apparent as the child gets older.

Response to sounds. May be normal except for certain high frequency sounds (such as the squeak of a rubber mouse).

Speech. Often little delay in attempting speech, but severe limitation in comprehension for speech (except through lip reading) and in the full use of language.

Articulation defective.

No interest in radio speech but may enjoy music.

In all cases of hearing loss the response to sounds and to speech, and the speech developed, is dependent on the degree and type of hearing loss, other conditions being equal.

Developmental aphasia

(*a*) *Receptive aphasia*

General development. Normal milestones.

Behaviour. Comparable to that of a child with partial hearing loss.

May be friendly and co-operative but with signs of shyness and feelings of inadequacy.

Response to sounds. Erratic and may be suggestive of hearing loss as result of auditory inattention.

Speech. Failure to understand speech and little interest in speech as a means of communication. Lip reading does not usually develop.

Development of speech severely retarded, and inadequate when development begins. Frequently jargon.

Gesture used for communication.

Articulation may be normal.

There is a tendency to use speech as in the vocal play of the young child for personal satisfaction rather than for communication.

Developmental receptive aphasia may be associated with some degree of hearing loss or mental defect to which the failure of comprehension for and use of articulation is not proportional.

(*b*) *Expressive aphasia*

General development. Normal milestones except for speech.

Behaviour. Normal social interests and play. There may be shyness and withdrawal when aware of disability, or frustration.

Response to sounds. Normal.

Speech. Response to speech apparently normal.

Comprehension for speech appropriate to age of child.

Failure to develop use of words or sentences within the normal time range.

Later, inadequate use of language.

Use of intelligent gesture or mime to assist communication.

SUMMARY

Our present experience of the delayed development of speech and its aetiology has been described for 280 children.

The four main causes of delayed speech development were found to be general mental retardation, psychotic ill health, severe or partial hearing loss and developmental aphasia, receptive or expressive.

General mental retardation and a severe hearing defect are the most common causes of delayed development of speech. Psychotic illness is rarely the cause of such delay in the children we have seen.

The use of language and articulation has been described in patients who are mentally defective. Although defective articulation occurs, the outstanding defect is a poverty of language with varying degrees of failure to comprehend speech.

The function of hearing has been briefly described in its relation to the appreciation of sound, and in particular to those sounds which constitute articulate speech.

Defects of hearing may be perceptive, conductive or mixed, and the effect of a hearing loss on the development of speech will vary according to its type and extent.

The causes of the hearing defect have been described in 110 children referred with delayed development of speech, and the relation of the degree of hearing loss to the age of speech development.

The extent of speech development was also studied in relation to the degree of the hearing loss and the findings presented in 112 older children.

Methods for the assessment of hearing have been described. Here we have considered the child with a hearing loss which is so severe that speech fails to develop or does so to a limited extent. The child with a partial hearing loss presents a somewhat different problem as the development of language may be adequate, but with defective articulation. This will be considered in Part III, Chapter XVI.

Developmental aphasia, transient or more prolonged, occurred in children with normal intelligence and hearing, and was the cause of delay in the development of speech beyond the normal age range.

Developmental aphasia is usually an expressive disability only, but it is possible that more children than one has realised have also had some degree of limitation in their understanding for speech in early life, and a small proportion will be found who have a severe disability, or developmental receptive aphasia.

Developmental executive dysphasia, with difficulty in the

	Mental Defect	Psychogenic Retardation	Hearing Loss		
			(*a*) Severe	(*b*) Partial for all frequencies	(*c*) Higher freq
General development.	Delayed.	Normal milestones.	Normal milestones except speech.	Normal milestones except speech.	Normal milestone
Behaviour.	Lack of interest. Poor concentration. May be destructive.	Abnormal, especially of emotional response.	Failure to respond to speech. Use of gesture. Otherwise normal apart from temper tantrums due to frustration.	Normal, apart from temper tantrums which may be more evident than in severely deaf child.	May be normal, b lack of confidenc awareness of disab
Response to sounds.	There may be inattention with failure to respond. Otherwise immediate response to familiar sounds, especially those associated with feeding (e.g. sweet-paper rustle, or rattle of crockery).	Normal, unless inhibited and there is refusal to co-operate.	Responds to very loud sounds only, if at all.	Responds to loud sounds.	Responds at onc sounds.
Response to speech.	Usually responds, but does not always understand.	Normal unless inhibited, with refusal to co-operate.	None.	Responds to a loud voice only. Partial understanding for speech.	Understands spec through lip readin
Lip reading.	Nil.	Nil.	A little, or none.	Usually lip reads well according to age.	Good lip reading a
Response to radio or stories.	Apparently normal or little interest.	Normal, no interest or inhibited.	Nil.	Likes increased volume. Appreciates music better than speech or stories.	Hears music at r No interest in radi stories if he can lip
Gesture.	Little or no gesture.	None.	Gesture and mime well developed.	Some gesture to supplement speech.	Used when speech
Onset of speech.	Delayed.	Usually normal.	Severely delayed, if any.	Some delay.	May occur at norr
Language.	Limited use.	Usually normal, but use may be inhibited or defective.	None or extremely limited.	Limited vocabulary and use of sentences.	Limited or full u depending on ext defect.
Articulation.	Normal, or persistent dyslalia, or associated with dysarthria or articulatory apraxia.	Normal, or regression to dyslalia.	Very defective if any attempt.	Defective.	Very defective.

recall of words or the use of the verbal symbols of speech may persist into school or later life. There may also be associated disabilities such as dysarthria, articulatory apraxia, or difficulties associated with the use of the written and printed symbols for speech in reading, writing and spelling.

The child who fails to develop speech faces a serious handicap, and the type of education most suitable for his needs will require special consideration.

The help which can reasonably be expected from speech therapy has been briefly outlined.

PART III

DEFECTIVE ARTICULATION

XI. Defects of Articulation and their Aetiology

During the development of speech many children pass through a period when the phonetic sounds, which in sequence constitute articulate speech, are not used normally. Omission of consonants, or the use of consonant sounds other than the correct ones, whatever the basic aetiology, may cause speech to be unintelligible. Defective use of the consonants [r] [θ and ð (th)] [j (y)] and [l] is common in young children but has little effect on intelligibility. The consonant [s], however, occurs frequently in speech, and omission or defective articulation of this one sound may cause a much more serious interference with the intelligibility of the child's speech. In general, the child has developed the use of only a limited number of consonant sounds, and he either uses these for those he has not acquired or omits them.

Such defective articulation may occur as a transient stage in the development of speech in infancy with spontaneous and steady improvement towards normal articulation, or it may be the result of a structural abnormality such as cleft palate, a partial hearing defect, or some failure of the neurological development for speech with or without other signs of brain injury (Morley *et al.*, 1950).

Incidence

As previously described (Chapter IV), the findings during a survey of the speech of 944 children in the normal population showed that 32 per cent passed through a period when articulation was so defective that speech was largely unintelligible, at least to strangers. The following table shows the ages at which these children used intelligible speech (Fig. 46).

These figures do not include those children with less severe defects of articulation whose speech was intelligible. The total percentage of children with persistent defects of articulation at four years nine months was 11 per cent and at six and a half years 3 per cent. In this group there were no children with a severe dysarthria, cleft palate speech nor a severe hearing defect.

Age in years	Percentage using intelligible speech
At 2	70
3 9/12	90
4 9/12	95
6½	99

FIG. 46

The age when speech became intelligible in 944 children

RELAPSING ARTICULATION

During progress towards normal speech there is in most children a period of unstable and relapsing articulation. Even when speech is apparently normal, or nearly so, being used easily and without conscious thought, previous faulty patterns of articulation recur at times of excitement and emotional stress. Clinical experience suggests that this is a temporary stage in speech development and one through which most of such children pass in their progress towards the use of stable, normal articulation. At six and a half years, four per cent of the children who used normal or at least intelligible speech relapsed occasionally into unintelligible speech.

Summarising the findings already described (Chapter V), such defective articulation was more common among boys than girls and persisted in the former to a later age. It occurred more frequently in second and younger children in the family, with a highly significant absence of defects of articulation among first children. We found no significant correlation between social status and defective articulation apart from a group of 44 children with unintelligible speech persisting until four years nine months, of whom 59 per cent were in social classes IV and V, nor with other environmental conditions.

PROGNOSIS

In many such children there is spontaneous improvement. In others the defective articulation may prove a serious handicap in school, and without adequate treatment may persist into adult life.

From the figures stated above it is clear that there is a certain type of defective articulation which occurs so frequently during the development of speech in young children that, if adequate means of communication are established by the age of three to four years, it may well be regarded as within the normal range. This temporary defective use of articulation is sometimes described as 'baby talk'.

It is also clear from these findings and from clinical experience that some children, approximately three per cent, encounter a much more persistent and handicapping disability in the process of acquiring speech. During speech therapy there is a marked difference in response to treatment. Whereas some respond quickly, others apparently have much greater difficulty, even in the absence of any obvious organic basis for the defective articulation, and progress may be slow or almost imperceptible. Some children may show little improvement for several months or even years until a stage is reached when progress becomes much more rapid with the final use of normal articulation developing perhaps within a few weeks. It does not seem possible to foresee, however, when this stage will be reached, and patient and persistent treatment will be required in the meantime.

In some children there may be spontaneous improvement in articulation after entry into school. The slow articulation of words whilst learning to read provides conditions under which the child may unconsciously develop the use of normal articulation through visual and kinaesthetic associations of the symbols of speech. This skill is acquired at a later stage of the child's development, and such associations may be normal when the auditory-kinaesthetic associations formed in earlier life were defective. Where, however, the organic basis for the defect is more severe and persistent, children may learn to read but still use their own defective patterns of articulation, and if such articulation then persists until seven or eight years of age, it will tend to become stabilised, improvement is less likely and it may then continue into adult life.

Developmental defects of articulation, therefore, do not constitute a simple group which can be adequately described as dyslalia, even when those occurring as a result of a hearing loss or of some structural abnormality are excluded. Such defects of articulation were studied over a period of six years by a team consisting of a paediatrician, a neurologist, a psychologist and a speech therapist (Morley *et al.*, 1954) and we found it possible to identify three types of such defective articulation.

It was first recognised that in some of these children the failure to develop normal articulation was probably the result of an organic condition. There was abnormality of movement of the muscles used in speech similar to that found in association with other more general signs of motor disability as in cerebral palsy, but sometimes isolated and occurring in the absence of any other detectable signs of brain damage. In others there appeared to be no abnormality of muscle tone, but consciously directed movements of lips and tongue lacked control and co-ordination, affecting the direction of such movements for the imitation of the articulate sounds of speech.

Factors which strongly suggested an organic basis for these types of defective articulation were the frequency of abnormal movements of lips, tongue or palate and the close similarity of the isolated dysarthrias to the dysarthria associated with cerebral palsy and with degenerative lesions in later life. In many there was a family history of speech defects, and the steady but slow improvement in response to time and treatment were also strongly in favour of an organic basis. The disability showed neither the intermittency and tendency to recurrence of a speech disorder such as stammering nor the rapid response to treatment which occurs in those cases of consonant substitution to which we have limited the use of the term dyslalia. We eventually classified these defects as follows:

CLASSIFICATION OF DISORDERS OF ARTICULATION

1. Developmental dysarthria.
2. Developmental articulatory apraxia.
3. Dyslalia.
4. Defective articulation due to deficient hearing.
5. Defective articulation due to various structural abnormalities.

When observing these children with defects of articulation the outstanding features of each group are clear, but the differential diagnosis is not always easy, and in some the response to treatment is the only means by which the diagnosis can be confirmed. If it can be ascertained, however, it is useful in assessing the prognosis and in planning the treatment of the individual child.

The types of defective articulation mentioned above may be briefly defined as follows:

Developmental Dysarthria

This disorder of speech occurs when there is difficulty in the movement and control of any of the muscles used for articulation, phonation or respiration. The outstanding picture is one of inadequate movement due to abnormal muscle tone, with poor control and co-ordination of the muscle groups used during speech when it seems apparent that the child has little or no difficulty in knowing what he should do to imitate the sounds he hears. He may be able to do so at slow speed, but has difficulty of varying degrees in accomplishing his end, especially at the speed of normal conversational speech. Other indications may be a history of sucking or swallowing difficulty in early life, or a laryngeal stridor.

Developmental Articulatory Apraxia

In contrast to those children with developmental dysarthria we find those who apparently have no difficulty in moving the tongue, lips or palate for spontaneous movements but have difficulty in directing them for voluntary imitation of movements or for the reproduction of the correct articulatory sounds when hearing is normal. In such children the disturbance of function probably originates at a higher level of the nervous system and may be described as an apraxic dysarthria or articulatory apraxia, or more commonly dyspraxia, according to the degree of severity. The child is able to carry out the movements necessary for articulation but may have acquired only a limited number of consonant sounds and has insufficient audio-kinaesthetic control to reproduce such sounds accurately when they occur in the long sequences of consonant and vowel sounds we call speech.

Dyslalia

In this group we have included those defects of articulation which appear to be functional in origin rather than attributable to any damage to the brain or failure of the neurological maturation for speech. In many there is spontaneous improvement or rapid response to guidance and treatment.

Defective Articulation due to Deficient Hearing

Defective hearing, other factors being equal, will affect articulation according to the degree of hearing loss and the frequencies of sound for which hearing is affected. The greatest difficulty is experienced when there is a hearing defect of the inner ear or perceptive deafness. The consonant sounds are then heard inaccurately and the child imitates them as he perceives them.

Defective Articulation due to Structural Abnormalities

This group includes children who have adequate neurological development for speech but in whom some structural anatomical defect renders normal articulation impossible or contributes towards the disability when, in addition, there is some degree of dysarthria or articulatory apraxia.

The most important of such conditions is the incompetent nasopharyngeal sphincter. Although this may occur as a result of paresis of the palatal and pharyngeal muscles, when the basic condition is a developmental dysarthria, it also occurs in those with a developmental failure of union in cases of cleft palate or other abnormalities of the palate and pharynx.

Structural abnormalities of the upper or lower jaw with malocclusion may in some children be the cause of the defective articulation of certain consonant sounds, especially if the child has also some degree of dysarthria or articulatory apraxia. The compensatory adjustments usually achieved, with resulting normal speech, are then rendered more difficult.

An excessively large tongue, or macroglossia, may hinder the development and use of normal articulation. A short fraenum may or may not interfere with the development of articulation, and the use of the nasal consonants [m] [n] and [ŋ (ng)] may be impossible when the nasal airways are obstructed as the result of enlarged adenoids or other causes.

In considering these defects of articulation it must always be remembered that the resultant speech disorder is determined not only by the basic neurological or anatomical condition but is necessarily affected by other conditions such as the intelligence and personality of the child. The various types of defective articulation described may exist in isolation or in combination one with another, as when a dysarthria, or anatomical condition such as cleft palate, is complicated by a hearing defect or some degree of articulatory apraxia. Treatment must be designed to meet the condition and need of each individual patient and should be available at the time when the child becomes aware of the frustrations associated with inadequate use of speech as a means of communication, and where possible before the stabilisation of faulty speech patterns renders the development and use of normal speech more difficult.

REFERENCES

Morley, M., Court, D., and Miller, H. (1950). Childhood Speech Disorders and the Family Doctor. *Brit. med. J.*, **1**, 574.

Morley, M., Court, D., and Miller, H. (1954). Developmental Dysarthria. *Brit. med. J.*, **1**, 8.

XII. Developmental Dysarthria

In children with developmental dysarthria there are obvious signs of interference with the movement and co-ordination of those muscles required for speech due to abnormal muscle tone. The tongue may appear thick, narrow, bunched and spastic, or broad at the tip, and movements may be clumsy with inability to elevate the tip or move it from side to side. Movements of the muscles of the soft palate and pharynx may be abnormal or there may be difficulty in moving the lips easily for the articulation of the bilabial consonants. Co-ordination of the various muscle groups may be affected, as for example co-ordination of the muscles of respiration with those of phonation, or of phonation with articulation. Expressive speech is used, but is inadequate for communication because normal co-ordinated muscle movements are impossible. Various abnormal movements for articulation may therefore have developed and these tend with time to become established.

There are many varying degrees of severity of developmental dysarthria. In some children the movements of one or more of the muscle groups used in speech are so severely affected that articulation is only partially achieved by the use of slow and laboured speech, the child making prodigious efforts to obtain the correct apposition of the tongue, lips and teeth for the production of the sounds he wishes to produce. In others the difficulty is less severe and may interfere only with the movements of one of the muscle groups used for articulation. Or again, muscular movements may be adequate for slow conversational speech and the defects of articulation chiefly noticeable when rapid and excited speech is used.

Although the exact aetiology of this condition at present remains in doubt, it is thought that in such children there is an organic defect or delay in the neurological maturation for the movement and control of the muscles required for speech as a result of cerebral damage or mal-development causing cerebral dysfunction. It is well known that defective articulation results from certain degenerative neurological processes, but we are concerned here with the failure to develop the normal use of the muscles adapted for speech so as to produce clear and accurate articulation in co-ordination with respiration and phonation.

It is generally accepted that in the formulation and expression of thought through the act of speaking the muscular movements involved are integrated at the cortical level and controlled through the lower portion of the motor cortex. Penfield (1954) has stated that to judge by the results of electrical stimulation of the cortex 'articulation and vocalisation can be controlled through the lower portion of the Rolandic motor strip'. He also found that this portion of the motor apparatus could be excised completely without interference with the ideational mechanisms of speech and without aphasia, even in the dominant hemisphere, but that such removal produced a severe anarthria or dysarthria which tended to improve after operation. He thought it likely that such a patient was able to speak by employment of the cortical motor mechanisms of the other hemisphere.

Developmental dysarthria can be of many varying degrees and is frequently seen in its most severe form in children with other extensive signs of cerebral trauma or mal-development, causing spasticity or athetosis. We have also found some children with a severe motor disability as the result of pyramidal and extra-pyramidal lesions who have normal or near normal use of the muscle groups required for speech and no obvious defect of articulation.

A severe dysarthria may also occur in children who have no obvious signs of cerebral injury, but full neurological examination reveals a general *minimal motor disability*. The speech defect, then, is out of all proportion to the general physical condition.

In other children a dysarthria has been found in the absence of any other signs of cerebral damage at the time of examination. The defect of articulation may be slight or severe and associated with inadequate movements of the lips, tongue or palate. We have used the term *isolated dysarthria* for this type of developmental dysarthria (Morley *et al.*, 1958).

Our observations of these children indicate that the severity of the general motor disability may bear little relationship to the degree of dysarthria, that the defective articulation would seem to depend on a focal cerebral dysgenesis essentially similar to but more limited in extent than that associated with more extensive signs of cerebral trauma, and that though widespread brain injury may involve the neurological mechanism for speech, a developmental dysarthria may occur in isolation.

Dysarthria will therefore be described, firstly, in children with general motor disability or cerebral palsy, secondly, in those children who have a minimal degree of cerebral palsy, and thirdly, where it occurs in isolation and without any other signs of brain damage. These divisions do not represent three different conditions but only clinical pictures of varying degrees of physical or motor disability occurring in association with developmental dysarthria.

DEVELOPMENTAL DYSARTHRIA IN CHILDREN WITH EXTENSIVE BRAIN DAMAGE AND GENERAL MOTOR DISABILITY OR CEREBRAL PALSY

In recent years what has come to be known as cerebral palsy has been recognised, investigated and described to an ever-increasing extent. Although this is a general term including a variety of motor and sensory disabilities, it is now generally accepted that it results from injury to or abnormal development of certain areas of the brain which control and co-ordinate muscle movements.

Asher and Schonell (1952) studied a series of 349 cases of congenital cerebral palsy, including 36 cases of athetosis, 31 of whom had a history of neonatal jaundice. They suggest that athetosis is usually the result of birth injury, asphyxia or neonatal jaundice, and that although some cases of spastic paralysis may be the result of birth injury, others are probably the result of genetic or intra-uterine factors.

According to Benda (1952), the term cerebral palsy denotes 'all those conditions in which interference with the motor system arises as a result of lesions within the brain'. Bronson Crothers (1951) states that 'a child has cerebral palsy when it has suffered injury to the brain, occurring during the period of rapid development from conception to three years of age which distorts orderly development and leads to abnormal motor control'. He also emphasises that 'most of the phenomena due to lesions in early life are evidence of failure of development and orderly integration rather than of destruction or distortion of matured patterns'. Ellis (1955) explains that the term cerebral palsy does not apply to one specific condition but that 'it is a comprehensive term covering a large number of conditions of varying degrees of severity but characterised by the presence of abnormal muscle tone, often associated with disturbance of sensation and impairment of intelligence. The group is a clinical one without any implication of aetiology. It may be recognised clinically as (*a*) spasticity, (*b*) athetosis and (*c*) ataxia.'

Bobath (1955) has described cerebral palsy as resulting from the persistence of abnormal postural reflex activity which 'results from the release of motor responses from the restraining influence of higher centres, especially of the cortex'. Such abnormal postural reflexes are the cause of abnormal muscle tone, the distribution of which changes with the position in which the child is placed and which interfere with the growth and development of the normal automatic righting reflexes and willed movements.

Righting reflexes determine the developing movements of the child and normally occur against a background of muscle tone which is sufficient to maintain posture against gravity but is not high enough to cause resistance to the increasing mobility of the child. The righting reflexes enable the child to raise the head when lying in supine, to turn the head, shoulders and pelvis as he rolls over, and gradually to progress through the normal stages of increasing mobility and muscle co-ordination to the development of cortical control and voluntary movements. These postural and righting reflexes have been described by Magnus (1926) in animals, and in children by Schaltenbrand (1928). In animals the righting reflexes are present at birth and enable a newly born calf, for example, to rise and stand on its four legs, somewhat unsteadily, soon after its arrival in this world. In the child, however, they develop gradually in early life.

As development progresses, the normal primitive reflex movements are not completely lost, but with the development of cortical control there is increasing selective inhibition of the earlier movements. In children with cerebral palsy such development is distorted and is inadequate for normal mobility.

Motor Disability and Speech

Expressive defects

(*a*) *Developmental dysarthria.* The general physical disability differs in its distribution according to the site and extent of the lesion. If the areas for the integration of those muscle movements used in speech are affected, namely those involved in respiration, phonation and articulation, there will be interference with the movements for speech and a resulting dysarthria.

(*b*) *Developmental aphasia.* Where there is damage to those areas of the cortex involved in the formulation of expressive speech, there will be varying degrees of failure to develop the use of language at the normal time, or developmental aphasia, in some of such severity that use of speech is limited to a few single words or phrases throughout life.

(*c*) *Apraxia.* Developmental articulatory apraxia of severe degree may also occur in these children, whether in isolation or in association with dysarthria or dysphasia.

Sensory defects

(*a*) *Hearing loss and auditory imperception.* Some children may have a partial failure of cochlear development, or of auditory perception with varying degrees of hearing loss, or of failure to understand spoken speech. It is possible that such interference with hearing or perception may not be constant and may be increased during moments of muscular spasm. It is common experience that sounds near the threshold of hearing may be entirely lost during the process of a normal stretch of the whole body, and in children with brain injury there may be increased and varying degrees of failure to understand speech at times of emotional stress, when fatigued, or during moments of increased spasticity, or of involuntary movements.

Various investigators have reported a high incidence of hearing defects in patients with brain injury. Fisch (1955) has tested the hearing ability in 89 children with cerebral palsy. These comprised 39 children in a special school for cerebral palsied children, 35 older children who had left school and were attending a school for vocational training and 15 children with cerebral palsy who were attending a school for physically handicapped children. In 18 (20 per cent) the hearing loss was sufficient to cause a serious disability. In six, four with a severe loss and two with a slight loss, it was unilateral, in one being due to wax in the auditory canal only. He states that in no child was there any disease of the middle ear, and that in 25 the hearing loss was perceptive and in five conductive.

Asher (1952) found a hearing deficiency in 26 out of 42 children with athetosis attending the Spastic Clinic at the Birmingham Children's Hospital. A hearing defect occurred in 22 out of 24 children in whom there was a history of neonatal jaundice, but was found in only four of the remaining 18 where jaundice had not been evident. She also states that deafness is uncommon among spastics, and she found only two in a group of 28 who had sufficient hearing loss to cause delay in the development of speech. In neither of these was it the typical high frequency hearing loss usually associated with athetosis.

Dunsdon (1952) tested the hearing of 27 children with cerebral palsy and found only two with what she described as 'normal' hearing. In four, however, the percentage loss was less than ten per cent and in 18 more it was less than 20 per cent. She estimated this percentage loss using Harvey Fletcher's method of multiplying by 0·8 the average hearing loss in decibels for the frequencies 512, 1024 and 2048 c.p.s. Therefore all these 22 children had an average hearing loss for that frequency range which is most important for speech of less than 25 decibels, and this may well have indicated hearing for speech which was within the normal range. Five children, four with athetosis and one with spasticity, had a hearing loss greater than this, although one of these showed adequate unilateral hearing up to 2048 c.p.s. but with increasing loss up to 70 db. at 8000 c.p.s. for the higher frequencies. Ineffective hearing for speech was therefore established in only four of the 27 children, or 15 per cent.

(*b*) *Auditory agnosia* describes the condition when there is failure to associate meaning with sounds heard, and also, of course, affects the recognition and meaningful interpretation of the sound symbols used for language. Sounds which have no meaning for the child will frequently be ignored. The auditory impulse (Gordon, 1966) fails to reach the cortex and cannot be endowed with meaning at the cortical level, and peripheral deafness may at first be suspected.

(*c*) *Visual and spatial perception.* Varying degrees of interference with visual and spatial perception, more extensive than is normal, may also occur in these children, and also in those with isolated disorders of speech, and where the variation from the normal is more pronounced it may prove a serious handicap, especially when learning to read.

(*d*) *Disturbances of sensation.* Various disturbances of sensation may occur and have been found to be more common in children with spastic conditions than in those with athetosis (Kenney, 1963). Tizard *et al.* (1954) studied disturbances of sensation in children with spastic hemiplegia and found an impairment of sensation to touch, pain, position sense, two point discrimination, stereognosis and other sensations in about half the children studied. He also noted that the severity of the sensory impairment was not proportional to the severity of the motor disability.

(*e*) *Sensation of movement.* Where there is defective movement for articulation due to dysarthria there will be interference with the normal patterns of feed-back, in that the abnormal muscle movements will inevitably cause sensori-motor experience to be abnormal with the tendency for these faulty patterns of movement to be perpetuated. Such abnormal sensations of movement affecting auditory, tactile and kinaesthetic perception through feed-back may contribute towards the articulatory apraxia which occurs in some of these children.

(*f*) *General mental retardation.* Failure of comprehension may be associated with general mental retardation, and it is not easy to assess how far it may have contributed to, or have been the result of, the general retardation of mental growth and development.

The usual sensory learning experienced by the normal child is also limited in these children who lack mobility, and visual learning may be confined to what the child is able to see from a supine position. Growing experience of his environment associated with growth of vocabulary is hindered if the child is immobile, perhaps spending most of his life in one room, and so many of these children, perhaps with adequate intellectual capacity, appear to be mentally retarded and fail to develop use of speech at the usual time when compared with the child who has no motor disability and has been able to learn through contact with and growing awareness of his environment. However, where there has been widespread cerebral damage it is not surprising that in a large proportion of these children there are also varying degrees of intellectual impairment.

A SURVEY OF DISORDERS OF SPEECH IN PATIENTS WITH BRAIN DAMAGE

The speech of children with brain injury and a general motor disability has been studied in 110 patients. They fall into three groups.:

1. Patients referred to hospital speech therapy departments.
2. Children attending a special school.
3. Young children attending an out-patient clinic.

1. Patients referred to Hospital Speech Therapy Departments

Fifty patients aged 4 to 27 years had been referred to hospital speech therapy departments. In 31 of these there was obvious interference of varying degrees with motor activity. In 19 there was a severe dysarthria but only minimal signs of cerebral palsy which had not previously been suspected until neurological examination revealed the true organic condition.

In three of these 50 patients there was some degree of hearing loss for pure tones on audiometric assessment. In each case it was of perceptive type with greater loss for the high than for the low frequencies of sound.

2. Children attending a Special School

Thirty-two children, aged 7 to 14 years, were attending a special school for children with cerebral palsy. These were a selected group in whom the general physical handicap was of such severity as to preclude education in a normal school but where the general level of intelligence was considered such as to justify special education.

Of these 32 children, 18 had no serious interference with the use of speech. Seven of these 18 children had normal speech, whilst in ten there was occasionally some degree of facial spasm affecting movement of the lips or some hypertension in the muscles of the tongue or jaw which did not interfere to any marked extent with articulation. One child had a slight tendency to stammer. The defects of speech in these 18 children were so slight that speech therapy was not considered necessary. They were regarded by the teaching staff as having normal speech, and this group of children will be referred to as the group with 'normal' speech.

Fourteen children had a much more extensive interference with the use of speech. In three there was a developmental dysphasia, with very limited expressive speech, whilst in 11 executive speech had developed but there was defective articulation. One of these children had a partial hearing loss. In none of the other 32 children in the school was a hearing deficiency proved.

3. Children attending an Out-patient Clinic

Twenty-eight children between the ages of 18 months and six years were attending the out-patient clinic attached to the special school. They attended for observation, physiotherapy and, where necessary, speech therapy. In these children it was possible to observe the development of speech over a period ranging from 6 to 12 months.

To summarise, we had therefore:

1. 50 hospital patients with severe dysarthria of whom
   31 had an associated obvious motor disability, and
   19 had a minimal and unsuspected motor disability.
2. 32 schoolchildren with a severe motor disability of whom
   18 had 'normal' speech, and
   14 had defective speech.
3. 28 young out-patient children with a general motor disability and varying degrees of speech development.

In these patients the following conditions have been considered:

(*a*) Hearing defects.
(*b*) The age of speech development.
(*c*) The relation of speech development to general motor development.
(*d*) Defects of speech in relation to the general motor disability.
  (i) The extent and distribution of the general motor disability.
  (ii) The type of disability, or function.
  (iii) General motor development.
(*e*) Lateral dominance.

The clinical findings concerning respiration, phonation and articulation will also be described for these patients.

(*a*) HEARING DEFECTS IN 110 PATIENTS

In these 110 patients a hearing loss was found in four, in three of those attending a hospital speech therapy department where the disability was chiefly athetosis associated with some degree of spasticity, and in one child attending the special school, where there was spasticity but no athetosis. The hearing loss in these patients contributed towards the defective articulation; and one boy aged 16 years had developed no speech, although he had some limited comprehension for speech through lip reading.

When testing these patients the response to pure tone audiometric assessment often showed some degree of loss of hearing up to 30 decibels, but it was considered probable that this may have been due to failure on the part of the patient to respond to sounds at threshold rather than to any significant hearing loss, as the hearing response for quiet speech was adequate without lip reading. Such a hearing loss, if in fact it did exist, is insufficient to affect seriously hearing for the conversational voice and hinder the development of speech. In only four, therefore, of 110 patients was there a proved partial hearing defect for pure tones which was sufficient to affect speech. In each case it was of inner ear type with greater loss for the higher than for the lower frequencies of sound. In three who had developed speech in spite of their hearing loss, a hearing aid provided some improvement for the understanding of speech.

T. B., a boy, was 16 years of age when first seen and had no expressive speech. He had been considered to be mentally defective. He had a spastic diplegia with some involuntary movements of legs, arms, head and facial muscles, and did not walk until eight years of age.

It was found that he had a hearing loss for pure tones ranging from 40 decibels loss at 256 c.p.s. and 512 c.p.s. to 70 db. at 1000 c.p.s. and 75 db. at 4000 c.p.s. He had a little understanding for speech through lip reading, but comprehension was very limited. A hearing aid failed over a period of 18 months to give him any improved understanding for speech, and although he liked to wear it he still made no attempt to use speech of any kind, continuing to communicate by means of gesture.

Although intelligence was probably subnormal, he had some practical ability, and at his present age it was impossible to assess how far his inadequacy was associated with his failure to hear and comprehend speech, and whether or not there was a receptive aphasia in addition to his general physical disability.

C. S., aged nine years when first seen, had a moderate degree of athetosis and some spasticity. He had a hearing loss ranging from 20 db. at 500 c.p.s. to 60 db. at 2000 c.p.s. and up to 12000 c.p.s. A hearing aid gave him some assistance and at 16 years of age he was maintaining a high standard of educational attainment at a well-known public school. Articulation was affected as the result of his hearing loss for the frequencies of sound important for speech, and in addition there was some dysarthria. He later gained entrance to, and studied mathematics at Cambridge University.

A.W., aged 22 years, with athetosis and spasticity had a hearing loss ranging from 20 db. at 250 c.p.s. to 75 db. at 3000 c.p.s. She found a hearing aid useful, especially at the theatre, where she was able to follow a play when previously she had had to have the events explained to her. Speech was defective but intelligible with dysarthria aggravated by inadequate hearing for the consonant sounds of speech.

E. D., aged ten years, attended the special school for children with cerebral palsy. Her hearing loss was not at first suspected, but it was noticed that she showed no interest in stories told by the teacher to the class, and there was inattention at other times. She had had a hearing aid for six months and her teacher reported that she subsequently listened with interest to stories. Articulation was also improving.

(*b*) THE AGE OF SPEECH DEVELOPMENT.

The age of speech development and of its relation to defects of speech will be considered first in patients with a general motor disability in:

(i) 50 who attended a hospital speech therapy department, and

(ii) 32 children attending a special school.

(*i*) *The age of speech development in* 50 *patients with general motor disability attending a hospital speech therapy department*

In many of the 50 patients referred for speech therapy the age of development of speech could not be ascertained with accuracy, as in older children and adults it could not be remembered. The three patients with defective hearing are also excluded from these findings as it was impossible to determine to what extent the age of speech development had been influenced by this factor.

In 35 patients, therefore, aged 4 to 27 years when first seen, the mean age for the first use of words was three and a half years (Appendix, Table XXVI). In 18 of these patients there was a severe motor disability whilst in 17 there were only minimal signs of cerebral palsy.

The age when phrases were first used in the case of 29 of these patients ranged from one to ten years, and six of them had used no word sequences whatever. The mean age was five and a half years for those who had used phrases.

In 15 of these 29 patients there was a severe general disability and in 14 it was only minimal. The mean age and the age range for the first use of words and phrases in this group of patients subdivided according to the degree of the general disability is shown in Figure 47.

Although there is a marked difference in the motor disability in these two groups of patients there is little difference in the mean age at which speech was first attempted. Many of these patients were also thought to have some degree of mental retardation, and this factor may have contributed to their late development of speech in some, and for the considerable age range for the first use of single words and phrases. There is, however, a marked retardation in speech development in these patients with developmental dysarthria as compared with the normal (Appendix, Table I).

First use of—		Motor Disability	
Words— 35 patients	 Mean age Age range	(*a*) Severe—18 3·9 years 1½-8 years	(*b*) Minimal—17 3·4 years 1½-5½ years
Phrases— 29 patients	 Mean age Age range	(*a*) Severe—15 6 years 2½-11½ years	(*b*) Minimal—14 4·8 years 1½-9½ years

FIG. 47

Age of speech development in patients with severe dysarthria.
Six patients used no phrases at the time of assessment.

(*ii*) *The age of speech development in* 32 *children with a severe motor disability attending a special school*

In this group of children, aged 7 to 15 years, who were all considered to be of sufficient intelligence for education in a special school, the mean age for the first use of words was two years, as compared with one year in the normal child. Fourteen of these children had a severe defect of articulation, including the one who was partially deaf, whilst in 18 speech was normal or nearly so. In two children with normal speech the age of speech development could not be ascertained. The findings are given, therefore, for 13 children with defective articulation, excluding the child with a partial hearing loss who first used words at three years and phrases at six and a half years, and for 16 children with normal speech (Fig. 48).

Phrases were being used by all but one boy aged 13½ years at the time of assessment, but in five of the children with defective speech, and in one of those with normal speech, word sequences were not attempted before five years of age. In these children with cerebral palsy there was a delay of approximately one year in the first use of words and of three years for the first use of phrases as compared with the findings for the children already described (Chapter III), representing the normal childhood population.

In the 18 children with normal speech the average age for the first use of words was 1·8 years, as compared with 2·2 years for the children with defective speech, the age range being eight months to five years, and ten months to six years respectively. In the children with defective speech there was, however, a more marked retardation in the first use of phrases. These were first used by the group of children with normal speech at the mean age of two and a half years, but not until four and a half years by those with defective speech (Fig. 48) (Appendix, Table XXVII).

First use of—		Speech	
		Normal—16	Defective—13
Words— 29 children	Mean age Age range	1·8 years 8/12 to 5 years	2·2 years 10/12 to 6 years
Phrases— 28 children	Mean age Age range	2·5 years 1 to 6 years	4·5 years 1 to 12 years

FIG. 48

The age of speech development in 32 children with a severe motor disability. One child had used no phrases at the age of 13½ years.

Eighty-seven per cent of the children with normal speech were using words by three years of age as compared with 50 per cent of those with defective speech, and at four years the comparative figures for the use of phrases were 86 per cent and 46 per cent respectively.

Although in almost all these children with cerebral palsy there was delay in the onset of speech, some developed the use of language within what we have considered to be the normal age range (Chapter III). In others there was a more severe delay in the development and use of language, and where intelligence was probably not below normal, the speech disorder may be described as developmental aphasia.

In addition, a dysarthria became evident in many of these children as use of language progressed, although, as previously described, one child, who did not attempt word sequences until five years of age, rapidly developed adequate use of language with normal articulation.

(*c*) Speech and general motor development

Normally, speech development occurs simultaneously with the development of other muscular movements and skills. The infants' vocalisation is frequently associated with movements of the legs and arms, babbling develops around the time at which the child is able to sit, and following a wider appreciation of his surroundings the child begins to associate speech sounds with objects, and develops the use of articulate sounds with meaning. McGraw (1952) has studied the motor development of infants and states that developmental changes in behaviour are associated with advancement in cortical maturation. This is reflected in behaviour by suppression or diminution of certain activities and by the emergence and integration of other neuromuscular performances. Gesell and Armatruda (1949) have described the various stages of development as a guide to the maturational level of the child and his intelligence.

General patterns of movement change from the turning of the head in supine to the rotation of the body into the prone position, ability to raise the head, to raise the head and shoulders supported by the arms, to sit unsupported and to change from lying into the sitting position. The child learns to get on to hands and knees and crawl, to pull himself into the standing position and finally to acquire the balance and co-ordination of movements involved in walking and other complicated patterns of activity common in childhood.

Similarly, the reflex movements involved in sucking and swallowing are extended to the making of sounds with the tongue and lips associated with vocal sounds. Penfield and Rasmussen (1950) state that 'control of vocalisation and of the lips and tongue is carried out according to what might be called an inborn pattern of neuronal connections'. In the adult the movements for crying, sucking and swallowing are represented in the cortex, and such movements may be produced by stimulation of certain areas of the cortex. Speech, however, involves a learned dextrous movement of certain muscles comparable to learned movements of hands and feet, and such movements cannot be reproduced by stimulation of the cortex, though arrest of speech may occur. As cortical control develops, these early movements become more independent as the result of selective inhibition. Tongue and lip movements which combine in the act of sucking become disassociated and may be used independently for the articulation of various consonant sounds. During the babble period of speech development the child is acquiring the voluntary control of the independent movements of the lips, tongue and palate associated and in co-ordination with those of phonation and respiration for eventual use in the cortically controlled and integrated audible expression of thought through speech. Again, development depends on normal proprioceptive sensations. Sherrington (1947) states that:

> there exists, therefore, two primary distributions of the receptor organs. The surface field is freely open to the numberless vicissitudes of the environment. This field, exteroceptive as it is called, is rich in the number and variety of the receptors which adaptation has involved in it. The proprioceptive (receptors) receive their stimulation by some action, e.g. a muscular contraction which was itself a primary reaction to excitation of a surface receptor by the environment.

The child who is unable to experience normal movements of the limbs, head, or muscles of articulation will have abnormal proprioceptive sensations again leading to the arrest or distortion of progressive development.

The relationship between general motor development and speech development has been observed in 29 children who were attending an out-patient clinic for observation and for physiotherapy, and it seems apparent that the child who does not develop the ability to sit unsupported and to walk, may learn to speak, and that development of speech may be to a large extent independent of the rate of maturation of other movements and muscular control in children with brain damage.

Speech development and general motor development in 29 children between the ages of two and six years who were attending an out-patient clinic

An attempt was made to ascertain if there were any relationship between the age of speech development in these children and their general physical condition and motor development.

Dunsdon [17] found a direct relationship between sitting and the use of first words, sitting balance being achieved just before words were first used, but we were unable to establish any significant correlation.

The children seen by us were observed over a period of 6 to 12 months, depending on the time of their referral for physiotherapy. They fell into three age groups, namely:

1. Eight children between two and three years of age.
2. Ten children aged three to four years.
3. Eleven children over four years and aged four to seven years.

The ages of the children and the stage of development described refers to the time when they were last seen.

Eight of these 29 children were between two and three years of age, the average age being two years seven months (Appendix, Table XXVIII). Five were able to maintain sitting balance, but no child did so before the age of 15 months. Two had attempted to walk with support when over two years of age. Two children who were still unable to sit without support at two years eleven months and two years eight months respectively had developed speech within the normal age range, one using words and phrases at 18 months and two and a half years, and the other at 14 months and 18 months respectively. Articulation was also normal. Four other children had used a few single words between 18 months and two years, but in two articulation was defective. Therefore, in this group of eight children aged two to three years, six had used single words and two of these had also used phrases or short sentences. Two had made no attempt to speak whatever, but had made vocal sounds.

Ten children were aged three to four years, the average age being three years seven months. Two of these walked without support at two and a half and three and a half years of age respectively, and two others were able to sit unsupported at two and three-quarter years and three years of age. Six children were still unable to sit without support. Three children were using phrases and sentences at two, three and three and a half years respectively. In the first two articulation was normal, but in the third there was some degree of dysarthria. Three other children were using a very few single words, and four made no attempt to use speech. Therefore, of these ten children, six had begun to use speech, three having developed the use of phrases. Two of these had normal articulation (Fig. 49).

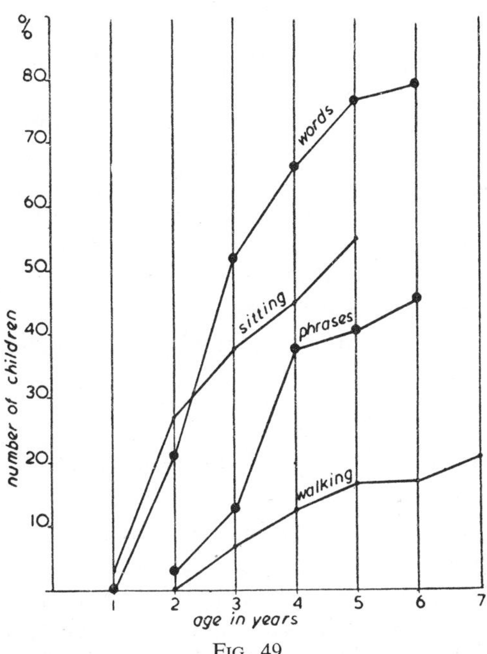

FIG. 49

The relationship between the development of motor activity and speech, as indicated by sitting balance and walking age, and the first use of words and phrases in 29 children with cerebral palsy aged two to seven years at the time of the assessment.

Eleven children were aged four to seven years, the average age being six years two months. One child in this group walked at six years of age, and two, aged three and a half and four and a half years, could sit and had attempted to walk with support. Four others could maintain sitting balance, but four more at the ages of six, four and a half years, four years eight months and four years seven months were still unable to sit without support. All these 11 children had attempted to use words, and eight also used phrases or sentences. In five, speech was normal except that one had defective articulation of the sound [r], and occasional facial spasms in another caused some interference with the articulation of the bilabial consonants. Two children had defective articulation, which in one was an articulatory dyspraxia and in the other a developmental dysarthria with some associated dyspraxia. In four articulation could not be assessed as there was insufficient development of speech. In the eight children with normal or near normal speech the diagnosis was spastic quadriplegia in two, spastic diplegia in four, spastic paraplegia in one and ataxia in one. It will be noted from the graph (Fig. 49) that although in a few children words followed the achievement of sitting balance as in normal development, the inability to sit did not restrict the onset in the use of words in many of these children. Similarly in the use of phrases; the majority of these children developed the use of word sequences and useful language before being able to walk. The details concerning these children are shown in the Appendix, Table XXVIII.

(*d*) Defects of speech in relation to the general motor disability

This is considered in 44 of the 50 hospital patients and in 32 children who were attending the special school.

Speech. Six of the 50 hospital patients had insufficient speech for assessment, but 44 patients were referred for speech therapy with useful language and developmental dysarthria or dyspraxia.

In the 32 schoolchildren, as previously described, there were 18 children with normal or near normal speech and 14 with defective speech.

Nine of these 14 children had a typical dysarthria. One had in addition an intermittent stammer. This was present when he entered the school two years previously, improved and was not noticeable for nearly one year, and then returned. The articulatory defect was of medium severity and showed steady but slow improvement, whilst the stammer was variable.

Three of these 14 children had a severe degree of developmental aphasia. At the ages of 14, 13½ and 13 years respectively, speech was limited to the use of short, incomplete sentences, and in one to single words with the addition of useful gesture.

One child had a marked articulatory dyspraxia associated with a severe dysarthria but no abnormal delay in the attempted use of speech. He had good language ability but often resigned himself to silence when aware of his failure to use articulation which was intelligible to others.

One child, already described, had a partial hearing loss in addition to a dysarthria.

In 18 children speech was adequate, articulation being clear and easily intelligible. In seven of these children no abnormality could be detected. In seven others there was at times a minimal degree of consonant substitution such as [f] or [v] for [p] or [b], which occurred when spasm of the elevators of the upper lip momentarily prevented the normal articulation of the bilabial consonants. At times, interference with the movements and rhythm of respiration caused use of speech to deviate from the normal but was insufficient to hinder clear articulation and intelligibility. In three others there was slightly more interference with articulation due to extensor spasticity of the lips, or to interference with co-ordination of respiration and phonation, and one child had an occasional slight hesitation or stammer.

Motor disability. We wished to know if any relationship could be established between defective speech in these patients and (*i*) the extent and distribution, (*ii*) the type of general disability and (*iii*) if it was in any way related to the development of general motor behaviour.

(*i*) *The relationship between speech and the extent and distribution of general motor disability*

For this purpose a simplified classification of cerebral palsy was used. This was based on distribution and function.

Distribution may be classified as follows:

1. Diplegia, where there is a symmetrical paralysis most marked in the lower extremities.
2. Paraplegia, where the lower limbs alone are affected.
3. Quadriplegia, where the four extremities are involved.

4. Hemiplegia, where there is spasticity in the limbs on one side of the body only.
5. Athetosis, according to the number of limbs affected.

Defects of speech in relation to the extent and distribution of the general motor disability were considered in

(*a*) 44 hospital patients with dysarthria, and
(*b*) 32 schoolchildren, 14 of whom had defective and 18 normal speech.

In 74 of these 76 patients the predominating condition was of varying degrees of spasticity from minimal to severe, in some associated with involuntary movements or athetosis, whilst in two there was athetosis with little or no detectable spasticity but of minimal degree. The relation between the general condition and speech is shown in Figure 50, for 58 patients with dysarthria and 18 with normal speech.

Distribution	No. of cases	Percent- age	Defective speech −58		Normal speech −18	
			No.	% of 58	No.	% of 18
Diplegia .	27	35·5	20	34·0	7	39·0
Paraplegia .	3	4·0	2	3·5	1	5·5
Quadriplegia .	36	47·5	27	46·5	9	50·0
Hemiplegia .	8	10·5	7	12·5	1	5·5
Athetosis in all four limbs .	2	2·5	2	3·5	0	0
	76	100	58	100	18	100

Fig. 50

The extent and distribution of general motor disability in 58 patients with defective speech and 18 with normal speech.

The exact diagnosis is not easy and we are unable to draw any definite conclusions from this group of patients, but our findings show no evidence of any marked difference in the extent and distribution of the motor disability between those patients with a marked disorder of speech and those who had acquired normal or at least adequate speech, or that the degree of speech disability was closely and directly related to the general motor disability.

(*ii*) *Defects of speech in relation to the type of disability or function*

In all these patients with brain injury there are, as described, varying degrees of abnormal muscle tone which varies in its distribution from patient to patient and also at different times in the same patient according to the position in which he is placed. Such abnormal muscle tone causes abnormality of posture and movements.

In spasticity there is increased muscle tone with exaggerated resistance to movement and abnormal reflex activity.

In athetosis the muscle tone fluctuates abruptly between hyper- and hypo-tonicity. Reciprocal innervation is abnormal, resulting in abnormal control and balance of the muscle groups for movement. Involuntary movements occur and are aggravated by effort or emotion, but tend to disappear when at rest and especially during sleep.

In ataxia the reflexes may be normal but muscle tone is too low. Reciprocal innervation is defective in that there is absence of a steady and progressive change of muscle tone between muscles and their antagonists, which results in jerky and inadequately controlled movements. Bobath (1954) states that she finds pure cases of ataxia are rare and that it is usually combined with some degree of athetosis or spasticity.

There are also other mixed disabilities. Some degree of spasticity is frequently associated with a condition which is predominantly one of athetosis, and many children in whom spasticity is the chief disability have also some degree of involuntary movement.

The type of motor disability has therefore been analysed under three headings: (1) predominantly spastic, (2) predominantly athetoid and (3) predominantly ataxic (Fig. 51).

Defects of speech were present in all the 44 hospital patients assessed and in 14 schoolchildren. Eighteen schoolchildren had normal speech.

All the patients with any degree of athetosis in this group had defects of speech, whilst 95 per cent of the normal speech group were predominantly spastic.

In 16 of the 58 patients with defective speech the general physical disability was minimal. Three of these had evidence of spasticity, 11 had mixed lesions and two had minimal signs of athetosis only.

Function	Total		Defective speech —58		Normal speech —18	
	No. of patients	% of 76	No. of patients	% of 58	No. of patients	% of 18
Predominantly spastic . .	62	81	44	76	17	95
Predominantly athetoid . .	9	12	9	16	0	0
Predominantly ataxic . .	5	7	5	8	1	5
	76	100	58	100	18	100

FIG. 51

Type of disability in 58 patients with defects of speech and 18 schoolchildren with normal speech.

Although this is not a random sample, it would appear from these findings that normal speech seldom or never develops where there is any degree of athetosis, but that in these patients approximately one-third of those with spasticity developed normal speech.

(*iii*) *The relation of defects of speech to general motor ability*

The development of speech in relation to general motor behaviour was observed in the children attending the out-patient clinic. Here we shall compare the general motor ability in the 32 schoolchildren, that is 14 of whom had defects of speech and 18 normal speech.

Motor ability was considered in relation to:

1. Lifting the head in supine.
2. Sitting balance.
3. Walking with or without support.

Lifting the head in supine. One of the early movements which a normal child acquires is to raise the head when lying in the supine position. It was found that only two of the 32 schoolchildren aged 7 to 14 years were able to raise the head normally, and both had normal speech. Sixteen children with normal speech and all the 14 children with defective speech failed to do so.

The relationship between speech and ability to raise the head is shown in Figure 52.

Head raising	Normal speech –18	Defective speech –14	Total
Normal . .	2	0	2
Minor abnormality .	7	2	9
Difficult and grossly abnormal . .	8	11	19
Not possible . .	1	1	2
	18	14	32

FIG. 52

Ability to raise the head when supine in the 32 schoolchildren with cerebral palsy.

Nine children, seven of whom had normal speech, showed minor abnormalities when attempting to raise the head in the supine position. These included hyperextension of the neck and head with protrusion of the lower jaw, and spasms of the facial muscles with extension of the lips, or with contraction of the elevators of the upper lip and consequent lifting of the lip.

In 19 children, eight of whom had normal speech, the head could only be raised with great difficulty. There was contraction of the pectoral muscles, protrusion of the shoulders and inability to raise the head independently of the shoulders. In many there was a general increase of spasticity throughout the trunk, arms and legs during the attempt.

Two children, one of whom had normal speech, were unable to raise the head when lying supine. The child with normal speech, aged eight years, had a spastic quadriplegia and was able to maintain the head position in sitting. The child with defective articulation aged nine years had a spastic diplegia with some degree of athetosis. He could walk, but only in an abnormal manner.

Sitting and walking. Some children could maintain the normal head position in sitting, but balance was precarious and some support was needed. Eleven of the 32 children could sit unsupported and three with support. Eight could walk with support and ten without support, but in an abnormal manner. It is natural for the intelligent child to wish to imitate others walking, and if he can maintain balance in the upright position he will walk, even if the movements are abnormal and tend to increase spasticity and postural deformity. Walking with support indicates that balance has not been achieved, but that the upright posture has been maintained through the use of support such as suitable furniture, a nearby wall or the hand of another person. Many of these children can ride a tricycle when they are unable to maintain the necessary balance for walking.

Of the 18 children who could walk with or without support, ten had normal and eight had defective speech.

The following table shows the relationship between ability to sit and walk, and normal and defective speech in this group of 32 children (Fig. 53).

Motor ability	Normal speech −18	Defective Speech −14	Total 32
Unable to sit without support	1	2	3
Sits unsupported	7	4	11
Walks with support	4	4	8
Walks unsupported but not normally	6	4	10
	18	14	32

FIG. 53
Extent of the general motor disability and speech.

Crawling. Some of the children were able to support themselves in a position on the floor which enabled them to move in a forward or backward direction. Some could do this before they could sit without support. In some only the arms were used for propulsion, the legs being passively drawn along the floor, or other abnormal methods of moving from place to place were used.

Although most normal children crawl before they walk, others omit this stage, which is not essential in the process of maturation leading to ability to balance in the upright position and to control the movements of walking. For this reason, and because the term 'crawling' as used by the mother includes a variety of abnormal movements in children with cerebral palsy, this stage in the development of motor disability has been excluded from our assessments.

According to the findings in this group of children defects of articulation did not appear to be closely associated with general motor development, and it would seem that only in so far as the movements for articulation are hindered will the ability to use clear, intelligible speech be impaired. Severe delay in the development of executive speech, or developmental aphasia, which occurred in three children, again was not necessarily associated with a general delay in motor development.

(*e*) Speech and lateral dominance

Tests of handedness are difficult to carry out in these patients, and in many the preferred hand could not be ascertained. The results tend to be unreliable owing to the combination of various factors. For example, one child held the pencil more easily in his right hand than in his left, yet because the right side was more severely affected than the left his actual ability to make clear marks on the paper was better when he used his left hand, which was obviously the more awkward for holding the pencil. These findings are also described in Chapter XXII on speech and cerebral dominance, and it is sufficient to state here that in these children we found a higher incidence of left-handedness than in the normal population, in the majority because the right hand was more severely disabled than the left, indicating damage to the left cerebral hemisphere.

In assessing the relationship of handedness to both speech and general disability the patients in whom this had been ascertained have been grouped as follows:

1. 33 in whom both the speech and general disability were severe.
2. 14 who had a severe speech disorder but only a minimal general motor disability.
3. 18 who had normal speech and a severe general motor disability.

The highest incidence of left hand preference was in 33 patients with both a severe speech and general motor disability, and to a much less extent, although still much higher than in the normal population, in those who had either a severe speech disorder or severe motor disability, but not both (Fig. 54). The preferred hand was therefore ascertained in 47 patients with defective speech, 14 of whom were attending a special school, and in 18 also attending a school who had normal speech. In 14 of the 47 hospital patients the motor disability was minimal.

	Right hand	Left hand	Ambi-dextrous	Total
Severe speech disorder and obvious motor disability .	17	15	1	33
Severe speech disorder and minimal motor disability .	6	7	1	14
Normal speech and severe motor disability . .	8	8	2	18
	31	30	4	65

FIG. 54
The preferred hand in 65 patients with general motor disability.

It was found that the incidence of left-handedness was 46 per cent. This is significantly higher than in the normal population, where it was found to be six per cent. The incidence of ambidexterity, or preference not established, was six per cent.

In the 32 schoolchildren, tests for the preferred eye were also carried out, and the findings for the preferred eye and hand were analysed according to whether the speech was normal or whether there was a developmental dysphasia or dysarthria (Fig. 55). Tests for the preferred foot were not carried out in these children.

We found, therefore, that eight (25 per cent) lacked a preferred side, or were cross-lateral. In the normal population this is usually associated with left eye preference in a right-handed individual. In all these eight children, however, there was a preferred right eye with use of the left hand, One per cent were ambidextrous, and lacked decided preference for the use of eye, hand or both. One such child had a severe defect of spatial perception. Thirty-three per cent were right sided, as compared with 70 per cent in the normal population.

These findings probably indicate that the inherited tendency towards establishment of left hemisphere dominance has been prevented as a result of brain damage or mal-development. In three children with developmental aphasia two were right sided and one left sided. One of the right-sided children may have inherited a tendency to left-sidedness from her mother, and the child's dysphasia, persisting in a severe form to her present age of 13 years, may have been associated with damage to the right cerebral hemisphere. The other right-sided child had a very severe spastic quadriplegia with only minimal development of speech at 13½ years of age and there may have been damage to the speech areas in both cerebral hemispheres. In 11 children with dysarthria in this group only one was right sided as compared with eight in the group of 18 children with normal speech.

Speech		Hand			Eye			Side			
		R.	L.	A.	R.	L.	A.	R.	L.	X.	A.
Normal	18	8	8	2	11	5	2	8	5	2	3
Developmental dysphasia	3	2	1	–	2	1	–	2	1	–	–
Developmental dysarthria	11	2	9	–	6	5	–	1	4	6	–
		12	18	2	19	11	2	11	10	8	3

R=right
L=left
A=no preference
X=cross-lateral.

FIG. 55
Speech and lateral dominance in 32 children with cerebral palsy.

RESPIRATION, PHONATION AND ARTICULATION IN CHILDREN WITH DYSARTHRIA

In many of these children respiration and the fluent use of speech is affected as a result of spasticity or of involuntary movements of the muscles of the diaphragm, or other muscles concerned in the processes of inspiration and expiration. Phonation may be forced, breathy or nasal, or may fluctuate due to inadequate control. Defective articulation is associated with clumsy and inadequate movement of the muscles of the jaw, tongue, lips and palate, although some children achieve intelligible articulation with varying degrees of abnormality in the movement of these muscle groups.

Unintelligible speech results when the muscles used for articulation are severely affected. Interference with respiration and phonation will affect the rhythm and fluency of speech, but, unless very severe, usually has much less effect on the intelligibility of speech. In many of these children attempts to speak are also associated with an increase of spasticity or of athetoid movements in certain parts of, or generally throughout, the body.

The muscles used for speech are in action at or immediately following birth for the reflex acts of breathing, sucking and swallowing if life is to be maintained. Where there has been brain injury or mal-development, the normal rhythm of respiration may not have been easily established at birth, or there may have been difficulties in sucking or inco-ordination in swallowing, and whilst these reflex acts may have been possible they may still have been accomplished in an abnormal manner. Abnormal reflex function may lead later to abnormalities of movement for speech, and the study of such abnormal reflex patterns in the more primitive use of the muscles used for speech, as in sucking, chewing and swallowing, and of respiratory movements when at rest in various positions, and during phonation and speech, may contribute to an understanding of dysarthria.

In order to recognise the abnormal it is first of all essential to study the normal, and because it would seem that in some of these children respiratory movements resemble those occurring in foetal life, the early development of this function is of interest and may lead to fuller understanding of the problems involved.

RESPIRATION

The first movements of the respiratory muscles have been described as occurring about the 16th to 20th weeks in the human foetus. At first there is only an occasional single movement of the chest, but between the 20th and 24th weeks true inspiratory and expiratory movements occur. In this pre-respiratory stage, of course, the lungs are not used for the interchange of oxygen and carbon dioxide, as in breathing, which is not established until birth.

Sir Joseph Barcroft (1942) described four stages in the development of such pre-natal respiratory movements in the foetal lamb, occurring between the foetal ages of 35 and 65 days.

Stage 1. *Spasm.* In this stage a tap on the face produced a single movement of the head and neck associated with movement of the diaphragm.

Stage 2. *Rhythm.* In the second stage, about the 40th day, a tap on the face produced a rhythmic series of spasmodic movements involving the whole body. Movements of the intercostal muscles were then associated with movements of the diaphragm.

Stage 3. *Segregation.* In the third stage, about the 48th day, the movements of the intercostal and diaphragm muscles had become separated from those of the rest of the body, and a series of prolonged rhythmic contractions of the respiratory muscles might occur following a general movement. At this stage the foetus was very sensitive to stimulation.

Stage 4. *Inhibition.* In the fourth stage, about the 60th day, this sensitivity disappeared and there was then inertia and inhibition of respiratory movements.

The change from one stage to the next is not sudden, but 'each stage as it develops imposes itself upon rather than replaces its predecessor'.

Normal adult respiration involves the simultaneous expansion of the chest wall and abdominal muscles with the contraction and downward movement of the diaphragm. In the newborn infant, however, and in early life, normal respiration depends mostly on movements of the diaphragm and abdominal muscles, and there is usually little expansion or movement of the thoracic cavity walls.

Neonatal respiration

Smith (1946) has described 'many grades of respiratory performance at birth'. He says that 'some infants commence to breathe almost before their bodies have left the birth canal and rhythmic inspiratory and expiratory movements are rapidly established'. He also described the infant who does not breathe at all for a minute or even longer, when respiration is at first 'an irregular and inefficient series of gasps'. He states that 'a newborn infant may be apneic for ten minutes after delivery and may be revived to an existence which proceeds normally'.

In some newborn infants and in children with cerebral palsy spasmodic contraction of the diaphragm may be so severe that there may be an indrawing of the chest wall and a furrow may indicate where the sternum and chest wall are retracted by the pull of the diaphragm. There may also be some inhibition of respiration and resistance to re-inflation of the lungs.

Gesell (1954) has described various forms of breathing such as 'double breathing' in which the thorax and diaphragm move in unison, 'reversed breathing' with fluctuation between costal and abdominal movements, and 'antagonistic breathing' in which the thorax expands on inspiration whilst there is simultaneously a sharp contraction of the abdominal wall.

Respiratory Movements in Children with Cerebral Palsy

Respiratory movements have been observed in 32 children with brain injury, with and without dysarthria, who are attending a special school and 28 children attending an out-patient clinic.

18 *children with normal speech*

Of the 18 children with normal speech, all had well-established rhythmic respiration when at rest. During phonation or speech, however, seven had some degree of interference with normal respiratory movements which was insufficient to affect speech to any marked extent.

14 *children with defective speech*

Of the 14 children with defective speech, dysarthria or dysphasia, eight had abnormal patterns of respiration when at rest and 12 had interference with normal respiration associated with phonation or speech. In all these children diaphragm movement was limited and respiration chiefly intercostal.

Respiratory movements in young children aged 18 *months to* 6 *years*

Respiratory movements were also observed in 28 children

aged 18 months to 6 years who were attending an out-patient clinic. One child had a marked indrawing of the abdominal wall on inspiration with hyperextension of the lower rib margins and with marked diaphragm spasm when crying or voicing. Six children used intercostal breathing with little or no obvious diaphragm movement. In one child the onset of speech at four years of age was associated with abnormal tension in the laryngeal and neck muscles with forced phonation. Three showed some fluctuation of the respiratory muscles with lack of co-ordination and balance between the abdominal, intercostal and diaphragm muscles. In 18 respiration was apparently normal, although in two of these there was some slight degree of abnormal expansion of the lower rib margins. The children in this group who used normal phonation when crying or vocalising, and those who had developed normal speech, all had normal patterns of respiration.

Abnormalities of Respiration

The chief abnormalities of respiration were as follows:

1. In some children the abdominal muscles were tense and the abdominal wall retracted and concave. There was abnormal expansion of the lower rib margins, sometimes with depression of the sternum, and little or no detectable movement of the diaphragm. Inhibition of the excessive outward movement of the lower ribs by hand pressure allowed a more normal pattern of respiration with spontaneous onset of diaphragm movement and expansion of the abdominal wall. This type of respiration may be similar to the early stages of foetal respiration and be what Gesell describes as antagonistic respiration.

2. In others there was spasm or contraction of the diaphragm with relaxation of the abdominal wall on expiration, also during phonation and speech, resulting in weak vocal tone and a tendency to speak on inspiration. This has been described as 'reverse' breathing. As in antagonistic breathing, it is associated with abnormal movements of the diaphragm, but it occurs on expiration rather than on inspiration.

3. Some children attempted to fix the chest wall and other

respiratory muscles during speech. The glottis was closed and the thoracic cavity expanded as for effort. Phonation was then accomplished by forcing minimal air through tense vocal folds with little use of expiratory breath. This pattern of phonation had been developed in association with speech and occurred as a result of muscular spasm or as a habitual response at or just before the onset of speech.

4. In cases of athetosis, or where this was combined with spasticity, involuntary movements of the diaphragm and other respiratory muscles made control difficult. Inability to control fluctuating degrees of tension in the larygneal muscles also contributed towards inadequate respiratory control during phonation and speech.

There were, however, in these children variations from week to week, and in at least one who at first had an abnormal breathing pattern use of the diaphragm improved with the eventual establishment of normal respiratory movements. It is not known yet how far abnormal patterns of respiration are encouraged and increased by the growing child's efforts to move and to speak, nor how far physical treatment in early life, as by reflex inhibition, may contribute towards the development of more normal respiratory patterns and their maintenance.

Phonation

Phonation is affected by the type and control of respiration, as described, and also by varying degrees of ability to control the degree of tension in the vocal folds and the rate of outlet of the vocal air stream. The voice may be forced, the larynx being fixed as for effort with the glottis almost closed. This occurred in seven of the 14 schoolchildren with defective speech. In three of these seven children it was associated with retraction of the tongue and severe spasm of the muscles at the base of the tongue. In three children there were fluctuations of volume and pitch, and in two poor co-ordination of phonation and respiration, with resulting weak vocal tone. In two phonation was normal.

In at least ten of the 14 children attempts to phonate or to speak produced increased spasticity or associated movements in other parts of the body. This might be limited to the neck, shoulder or arm muscles or produce an extensor spasm throughout the body.

In 13 of the 18 children with normal speech phonation was normal. In five there were minor signs of inadequate vocal control at times, with breathiness, or some slight inspiratory spasm, and in one a slight and very occasional tendency to stammer. The defects were chiefly the result of inco-ordination or lack of balance between the various muscle groups involved, namely those of the neck, laryngeal, mandibular and hyoid muscle groups. In two respiration was mainly intercostal, and two had some degree of contraction of the diaphragm during speech. None of the children in this group had any obvious degree of athetosis.

Articulation

The muscles used in the movements of the jaw, lips, tongue, palate and pharynx for speech are used primarily for the purpose of sucking and swallowing, although, as Kinnier Wilson (1921) stated that as 'the same motor cells of the cortex, say innervating the mouth, lips, tongue and palate, are used at one time in the function of speech and at another in totally different physiological combinations, and since the function of motor speech may be grossly disturbed while the cells can be utilised for other functions, we cannot suppose the physiological defect to be localised in the cell groups concerned . . . disorders of speech must be, physiologically, disorders of higher mechanisms which play on those of a lower physiological level'.

In many children with severe dysarthria there may also be interference with the normal processes of sucking, chewing and swallowing, and persistence or exaggeration of certain lingual, palatal or maxillary reflexes may cause these functions to be accomplished in an abnormal manner. Interference with the movements required for intelligible speech is chiefly associated with disturbances of control and movement of the tongue, but spasticity or involuntary movements of the lips and other facial muscles, of the jaw, palate, larynx or respiratory muscles also contribute to the dysarthria.

Tongue movements

The muscles of the tongue are evolved by forward extension of the ventral neck musculature into the floor of the mouth and are innervated by the hypoglossal nerve. Tongue movements in particular are therefore associated closely with those of the ventral muscles of the neck.

R. J. Last (1955) has recently described the muscles of the head and neck as functioning in three groups and controlling (1) movements of the skull on the cervical spine, (2) movements of the mandible on the skull and (3) movements of the floor of the mouth on the mandible. Movements of the tongue on the floor of the mouth are then controlled by the extrinsic and intrinsic muscles of the tongue.

Movements of the skull

Extension of the neck and head is through the action of post-vertebral muscles, and flexion through gravity, the pre-vertebral muscles and the sternomastoid.

Movements of the mandible

Last describes the rest position of the mandible as being *produced* by tonus of the mandibular muscles and *determined* by the tension in the joint capsule. Closure of the mandible occurs through the action of the temporal, masseter and median pterygoid muscles, and the mandible is lowered and the mouth opened by the rotational pull of the lateral pterygoid and the digastric muscles (Fig. 56). There are differing opinions concerning the action of the digastric muscle, but Last believes that it works as on a pulley attached to the hyoid cartilage and is held down by the action of the infrahyoid muscles, and he considers that contraction in this muscle assists the opening of the mandible. Lateral and antero-posterior movements of the mandible used particularly in chewing are achieved by asymmetrical contraction, especially of the pterygoid muscles.

Movements of the floor of the mouth

The floor of the mouth is elevated by its own contraction, that is contraction of the mylohyoid muscles (Fig. 57). It is lowered by the infrahyoid group of muscles, lengthened by the stylohyoid and shortened by the geniohyoid. These muscles move the hyoid bone and assist the extrinsic muscles of the tongue, particularly in swallowing, and to some extent in articulation.

MOVEMENTS OF THE MANDIBLE

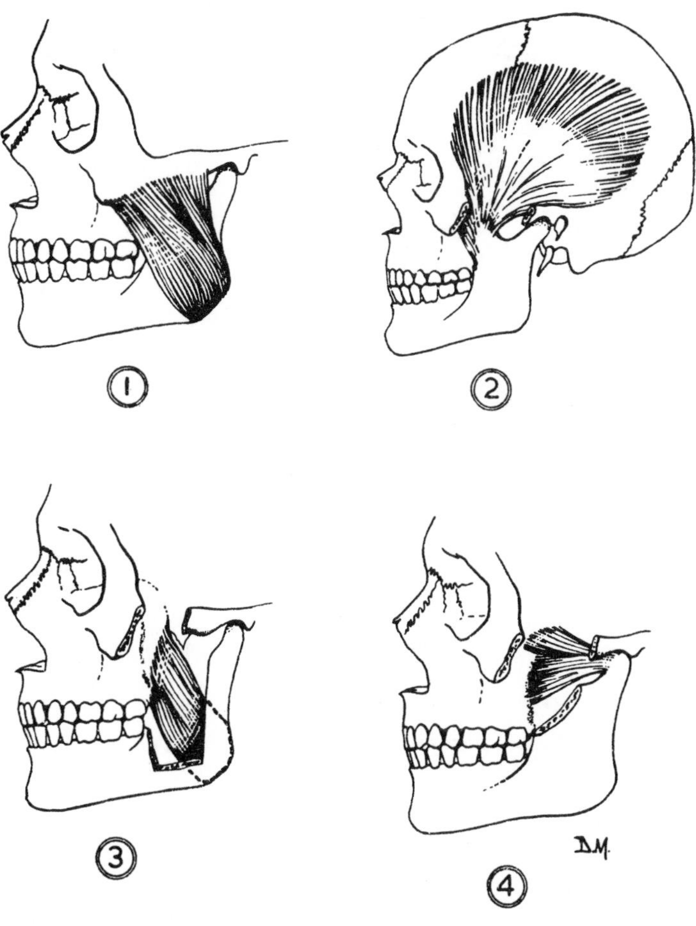

FIG. 56

1. The masseter—raises the mandible.
2. Temporalis—raises and retracts the mandible.
3. Median pterygoid—raises and protrudes the mandible.
4. Lateral pterygoid—protrudes and opens the jaw with the digastric.

MOVEMENTS OF THE HYOID BONE AND THE FLOOR OF THE MOUTH

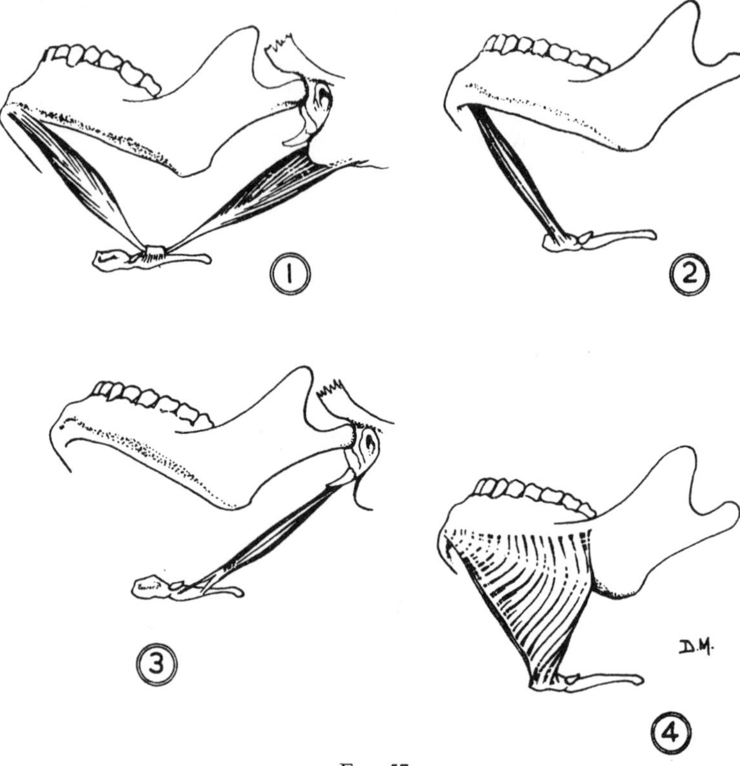

FIG. 57

1. Digastric—raises the hyoid bone and the floor of the mouth, and assists the lateral pterygoid in opening the mouth.
2. Geniohyoid } —raise the hyoid bone and floor of the mouth.
3. Stylohyoid }
4. Mylohyoid—forms the floor of the mouth, which is raised on contracture in conjunction with the hyoid bone and the base of the tongue.

Movements of the tongue

The mylohyoid, the digastric and the hyoid bone support the tongue as on a mobile shelf, raising or lowering its position in the mouth and increasing its mobility. The position of the tongue is then stabilised and controlled by the extrinsic muscles of the tongue which connect it to the hyoid cartilage (hyoglossus), the palate (palatoglossus), and the styloid process (styloglossus)

MOVEMENTS OF THE TONGUE

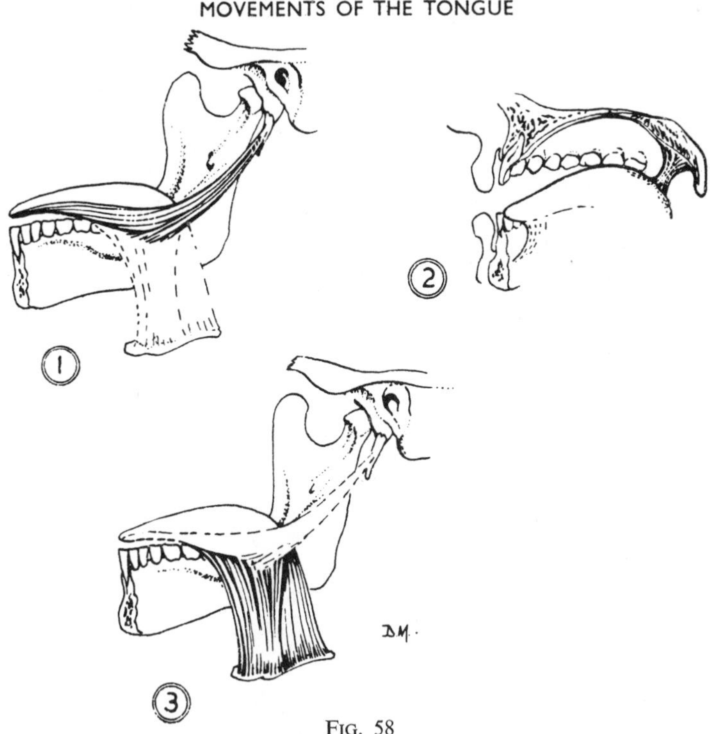

FIG. 58

The extrinsic muscles.

1. Styloglossus—assists the genioglossus to retract the tongue and the palatoglossus to elevate the tongue.
2. Palatoglossus—elevates the back of the tongue and narrows the oropharyngeal isthmus.
3. Hyoglossus—draws down the sides of the tongue and assists the genioglossus in depressing the tongue.

(Fig. 58). The intrinsic muscles of the tongue determine its shape and control the fine movements required for sucking, swallowing and for articulation. The genioglossus forms the main part of the tongue, some of its lower fibres being attached to the hyoid bone, and together with the longitudinal, vertical and transverse muscle fibres of the tongue, forms its intrinsic musculature (Fig. 59).

The hyoid bone

The hyoid bone is also attached to the styloid process (stylohyoid) and to the mandible (geniohyoid), to the sternum

MOVEMENTS OF THE TONGUE

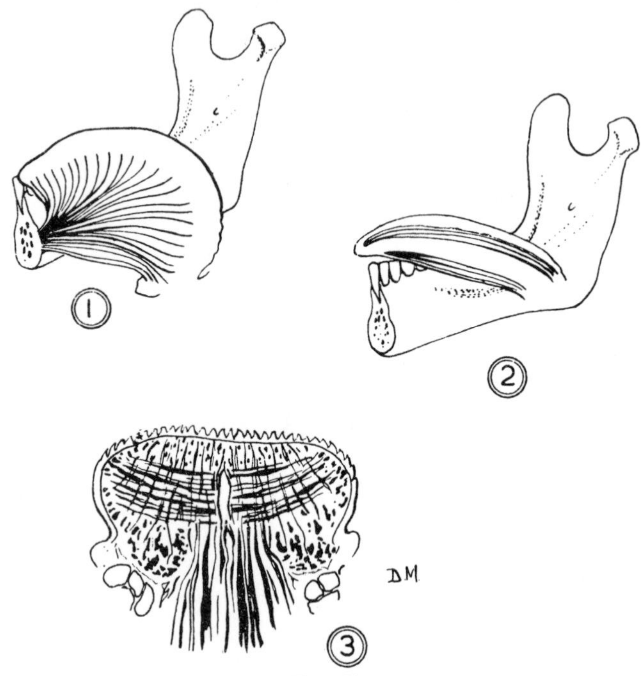

FIG. 59

The intrinsic muscles.

1. Genioglossus. Posterior fibres protrude the tongue and the anterior fibres retract it. Also depresses the tongue.
2. Longitudinal muscle fibres—inferior and superior. Modify the shape of the tongue. Superior fibres elevate the tip, inferior turn the tip downwards. Both cause shortening of the tongue.
3. Transverse and vertical fibres. Transverse fibres narrow and elongate the tongue. Vertical fibres flatten and broaden it.

(sternohyoid), to the thyroid cartilage and sternum (thyrohyoid and sternothyroid) and to the scapula (omohyoid) (Fig. 60). These muscles form the infrahyoid group and depress the hyoid bone. The diagastric, the geniohyoid and the stylohyoid are elevators of the hyoid, their upward pull being resisted by the infrahyoid group.

Abnormal muscle tone in any of these muscle groups may therefore directly or indirectly affect the movements of the tongue for articulation. It will also affect the position of the hyoid bone and of the larynx and may contribute to abnormal tension in the intrinsic muscles of the larynx and vocal folds.

MOVEMENTS OF THE LOWER JAW

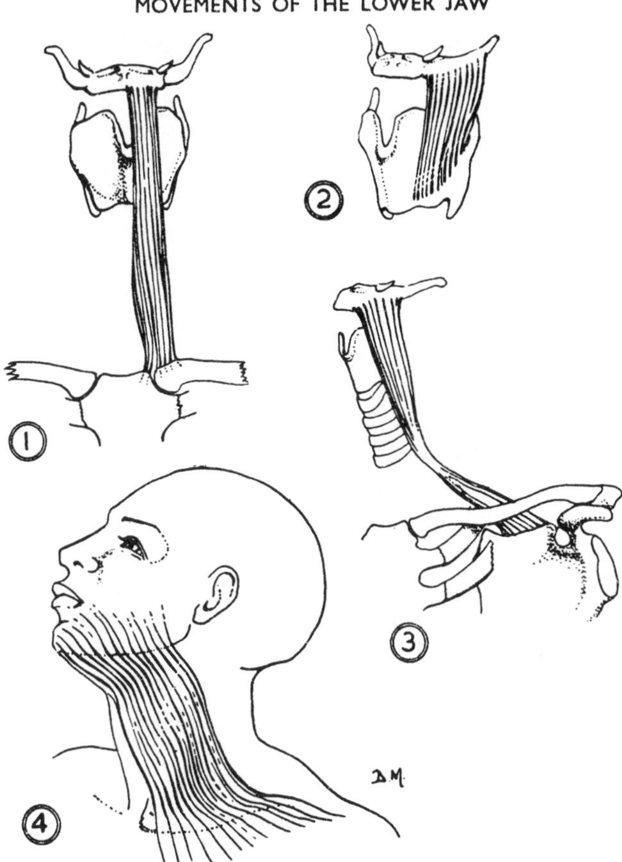

FIG. 60

Movements of the hyoid bone, floor of mouth and lower jaw.

1. Sternohyoid } —depress the hyoid bone and the floor of the mouth.
2. Thyrohyoid }
3. Omohyoid—depresses the hyoid bone.
4. Platysma—depresses the mandible and lower lip.

To what extent abnormal muscle tone in these muscles of the jaw, tongue and neck can be attributed to abnormal reflex activity is not yet fully understood, nor how far reflex inhibiting postures can contribute to more normal muscle tone and the control of the fine muscles of the tongue itself which are required for articulation. This will be discussed more fully in the chapter on the treatment of dysarthria.

Movements of the tongue in sucking and swallowing

In the newborn infant, sucking and swallowing are thought to be entirely reflex or automatic acts. Sucking is a response to the sensory stimulation of certain areas of the lips and mouth. Bieber (1940) studied sucking reactions and found that a rubber nipple brought into contact with the lips was insufficient to elicit sucking movements if the infant had no previous experience of sucking, but that contact of the nipple with the tongue and mucous membrane inside the mouth was necessary to initiate it. Later, but still during the first few days of life, contact of the nipple with the lips, corners of the mouth, chin or cheeks produced a response, the mouth being turned towards the stimulus. He also found that the grasp reflex was interrelated with the sucking reflex in the newborn, so that the presence of one facilitated the other and enhanced its intensity.

Whillis (1950) states that in infants the lips are atonic and the nipple is pressed by the tongue against the upper gum pad. The soft palate is depressed, the nasopharyngeal sphincter being open, and negative pressure can be brought about by tongue movements alone. Breathing continues during sucking and alternates with or is simultaneous with swallowing.

In the older child the posterior oral isthmus is closed by the back of the tongue, the lips and tongue enclose the object and the mouth is a sealed cavity. The mandible and the floor of the mouth are then depressed whilst the tongue is depressed and grooved by contraction of some of its intrinsic muscles and the anterior part of the genioglossus, thus creating a negative pressure in the mouth so that fluid may be drawn into the mouth. In infantile swallowing the tongue usually makes contact with the lips and cheeks and not with the alveolus.

Tongue movements play a considerable part in swallowing, and Ardran and Kemp (1951) have described these movements following a detailed radiographic study. Whilst food is being taken into the mouth, the forepart of the tongue is depressed whilst the dorsal surface of the tongue is arched posteriorly, closing the oropharyngeal isthmus. The tongue moves the bolus in the mouth during the process of mastication and finally the tip presses against the incisor teeth or alveolus and hard palate as the arched dorsal surface is lowered and the bolus is transferred backwards. As the tongue becomes further depressed, the soft palate rises, and the bolus passes between the pillars of the fauces into the pharynx. The tongue then arches backwards into the pharynx whilst the posterior pharyngeal wall comes forward to meet it. The bolus is gripped by the constrictors of the pharynx and the involuntary movements of peristalsis assist the passage of the bolus into and through the oesophagus. Re-inflation of the airways takes place from the larynx below and through the mouth or nasopharyngeal sphincter above.

Where tongue movements are limited, as in children with cerebral palsy or isolated dysarthria, swallowing and sucking may be accomplished in an abnormal manner with varying degrees of difficulty and inco-ordination.

Abnormal movements of the tongue

Protrusion. Failure to protrude the tongue may be associated with spasticity in its intrinsic muscles (particularly the genioglossus), in the supporting muscles (the mylohyoid and digastric), or in those muscles attached to the hyoid bone. Many children had difficulty in protruding the tongue. In some the tip was not pointed, whilst in others the whole tongue appeared to be thick, narrow and bunched, with spasticity of the intrinsic muscles, or the tip might be somewhat pointed but movements were stiff and clumsy, perhaps associated with spasticity in one or more of the extrinsic muscles of the tongue. In four of the young children rhythmic protrusion of the tongue tip was frequently observed with forward thrusting movements to the lip margin resembling sucking movements. In the group of 14 schoolchildren with defective speech, only five were able to protrude the tongue fully, and some could not protrude the tongue tip beyond the lip margins.

Elevation of the tongue tip. Only one of the 14 schoolchildren with defective speech could fully elevate the tongue tip towards the nose, whilst 13 of the 18 children with normal speech were able to do so. In 21 of the 29 young children seen in the Out Patient Department, where tongue movements could be observed, six were able to raise the tongue tip over the upper lip at this time. Some children attempted to assist the upward movement of the tongue tip by pressing it upwards with the lower lip or fingers, but there was a lack of normal flexibility and control of the muscles at the tip of the tongue and probably in other intrinsic and extrinsic muscles which may assist this movement in addition to those required for protrusion.

Lateral movements. Many children had difficulty in moving the tongue from side to side when partially protruded. Only two of the 14 schoolchildren with defective speech could do this fully, three could make no attempt whatever, and nine could move the tongue a little, or to one side only. Six of the 28 out-patient young children could move the tongue from side to side only, and four could make no lateral movements whatever. In the remainder it was doubtful. Some were able to move the tongue involuntarily but not on request, and others did not wish to, or were too young to co-operate. Even where possible, tongue movements in these children were in general slow and more clumsy than in the normal infant.

In some children the posterior part of the tongue and base was more spastic than the tip. Attempts to move the tip increased the spasticity and a spastic contraction of muscles could frequently be felt beneath the lower jaw, especially when the child attempted to protrude the tongue. The appearance of tongue movements suggested that the tongue might be anchored at the base. Whether this is the result of spasticity in the lower fibres of the genioglossus attached to the hyoid bone, or of other extrinsic or supporting muscles of the tongue, or even the result of spasticity in other muscles attached to the hyoid bone and to the sternum or thyroid cartilage, preventing free upward movement of the hyoid bone, cannot be stated with confidence.

Movements of the tongue have been analysed in 32 school-children with cerebral palsy, 18 of whom had normal and 14 defective speech (Fig. 61).

Movement	Normal speech (18)			Defective speech (14)		
	Full	Partial	Impossible	Full	Partial	Impossible
Protrusion	17	1	0	5	9	0
Elevation of tip	13	3	2	1	1	12
Lateral movements	16	1	1	2	9	3
Spasticity of muscles at base of tongue	1 (with partial protrusion)			11		

FIG. 61
Tongue movements in 32 children with cerebral palsy.

In this group of children there was a relationship between articulation and ability to move the tongue. Eleven of the 18 children with adequate speech had normal tongue movements and in only three was there a marked limitation of movement, whilst only one child with defective speech could move the anterior part of the tongue fully, and he had a considerable degree of spasticity at the base of the tongue.

Jaw movements

Biting and chewing involve movements of the masseter muscles, the temporalis, pterygoid and digastric muscles. Relaxation of the masseter and temporalis allows the mandible to be lowered and the mouth to open as the result of gravity assisted by the rotational pull of the digastric and lateral pterygoid muscles (Figs. 56 and 57). The jaw is protruded by the simultaneous action of the pterygoid muscles, whilst the posterior horizontal fibres of the temporalis cause retraction of the mandible. Chewing movements vary in individuals, and when there is spasticity or limitation of movement of the muscles concerned, chewing may be impossible and the food may then be sucked, or chewing may be limited or grossly abnormal.

The buccinator and orbicularis oris muscles assist chewing and aid the action of the tongue by maintaining the food in the cavity enclosed by the teeth.

Oral reflexes. Certain oral reflexes have been described whereby electrical stimulation of the mucous membrane of the tongue produced a reflex opening of the mouth, the linguomaxillary reflex. The palato-maxillary reflex also caused opening of the mouth when the hard palate was stimulated, but mouth closing movements when the soft palate was stimulated.

In some children with cerebral palsy certain abnormal reflexes tend to persist or be exaggerated. Touching the incisor teeth or hard palate with the finger may produce a strong bite reflex with injury to the intruding finger, and such reflexes may contribute to difficulties in chewing and swallowing, and perhaps articulation.

Abnormal jaw movements

All the 14 schoolchildren with defective speech had abnormal movements of the mandible during speech. Attempts to phonate or to speak were associated with abnormal positions of the head and jaw, or with abnormalities of muscle tone. In three there was spasticity in the muscles of the neck and masseter muscles which was increased during phonation. In 11 there were varying degrees of hyperextension of the neck and head, in seven associated with retraction of the mandible. In other children observed spasticity of the muscles of the neck hindered upward movement of the mandible and closure of the mouth, in some producing a permanent deformity. In a few there was forward protrusion of the mandible or deviation to one side. These movements were not always constant and varied in some children according to the position in which they were placed or with the degree of ease or emotional stress at the time of observation.

Eleven of the 18 schoolchildren with normal speech had normal movements of the mandible during speech, but in seven there were minor degrees of abnormal muscle tone associated with some degree of extension or retraction of the mandible which did not interfere with articulation to any noticeable extent (Fig. 62).

Movements of—		Normal speech (18)	Dysarthric speech (14)
Facial muscles and lips	(*a*) Normal range (*b*) Defective	8 10	0 14
Mandible	(*a*) Normal range (*b*) Defective	11 7	0 14
Tongue	(*a*) Normal range (*b*) Defective	11 7	1 13

FIG. 62

Movements of lips, mandible and tongue in children with dysarthric and normal speech.

Lip and facial movements

Last (1955) describes the facial muscles as constituting four sphincter and dilator groups, those of the lips and eyes, and those of the nostrils, and especially of the external auditory meatus, which are vestigial in man. Those concerned chiefly with articulation are the orbicularis oris which closes the mouth and the elevators, depressors and extensors of the lips which oppose its action (Fig. 63).

In all the 14 schoolchildren with defective speech there was abnormal tone in the muscles of the face and lips during speech. The chief defects observed were: (1) unilateral facial paresis with one angle of the mouth drawn back more than the other; (2) extension of the orbicularis oris due to spasticity in the buccinator and risorius muscles, which retract the corners of the mouth; (3) contraction of the orbicularis oris with spasticity and puckering of the lips; (4) spasmodic lifting of the upper lip due to spasm in the elevators of the lip, sometimes requiring voluntary effort to obtain closure against the pull of opposing spastic facial muscles; (5) depression of the corners of the mouth and lower lip due to spasticity in the depressors of the lower lip, spasm in the mentalis or superficial muscles of the neck, the platysma; (6) generalised facial tensions and fluctuating muscle spasm, or twitching associated with involuntary movements of the lips and other facial muscles.

In eight of the 18 schoolchildren with adequate speech there were no obvious abnormalities of movement of the face or lip muscles during speech, but in ten there was some degree of abnormal tension which affected articulation only at such times as these contractions prevented the approximation of the upper and lower lips for articulation of the bilabial consonants when [f] or [v] might be substituted for [p] or [b].

In Fig. 62 the movements of the lips and facial muscles, jaw and tongue are analysed as defective or of normal range in 32 schoolchildren, 18 of whom had normal and 14 defective speech.

Some of these children had difficulty in co-ordinating articulation with phonation. This may also occur in cases of cleft palate or other defects of articulation where faulty neuromuscular patterns of phonation and articulation have been acquired. In these children with dysarthria such inco-ordination tends to occur chiefly where control of the movements of the soft palate and closure of the nasopharynx is inadequate as a result of spasticity or paresis in the muscles of the lingual, palatal, pharyngeal or other muscle groups.

The important factor restricting the use of normal articulation in dysarthria is not the inability to imitate the sounds of speech

MOVEMENTS OF THE LIP AND NOSE

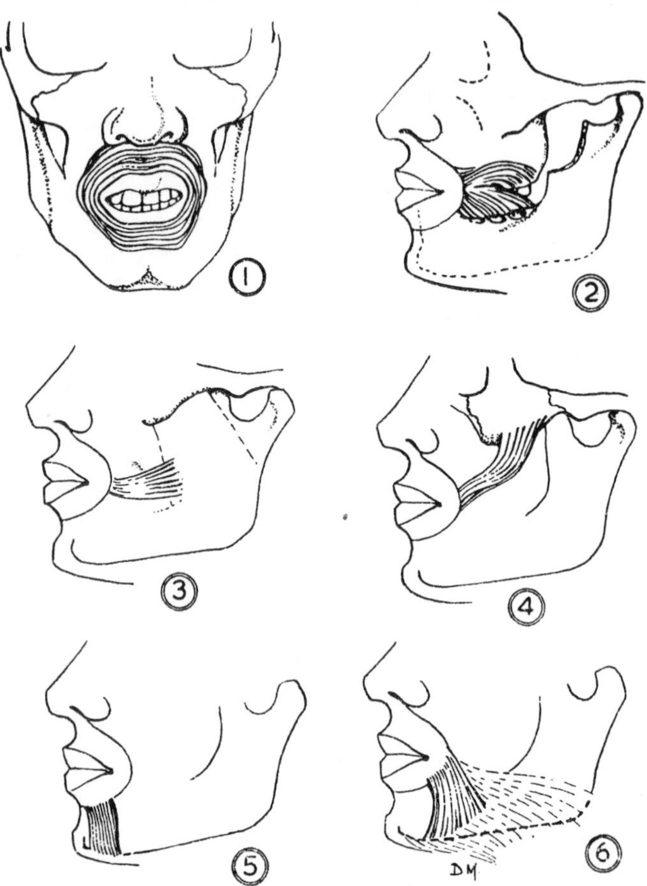

FIG. 63

The facial muscles concerned with movements of the lips and nose.

1. Orbicularis oris—closes the lips.
2. Buccinator—compresses the cheeks.
3. Risorius—retracts the angle of the mouth.
4. Zygomaticus—draws angle of mouth backward and upward.
5. Quadratus—depresses lower lip.
6. Triangularis oris—depresses angle of mouth.

but the limitation of movement, and of the speed of movement, of those muscles required for articulation. In patients with such a dysarthria, therefore, the imitation of consonant sounds may be accurate in isolation, in a single word or in slow speech, according to the degree of the disability. During speech at

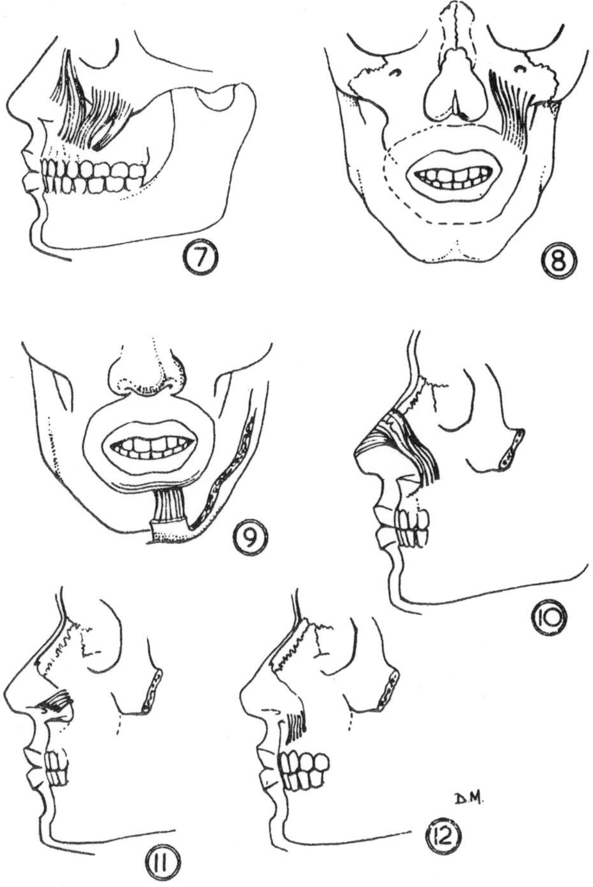

FIG. 63 (*continued*)

7. Levator labii superioris—elevates the upper lip.
8. Caninus—elevates the angle of the mouth.
9. Mentalis—raises and protrudes lower lip.
10. Nasalis—compresses nostrils.
11. Dilator naris—enlarges the nasal aperture.
12. Depressor septi—narrows nostrils and draws the septum down.

normal speed consonants tend to be omitted or used only in the initial position in words. Consonant substitutions may be used, and these may depend on the group of muscles chiefly affected, lips, tongue tip, back of tongue and so forth, or where there is in addition some degree of articulatory apraxia. Combinations of consonant sounds are usually more difficult than a single consonant and vowel combination, especially the co-ordinated movements required for the combination of a fricative and a plosive sound, as [sp] in spoon, or [str] in street, necessitating rapid and involved movements of the tongue. Diphthongs may be defective in a word such as 'boy' [bɔ:i] which becomes [bɔ:], the final rapid movement upwards of the mid part of the tongue being omitted.

The following case histories illustrate some of the points described:

Severe general motor disability and dysarthria

1. R. D. has a spastic diplegia with some involuntary movements or athetosis. He sat up at 12 months but did not attempt to walk until he was four and a half years. At six years he could walk without support, but in a grossly abnormal manner. He was first seen at four years of age. He had used single words by two years and sentences from three and a half years. Speech was unintelligible, and because he spoke only with great effort he did so as little as possible. Understanding for language was well developed. He was right handed and right eyed. The difficulties associated with attendance at the hospital as an out-patient outweighed the possibility of improvement from frequent visits for speech therapy, and this was carried out at home by the mother under guidance.

At eight years he was admitted to a special school for children with cerebral palsy, and regular speech therapy was then possible. He had a severe dysarthria and even then progress was slow, but he gradually became more intelligible.

It was found that attempts to speak produced increased spasticity throughout the trunk and limbs. Respiration was apparently normal until he attempted to phonate or to speak. He then fixed the vocal folds and larynx as for effort and breathing became very limited and shallow. Phonation was forced. Movements of the jaw were not noticeably abnormal except on phonation and speech when there was hyperextension associated with rigidity of the neck muscles, the head being extended backwards. The lips were normally relaxed at rest, but during speech there was sometimes variable degrees of abnormal tension in the mentalis or in the facial muscles of the forehead and around the eyes. Tongue movements varied according to his position. In the supine position with arms and legs flexed all movements of the anterior and posterior parts of the tongue were easy, as also in side-lying. In the prone position these movements were much more difficult, and when sitting or standing he was unable to elevate the tongue tip, attempts to do so being associated with spasms of the whole body musculature and of the facial muscles. At the base of the tongue there was severe tension with contraction of the muscles of the floor of the mouth and base of the tongue. This spasticity appeared to be least when he was in the side-lying position. At times there was some inco-ordination and limitation of palatal movement with nasal speech. He could articulate all consonants ([k] and [g] only with difficulty) when in isolation, but could not use them in speech.

Less severe motor disability but severe dysarthria

2. M. C., now aged eight years, was first seen at four years ten months. He sat up at one year and walked at three and a half years. At two years of age he had had a series of fits, and these continued occasionally until five years. He made no attempt to speak until four years, and was just beginning to use short phrases and say nursery rhymes when first seen. He had had difficulty in swallowing in infancy, with some nasal regurgitation.

Movements of the lips and jaw were normal, but tongue movements were limited. He could protrude it only just beyond the lip margins with deviation to the right. He could not move it to the left side at all. The tip was rounded and he could not elevate it. There was also spasticity of the muscles at the base of the tongue with palatal inco-ordination and nasal speech at times. Speech was not associated with any apparent increase of muscle tone throughout the body. Walking was, however, somewhat clumsy and he tended to fall easily, especially if he tried to run.

He attended for speech therapy and at five and a half years could articulate four plosive consonants and [l] [w] and [j (y)]. At six and a half years the only consonants he could not articulate were [k] and [g], although the dysarthria was obvious and hindered the use of consonants in speech. By seven years of age speech was intelligible, and at eight years the only consonants not used in speech were [k] and [g]. This boy was able to attend a normal school in spite of some degree of general physical disability which was gradually decreasing with improving compensation and control.

Moderate degree of motor disability with severe dysarthria persisting into adult life

3. T. C. This patient had no speech therapy until the age of 39 years, when he was first seen. He had an asymmetrical quadriplegia, worse on the right side than on the left. The early history could not be ascertained, but he could walk and travel alone by bus. He had, however, obvious difficulty, with spasticity and

involuntary movements in particular of the arms, head and facial muscles. He had attended a normal school but had been considered mentally defective, and he could not read or write. Speech was not intelligible. He lived alone and earned a little money growing and selling tomatoes and bedding plants. At 39 years his intelligence quotient on the performance scale of the Weschler Bellevue test was 97.

There was some spasticity of the jaw and lip muscles, but the chief difficulty was in movements of the tongue. It protruded with difficulty and there was a fine tremor. He could not elevate the tip, and lateral movements were only just perceptible. Speech therapy aimed to provide articulatory practice through association of the auditory and visual symbols of speech, and 18 months later he could read up to the seven-year level on the Burt Reading Scale. He also learnt to write, and when discharged after two years he could write a simple letter, or a description, for example of the culture of sweet peas or tomatoes, in which he was interested. He was then sent for a short course of training in horticulture. Speech remained dysarthric but was easily intelligible.

It is not known yet how far abnormalities of respiration, phonation and articulation, as described, are associated with, or are the result of, abnormal postural reflex activity persisting and producing abnormal muscle tone, such as the tonic neck and labyrinthine reflexes, nor how far they may be the result of central specific lesions occurring simultaneously with or without those causing extensive motor defects. Where attempts to speak have an adverse effect on the general distribution of muscle tone, either localised or throughout the body, it seems clear that this must be treated first, or simultaneously, by a method such as that of reflex inhibition as described by Bobath (1955). To attempt speech therapy in such patients, especially in young children, regardless of the general condition, may lead to an increase of spasticitv or of athetosis with little improvement in speech.

However, with repeated improved motor experience, requiring regular periods of treatment over a period of time, even years, the child may be able to take over to some extent the control of his own bodily movements and tensions with improved control of the movements for articulation, always within the limits of his neurological development at any one stage of progress.

Results of treatment are slow to obtain where the defect of

articulation is severe, but the aim must be to help each child to acquire speech which is intelligible where possible, and useful for purposes of communication. Treatment will be discussed in more detail in Chapter XV.

DEVELOPMENTAL DYSARTHRIA AND MINIMAL MOTOR DISABILITY

A severe dysarthria may occur in children who have no other obvious signs of cerebral injury, the true underlying condition being ascertained only on full neurological examination. In some there may have been difficulties associated with birth or with sucking and swallowing in early life, and the history may also indicate delay in motor development, instability or awkward running, and less agility than is usual in children. There may be a tendency to wear out the toes of the shoes, or to wear out one more quickly than the other.

In these children the disability is chiefly confined to the muscles of articulation, although abnormalities of phonation and respiration may also be present, and the existence of a general motor disability has usually not been suspected. The defective articulation is out of all proportion to the general condition and may be so severe that it resembles the dysarthria already described in children with obvious cerebral palsy. Neurological examination, however, reveals minimal signs of spasticity, of involuntary movements or of ataxia.

When these children speak, their attempts are usually not associated with any increase in muscle tone throughout the body, although in some a slight increase may be detected on careful examination. The movements of the tongue and other muscle groups used for articulation are severely affected, and the child is referred for treatment because of the speech disorder. The tongue movements may be clumsy and limited, the upper lip tight and immobile, there may be incompetent nasopharyngeal closure, or inco-ordination of respiration with phonation, or of phonation and articulation.

4. E. S. This girl was born normally at term and weighed six pounds six ounces. She had some difficulty in swallowing during early infancy, but at one year her general development seemed normal and she could take solid food. She sat up at ten months,

walked at 18 months, but was always somewhat 'clumsy on her feet'. She played normally and was not clumsy with her hands, was fond of books and pictures and was doing well in school. She was referred for speech therapy at six years of age because her speech had a nasal quality and resembled that of a child 'with a cleft palate'.

Speech Development. She talked freely from 18 months onwards, but speech was not intelligible at first, although there was a tendency towards slow improvement. At four years she had otorrhoea, followed by a thick nasal discharge intermittently for the next two years. Tonsils and adenoids were removed at five years and speech was thereafter more nasal and less intelligible.

On examination. She had an incompetent nasopharyngeal sphincter with limited palatal movement, and although she made the correct tongue and lip movements for all consonants there was insufficient air pressure in the mouth for normal articulation. The tongue was small and rather thick and firm and did not protrude well. There was occasional regurgitation through the nasopharynx when drinking. Blowing was weak, with nasal escape of air. Neurological examination revealed a spastic diplegia with both plantars extensor and with involvement of the muscles of the soft palate and tongue.

Three years later there was some improvement in the diplegia and the leg signs seemed to be slowly clearing. The tongue movements had also improved though there was still some spasticity. Speech was now intelligible and palatal movements had increased. Speech deteriorated, however, when she was nervous or excited. In this case the speech defect was more obvious than the spasticity of the legs, so that until six years of age the diagnosis of spastic diplegia had not been suspected.

5. E. F. was referred at the age of 25 years by the Ministry of Labour because he could neither read nor write and speech was unintelligible. It was stated that during boyhood he had suffered from 'asthma and a severe speech defect which combined in his youth to make him miss a great deal of school, with the result that he is largely illiterate'. The early history could not be obtained, but on examination he had a marked dysarthria and was largely unintelligible, although the only consonants he could not articulate were [s], which approached [ʃ (sh)], and [l] and [r], for which he substituted [j (y)]. Diphthongs were also defective. He was left handed, left footed and left eyed. The right hand was somewhat clumsy, but, when first seen, walking was normal. The neurological report stated that there was a spastic quadriplegia more marked on the right but

clearly present on the left, both plantars were extensor; the right arm was more spastic than the leg. There was no evidence of subnormal intelligence.

Respiration was upper costal with indrawing of the abdominal wall and there was little movement of the diaphragm. Phonation was approaching normal, but intonation was monotonous and speech lacked rhythm, being slow and laboured. Movements of the lower jaw were somewhat stiff, and there was deviation to the right on opening the mouth. He could elevate the tongue tip, but lateral movements were almost absent apart from a slight movement to the left. On protrusion the tongue deviated to the left. There was considerable tension in the muscles at the base of the tongue and in the ventral muscles of the neck.

Speech therapy aimed to obtain intelligible speech and to improve the rhythm and intonation, with instruction in reading and writing. He made slow but steady progress, treatment being continued for a period of five years.

6. J. G. This boy was first referred at the age of three years because he was not talking. He was the second of two children. The mother said that he had been late in talking, as had her first child, but in the latter speech had been adequate by three years. Delivery was normal, the birth weight was seven and a quarter pounds, he was breast fed and sucked well. He sat up at six months, walked at 17 months, fed himself from two years and at three years could undo his buttons and take off and put on his shoes and socks. Comprehension for speech was normal. Speech was limited to the use of a few isolated words or vowel sounds, but he had recently said one phrase, 'Train go on lines'. The mother said that he had had to 'take his time and think of each word'.

Three months later language was developing rapidly and he was using three- or four-word sentences. Articulation was very defective and he was dysphonic with forced phonation. Tongue movements were slow and he could not elevate the tip. Neurological examination revealed a minor degree of right hemi-paresis. His intelligence quotient at four years on the Drever Collins performance scale was 128. Use of consonants was acquired slowly over a period of 18 months, and speech therapy was discontinued when he was five years of age as articulation was then adequate except when he was in a hurry or when excited.

Congenital Facial Diplegia

Recently Evans (1955) has described cases of congenital facial diplegia, some of whom had an associated developmental dysarthria. Möbius in 1892 had recognised facial palsy combined with other cranial neuromuscular weaknesses, and the syndrome has since borne his name. The paralysis may be total or partial, bilateral or unilateral, and was presumed to be due to agenesis of the appropriate nuclei. Evans considers that the signs are not always in agreement with this theory and attributes it to 'interference with the development of the muscles of the mandibular and hyoid arches' which are differentiated about the same time, at the end of the second month of intra-uterine life. He describes nine cases with associated symptoms of persistent dribbling, sucking and swallowing difficulties in early life, laryngeal stridor, and in one a persisting dysphonia, and poor palatal and tongue movements with defects of articulation. He also considers that there is a tendency towards improvement in the condition with age, and there may therefore be spontaneous improvement in speech. Some degree of optimism in undertaking speech therapy may also be justified.

ISOLATED DEVELOPMENTAL DYSARTHRIA

In other children a similar dysarthria occurs in the absence of any other neurological signs at the time of referral for speech therapy. The defect of articulation may be slight or severe and would seem to depend on a focal cerebral dysgenesis essentially similar to, but less extensive than, that associated with more general signs of cerebral trauma. Motor development may have been normal and appropriate to the age of the child, or there may have been a history of a minor degree of awkward and inco-ordinated movements in the early stages of development. The movements of the muscles used for articulation, however, may resemble those of the child with a general motor disability, resulting in a severe dysarthria. Worster Drought (1953) has also described this condition of developmental dysarthria as being associated with, or the result of, cerebral agenesis, possibly due to lesions caused by head injuries at birth or by post-natal disease and has used the description 'infantile suprabulbar paresis'.

Lesser degrees of disability due to minimal disorders of cerebral function have been described by Mitchell (1966) as not differing in kind from the overt clinical disorders as in cerebral palsy. They represent, rather, one end of a range of severity which has no abrupt line of demarcation from the normal. Paine (1966) has estimated that between 4 per cent and 5 per cent of schoolchildren in America are so affected.

During the period 1947-53, 18 children with isolated developmental dysarthria were observed for periods ranging from one to six years. Twelve were boys and six were girls. They came from all social classes and covered the range of normal intelligence. Hearing was also normal.

Twelve of these 18 children had abnormal movements of the lips, tongue or palate under all conditions. The tongue was often thick and firm, lateral movements were slow and clumsy, and there was inability or difficulty in pointing the tongue and in elevating the tip over the upper lip.

When these children were first seen, the term isolated dysarthria was applied to all those where it was thought that there was an organic basis for the defective articulation. On further observation, however, it became clear that in some of these children the term articulatory apraxia or dyspraxia was more appropriate. In six children movements of the lips, tongue and palate appeared normal for gross movements but showed varying degrees of inadequate control for the imitation of the consonants of speech requiring more complex and rapid automatic movements. In some there was inability to imitate easily movements of lips or tongue, apart from articulation. We considered these children to be cases of isolated 'dyspraxic dysarthria' or articulatory dyspraxia.

In the 12 children described below there was obvious dysarthria, but it is possible that in seven of them there may have been in addition some degree of articulatory dyspraxia which contributed towards the total disability.

Age and sex

The ages of these patients ranged from 4 to 20 years at the time of referral, and from 5½ to 23½ years when last seen. They were observed for periods ranging from 18 months to 9 years. Nine of these were boys and three were girls.

Family tendency

There was a history of speech defect in seven of the 12 families. We were not able to interview all the affected relatives personally, but it was clear from accounts given by the parents that the difficulty had been considerable and had, in some instances, continued into adult life.

Birth injury

In only three cases was birth injury suspected from the history, and in none was there definite evidence.

Position in family

Only one of the 12 children was first born, and one was a second pregnancy, but the first surviving child. Six were second children and three were third or later births. This deficiency of defects in first children agrees with our findings during the investigation of speech development in the normal child population (Chapter V) and is in agreement with the findings of absence of birth injury which is more likely to occur in the first born than in subsequent children.

Prematurity

One of the 18 children was born prematurely, and this incidence is in accordance with that for Newcastle-upon-Tyne in recent years.

Intelligence

Apart from one child whose intelligence quotient was 75, intelligence was within the normal range and varied from 87 to 148.

Muscle movements

Ten of the 12 children had clumsy and difficult tongue movements. Three had in addition limited movements of the soft palate, although in only two of these was articulation affected and resonance nasalised. In two, movements of the lips were abnormal with some extension of the upper lip and less mobility than is normal.

Articulation and phonation

Of the five children with isolated dysarthria and no dyspraxia, two, as just described, had insufficient movement of the palatal and pharyngeal muscles for nasopharyngeal closure and normal articulation. The balance of resonance was disturbed, consonants were weak and vowels nasalised. In the remaining three, most consonant sounds could be articulated in isolation but not used in conversational speech at normal speed. In seven children there was in addition difficulty in directing movements for articulation or some degree of articulatory dyspraxia.

Associated disorders of language

Developmental dysarthria may be associated with articulatory dyspraxia as described and also with developmental dysphasia or aphasia. Later in childhood there may also be developmental alexia or dyslexia. Where developmental dysarthria and dyspraxia co-exist, they contribute towards a speech disability which is the result of these combined basic conditions. Three of these children also had a slight and temporary stammer.

Six of these 12 children had some delay in the development of expressive language. This varied in extent. In one boy (R.L.S.) the delayed development of speech was followed by a limitation of vocabulary, alexia and agraphia throughout school life, persisting until 20 years of age. In five others, although there was no appreciable delay in speaking, there was, later, difficulty in learning to read, with a dyslexia which persisted at eight, eight and a half, nine, ten and 14 years of age.

Prognosis

The less severely affected child, particularly when endowed with high intelligence, can make good progress and achieve normal or at least useful and intelligible speech. In severe cases of isolated developmental dysarthria the faulty neuromuscular patterns of articulation may continue until six or seven years of age and become so firmly established that they may then persist into adult life even where neurological maturation has continued and near normal speech may be potentially possible. This may also happen in cases of structural abnormality such as cleft palate, where operation has provided the necessary anatomical mechanism for normal speech, but not before speech has been stabilised with the use of faulty patterns of articulation and of neuromuscular co-ordinations. These then persist unless changed by some degree of conscious effort which may not be possible without the help of speech therapy. In other children with isolated developmental dysarthria normal speech may never be possible, and the aim of therapy must be to achieve speech that is useful for the purpose of communication and with as little obvious abnormality as possible. The following table gives details of 12 children with isolated developmental dysarthria (Fig. 64).

Representative Histories

Dysarthria with clumsy movements of lips, tongue and palate

J. C. This boy was aged seven years nine months when last seen. He was the second child in the family, was born before the arrival of the nurse, and weighed 12 lb. 10 oz. (5·7 Kg.). He breathed and cried immediately after birth, was successfully breast fed for seven months, and was walking on his first birthday. Words were used between 12 and 18 months and sentences from two years onwards. On his first visit at the age of five years his mother complained that 'he dribbled when excited, sucked instead of chewing his food and could not talk properly'. His intelligence quotient on the Drever Collins performance scale at five years of age was 111. No abnormality could be found in the nervous system except that speech was slow and clumsy, the tongue bunched and writhed on lateral movement, and the soft palate deviated towards the right. Two years after beginning treatment he could use all consonant sounds except [s] and speech was intelligible when spoken slowly though some final consonants were still omitted. Although it may be some years before speech is satisfactory under stress, it seems likely that this boy will eventually achieve normal speech.

Dysarthria with clumsy movements of the soft palate

B. F. This 15-year-old girl was the second of four children. There was a history of language delay in her father until the age of seven, and of an unspecified speech difficulty in a cousin persisting into adult life. She was born normally and weighed 11 lb. 4 oz. (5·1 Kg.).

	Sex	Position in family	Age period of observ. Years	Movements of			Age of speech dev.		Artic. defects	Assoc. lang. dis.	Family History	General Remarks
				Palate	Tongue	Lips	Words	Phrases				
M.B.	F	4	8½-14½	Normal.	Slow and clumsy.	Normal.	Not known 'early'.		k.g.f.v.s.sh.ch.j.r.l. th. Diphthongs. Transposes and perseverates.	Dyslexia. C.A. R.A. 11 yrs 5·7 yrs 14 yrs 7½ yrs	+	Speech almost normal with care at 14 years.
J.C.	M	2	6-8	Drawn to right on elevation, no nasality.	Stiff and clumsy	Normal.	18/12	2-2½ yrs.	Initially-k.g.s.f.sh. th.r. Finally-k.g. f.s.sh are normal.	Dyslexia; at 8 yrs R.A. 5½ yrs. Slight stammer.	+	Speech intelligible at 8 years. Use of [s] erratic—omits some final consonants at speed.
K.C.	M	2	4-13	Normal.	Poor movement.	Tense upper lip.	Before.	3 yrs.	f.v.th.s.r.w. Omits medial and final consonants. Erratic substitutions.	Nil.	+	Treatment for four years. Slow improvement. Normal at 13 yrs.
D.H.	M	2	10½-13	Poor movement in speech. Adequate for blowing.	Normal.	Normal.	'Normal age'.		Dysphonia assoc. with inco-ord. of articulation and phonation. No consonants used except nasal resonants.	Nil.	–	Final report—almost normal, but deteriorates at speed.
R.J.	M	2	4½-7	Normal.	Limited and clumsy.	Normal.	18/12	3 yrs.	All consonants defective except p and b.	Nil.	+	Final report—not always intelligible at speed.
C.P.	M	2	6 8/12-12	Normal.	Poor movement.	Normal.	'Not late'.		t.d.th.r. Omits medial and final consonants. Difficulty with double consonants, e.g. sp. fl. Poor artic. movements.	Dyslexia; at 12 yrs R.A. 8½ yrs.	–	Speech therapy for 18 months. Slight residual dysarthria at 12 years.
J.S.	M	2	4-8	Normal.	Limited protrusion, elevation and lateral movements.	Normal.	1 yr.	18-24/12	Omits medial and final consonants.	No dysphasia—Reading age at 7 yrs.= 10 yrs.	–	Normal at 5½ years.
R.L.S.	M	5	20-23½	Normal.	Poor movements, no elevation.	Some facial apraxia.	Not known but 'late'.		p.t.s.sh.ch.j, th.f.r.	Dysphasia Alexia; at 20 yrs.=nil. at 23 yrs.= 9 yrs.	+	When last seen, speech intelligible and almost normal when reading, conversational speech still unintelligible.
G.T.	M	1	8-9½	Normal.	Stiff and clumsy, no elevation.	Normal.	18/12 to 2 yrs.	3 yrs.	k.g.f.s.sh.th[θ & ð] consistent substitutions, but omits them in medial & final positions.	Dyslexia at 9 yrs. Not assessed. Slight stammer.	+	At 9½ years still omits some final consonants at conversational speed.
J.T.	F	3	4-6	Normal.	Spastic and very limited movements.	Normal.	2	3	k.g.s.sh.ch. th[θ & ð].	Nil.	–	Treatment and progress complicated by acquired middle ear hearing loss at 5½ years. At 6 years articulation was good at slow speed.
T.W.	M	1 (2nd pregnancy	4-5½	Normal.	Poor elevation and lateral movement.	Normal.	10/12	18/12	th[θ]v.f.ch, but poor articulation of all consonants in speech.	Slight stammer.	+	
B.F.	F	2	11-15	Poor movement. Incompetent sphincter.	Normal.	Normal.	2	3½	ch.j., other sounds weak.	Dysphonia.	+	Normal at 15 years apart from occasional audible nasopharyngeal escape of air due to incoordination of movements at speed.

FIG. 64
Details concerning 12 children with isolated developmental dysarthria.

Her mother did not remember the child's early years clearly, but she did not take the breast or bottle well and was slow in gaining weight. She was walking just before her first birthday.

Speech development. She was almost silent until two years, and then words came slowly. Articulation was defective when first seen at 11 years, with weak, nasalised consonant sounds and abnormal vowel resonance. She also had a marked dysphonia associated with attempts to co-ordinate phonation and articulation. Speech was unintelligible. There was no structural abnormality of the soft palate or pharynx, but the nasopharyngeal sphincter was incompetent. She attended for therapy for only three months, but returned at the age of 14 years 10 months. The dysphonia persisted and there had been no improvement in articulation during the interval of nearly four years. At 15 her reading age was 12 years 8 months and her intelligence quotient on the Wechsler Bellevue Scale was 96. During a further course of treatment a transient increase in the dysphonia occurred, but four months later she had made considerable progress and speech was normal except for an occasional audible nasopharyngeal leak due to inco-ordination under stress. Her school teacher reported that she was 'a co-operative, well-behaved girl who, without outstanding qualities, had reached a fairly good standard of general attainment'.

Dysarthria with clumsy movements of the tongue

J. S. This boy, aged six years nine months was a second child. Birth was normal and he weighed 10 lb. (4·5 Kg.). There was no difficulty with feeding or swallowing, and he walked at the age of 14 months. His father had had a speech difficulty which persisted into school life. This boy began to use words at one year and sentences followed quickly. When first seen at the age of five and a half years he was a well-developed boy of high intelligence with an intelligence quotient on the Alexander Performance Scale of 150. The nervous system was normal apart from a thick and clumsy tongue with especially poor lateral movements. Speech was unintelligible.

Sixteen months later he could speak clearly in rhymes and repetition, but articulation lapsed in its more rapid use in conversational speech. The abnormal appearance of the tongue was unchanged. We have regarded this boy as a case of dysarthria uncomplicated by dysphasia in whom the results of treatment have been facilitated by high intelligence.

REFERENCES

Ardran, G. M., and Kemp, F. H. (1951). The Mechanism of Swallowing. *Proc. R. Soc. Med.*, **44,** 1038.

Ardran, G. M., and Kemp, F. H. (1952). The Protection of the Laryngeal Airway during Swallowing. *Brit. J. Radiol.*, **25,** 406.

Ardran, G. M., and Kemp, F. H. (1955). A Radiographic Study of the Tongue in Swallowing. *Dent. Practit.*, **5,** 8.

Asher, P. (1952). A Study of 63 Cases of Athetosis with Special Reference to Hearing Defects. *Arch. Dis. Childh.*, **27,** 475.

Asher, P., and Schonell, F. E. (1950). A Study of 63 Cases of Athetosis with Special Reference to Hearing Defects. *Arch. Dis. Childh.*, **25,** 360.

Barcroft, Sir Joseph (1942). The Onset of Respiration at Birth. *Lancet*, **2,** 117.

Benda, C. E. (1952). *Developmental Disorders of Mentation and Cerebral Palsies.* New York, Grune & Stratton.

Bieber, I. (1940). Grasping and Sucking. *J. nerv. ment. Dis.*, **91,** 31.

Bobath, B. (1954). A Study of Abnormal Postural Reflex Activity in Patients with Lesions of the Central Nervous System. *Physiotherapy*, **40,** 259, 295, 326, 368.

Bobath, B. (1955). The Treatment of Motor Disorders of Pyramidal and Extrapyramidal origin by Reflex Inhibition, and by Facilitation of Movements. *Physiotherapy*, **41,** 146.

Crothers, Bronson (1951). Clinical Aspects of Cerebral Palsy. *Quart. Rev. Pediat.*, **6,** 142.

Drought, Worster (1953). Failure in Normal Language Development. *Folia phoniatr., Basel*, **5,** No. 3.

Dunsdon, M. I. (1952). The Educability of Cerebral Palsied children. London, Newnes.

Ellis, R. E. (1955). Cerebral Palsy. Unpublished Thesis for M.D., Camb. Univ.

Evans, P. R. (1955). Nuclear Agenesis. Möbius Syndrome. The Congenital facial diplegia syndrome. *Arch. Dis. Childh.*, **30,** 151, 237.

Fisch, L. (1955). Deafness in Cerebral Palsied School Children. *Lancet*, **2,** 370.

Gesell, A. (1954). *The Embryology of Behaviour.* New York and London, Harper.

Gesell, A., and Armatruda, C. S. (1949). *Developmental Diagnosis.* New York and London, Harper.

Gordon, N. S. (1966). The child who does not talk. *Brit. J. Dis. Commun.*, **1,** 78.

Kenney, W. (1963). Certain Sensory Defects in Cerebral Palsy. *Clinical Orthopaedics and Related Research*, **21,** 193–195.

Last, R. J. (1955). The Muscles of the Head and Neck. *Int. dent. J.*, **5,** 3.

Lucas Keene, M., and Whillis, J. (1950). *Anatomy for Dental Students.* London, Arnold.

McGraw, M. B. (1952). *The Neuromuscular Maturation of the Human Infant*. New York, Columb. Univ. Press.

Magnus, R. (1926). Some Results of Studies in the Physiology of Posture. *Lancet*, **2,** 531.

Marland, P. (1953). Speech Therapy for Cerebral Palsy based on Reflex Inhibition. *Speech*, **17,** No. 2, p. 65.

Mitchell, R. G. (1966). Minimal disorders of cerebral function. *Brit. J. Dis. Commun.*, **1,** 109.

Morley, M., Court, D., and Miller, H. (1950). Childhood Speech Disorders and the Family Doctor. *Brit. med. J.*, **1,** 574.

Morley, M., Court, D., and Miller, H. (1954). Developmental Dysarthria. *Brit. med. J.*, **1,** 8.

Paine, K. S. (1968). Promoting sensori-motor learning patterns for reinforcement. *Der. Med.*, **10,** 505.

Penfield, W. (1954). The Mechanisms of Voluntary Movements. *Brain*, **77,** 1.

Penfield, W., and Rasmussen, T. (1950). *The Cerebral Cortex of Man*. New York, Macmillan.

Schaltenbrand, G. (1928). The Development of Human Motility and Motor Disturbances. *Arch. Neurol. & Psychiat.*, **20,** 720.

Sherrington, C. S. (1947). *Integrative Action of the Nervous System*. Camb. Univ. Press.

Smith, C. A. (1946). *The Physiology of the New Born Infant*. Illinois, U.S.A., Thomas.

Tizard, J., Paine, R., and Crothers, B. (1954). Disturbances of Sensation in Children with Hemiplegia. *J. A. M. Assoc.*, **155,** 628–632.

Wilson, Kinnier S. (1921). An Introduction to the Study of Aphasia. *Lancet*, **2,** 1143.

XIII. Developmental Articulatory Apraxia

DEVELOPMENTAL articulatory apraxia, or dyspraxia in its less severe form, has been described as an inability to perform voluntary movements of the muscles involved in articulation although automatic movements of the same muscles are preserved. It may also be described as a defect of articulation which occurs when the movements of the muscles used for speech, that is of tongue, lips, palate or cheeks, appear normal for involuntary and spontaneous movements, such as smiling or licking the lips, or even for the voluntary imitation of movements carried out on request, but the control and direction of articulatory movements is inadequate for the complex and rapid movements used for articulation and the reproduction of the sequences of sounds used in speech. There are then varying degrees of defective use of the phonemic patterning, yet neuromuscular control appears to be adequate for all purposes other than for these highly integrated movements.

The condition may be developmental or acquired. The difficulties in the acquired condition have been vividly described by Darley (1967)—'the gropings of the patient for the correct positioning of his articulators, his clumsiness in finding the correct pattern of movement to produce a sequence of phonemes in a word, his near misses phonemically and his retrials'. This is coupled with no reduction in auditory comprehension, and no disability in fluent expression in writing. He describes it as a motor impairment, not a failure of language ability, nor is there any speech problem due to paralysis, spasticity or weakness of the muscles involved.

Geschwind (1965) using the term 'facial apraxia' describes it as 'disorders which intervene in the expression of phonemes at a pre-articulatory stage of word formation, that is at the level of the mechanism through which phonemes to be uttered are chosen among the repertoire of phonemes afforded by spoken language. However, the majority of such children are able to understand speech and appreciate the difference between the sounds of speech, as spoken by others, immediately and without difficulty.

Such a failure to reproduce accurately the accepted phonological system may be comparable to inability to control the frequency of vibration of the laryngeal air stream in order to reproduce the pitch of the sound sequences accurately as in singing a tune, or even the frequency of vibration as in whistling, yet associated with ability to recognise a tune when heard. Some individuals may also be unable to distinguish notes of varying frequency and are unable then to recognise familiar tunes. This failure of discrimination for musical sounds would seem to be of more common occurrence than the failure to discriminate the sounds of speech, and has been known to occur in those who have excellent ability to mimic dialectal speech with facility and accuracy.

Awkwardness of physical performance in children relating to general bodily movements and skills, described as 'the clumsy child syndrome' has been described by Orton (1937), Walton *et al.* (1962), Illingworth (1963) and Gubbay *et al.* (1965). They use the term dyspraxia, which, they say, is clearly distinct from clumsiness arising from brain damage affecting pyramidal, extrapyramidal or cerebellar dysfunction. The child is awkward rather than lithe and graceful. He may have difficulty in dressing, tying his tie, with buttons and zippers, and in the normal skills which most children rapidly master, such as running, climbing and skipping.

Certain learning difficulties also occur as in reading and spelling, or problems affecting behaviour at home and in school. Whilst some of these difficulties may be attributed to cerebral dysfunction, others may be related to delayed maturation or abnormal development. There may be perceptual difficulties, visuo-motor, spatial and lateralisation disorders and disorders of body image. Gubbay *et al.* (1965) found that apraxia or agnosis accounted for clumsiness in 14 of 21 children, the remaining seven showing evidence of minimal cerebral palsy.

Apraxia and Dysarthria

Apraxia may result from a degenerative or traumatic cerebral lesion in adult life, or may occur in its developmental form in children with severe brain damage and a general motor disability. It may be associated with dysarthria, as previously

described, and it may then not be obvious how far each contributes towards the total disability. It may also occur in association with a minimal motor disability, or as an isolated disorder of articulate speech.

Apraxia and Receptive Aphasia

As previously described, developmental receptive dysphasia may occasionally occur and result in the delayed or distorted use of language, even when hearing for and imitation of the actual consonant sounds of speech are not defective. It is possible that some degree of perceptive difficulty may contribute to the defective reproduction of articulation in some children, or that oral tactual and kinaesthetic sensations may be abnormal, but so far as we have been able to ascertain articulatory dyspraxia is not necessarily associated with receptive aphasia, the jargon used by these children being a language or syntactic disability, paraphasia or paragrammatism, rather than an articulatory disorder.

Apraxia and Expressive Aphasia

Brain (1952) defines apraxia in general as an inability to carry out a purposive movement, the nature of which the patient understands, in the absence of severe paralysis, sensory loss or ataxia. It is clear that such a disturbance of speech must be closely akin to expressive aphasia, and indeed Brain and Kinnier Wilson (1921) have suggested that motor aphasia might justly be regarded as an apraxia of the purposive movements concerned in speech. Head (1926), however, regarded anarthria, verbal apraxia and motor aphasia as descriptive terms for three different forms of abnormal speech which could occur separately or in combination.

In many of the children we have seen there was an evident articulatory apraxia without the marked delay in the development of speech which appears to us to be an essential feature of developmental aphasia. There was also no lack of fluency, and no evidence of impairment in the developing use of language. In the acquired condition it has been described as a defect in co-ordination of the movements of phonation, or a loss or disturbance of articulate speech with preservation of inner speech. It would seem that in these cases of articulatory apraxia the lesion must be at some point intermediate between that responsible for the spastic dysarthria which is evident on objective examination and the global failure of language which is encountered in true developmental dysphasia. For the present, therefore, we have considered articulatory apraxia and expressive or motor aphasia as separate though closely related disorders.

Nathan (1947) defines apraxia as a disorder of voluntary movement with retention of automatic movement and has described cases of 'apraxic dysarthria' or articulatory apraxia following cerebral trauma and associated with varying degrees of facial apraxia. He found that syllables could be fairly well pronounced, but that conversational speech became incomprehensible. He believes that in apraxia 'movements remain, but willed purposive movements are lost', and that 'a lesion of one hemisphere, and it is immaterial which, may suffice to cause bilateral apraxia of the face and of the movements of speaking'. 'In the usual cases', he says, 'apraxia affects only those acts which have been learnt with the aid of consciousness. In the rare most severe cases apraxia affects those movements which are so organised that, although they had to be learnt, they were learnt in babyhood before consciousness was much developed', that is the movements of articulate speech. He describes some patients who were at first aphonic but later 'the ability to phonate and produce vowel sounds returned before the use of consonants'. Again, Nathan describes how the patient with an apraxia 'has not at the command of his will some movements co-ordinated into purposive actions which he and his species have developed. He retains the will to perform the act and he retains a neurological apparatus capable of performing the movements involved, but between them there is a gap which he cannot bridge.'

Brain (1952) states that 'normal purposive movements depend on the integrity not only of the cortico-bulbar and cortico-spinal tracts but also of association tracts whereby these efferent paths are excited. The idea of the movements, whether formulated spontaneously or in response to an external command, then passes into action. Apraxia is the result of interruption of the transcortical fibres thus acting as ideomotor links.'

In the child with developmental apraxia or dyspraxia it is possible that there is delay in the development of such association tracts, faulty patterns of articulation are then laid down which if they persist until six or seven years of age may become stabilised and continue into adult life.

It is also possible that some intelligent children may attempt the use of well-developed and mature language before the neurological pathways for accurate imitation of articulation are complete. Such faulty patterns of articulation, once established, may resolve spontaneously but are frequently persistent. The child continues to associate the articulatory sounds he himself produces and incorporates into his developing use of language with those he hears used by others. Even in adult life he will probably be unaware of the difference between his own speech and that of others unless he hears it reproduced through a recording, or imitated by another, when it is at once obvious to him. Very few people appreciate their own dialectal variations except under similar circumstances.

This also applies in those with other types of defective articulation, whether these be the result of a neurological defect, hearing defect, or structural abnormality, unless the patient has previously had normal speech.

B. P., aged three years two months was referred because speech was not intelligible. She had begun to use words at ten months and sentences at 18 months. She could articulate most consonants correctly in single words but omitted some initial and all final and medial consonants in speech. She had recently gone to live in another part of the country with an aunt who reported that 'although she seems to be unaware of her own defective speech she will correct an adult using a dialect to which she is unaccustomed'.

Articulatory Apraxia and Verbal Memory

The part that verbal memory plays in apraxia is difficult to assess, and what we have described as articulatory apraxia has, in the past, been attributed to defective verbal memory. Bastian (1897), writing in the *Lancet*, described memory as 'the power of retaining knowledge in the mind but out of consciousness' and recollection as 'the act of bringing back what is retained into consciousness', and stated that loss of memory for the sound of words may result from loss of memory in addition to loss of recollection, or loss of recollection alone. More recently Schuell (1954) has used the term re-auditorisation for the ability to recall the sound of words. Bastian (1897) described four types of word memory: (1) visual for the symbols of speech; (2) auditory; (3) kinaesthetic, or the memory of sensory impressions resulting from movements of the vocal and articulatory organs during the utterance of words; and (4) writing, where memories associated with sensations from the muscle joints and skin are associated with visual memory for the written letters and words.

Macdonald Critchley (1952), describing articulatory defects in aphasia, states that:

> among the hypotheses which have been brought forward to explain paraphasic errors we may mention Wernicke's idea of the loss of sensory word images. Kussmaul believed that the basic disturbance was one of attention. Pieron blamed an imperfect control of sensory over motor aspects, the sensory control including both acoustic and kinaesthetic factors. Pick, however, thought that incorrect division of attention played a role, and he said that distraction often provoked paraphasic errors even in normal people, but he considered that the essential cause of the defect in aphasic patients was a lack of inhibition.

Critchley defines paraphasia as including either literal paraphasia where one sound is substituted for another, or verbal paraphasia where one word, a fragment of a word or explanatory words are substituted for another as 'chair' for 'table' 'sit on' for chair, and 'cut with' for scissors. Although such verbal paraphasia occurs in children with developmental aphasia, literal paraphasia may be a description of what we have termed articulatory apraxia. This is a very complex subject and the precise relationship between apraxia and aphasia is not yet clear.

Articulatory Apraxia and Facial Apraxia

There are varying degrees of articulatory apraxia. It may be associated with some degree of facial apraxia when the imitation of such movements such as licking the lips may be impossible although the action can be carried out spontaneously when the need is present. A child may have no idea how to imitate such movements as touching the upper teeth with the tongue tip, even when watching the therapist, moving the tongue tip from side to side on request, or making contact between the upper teeth and lower lip as for [f]. In others there is no apparent facial apraxia but the child has difficulty in controlling and directing the movements for articulation on auditory stimulus alone for the imitation of the sounds of speech. Yet understanding for language is normal and there is no hearing loss for any of the frequencies of sound required for speech. There would seem to be dissociation between the ideational and motor processes involved in articulate speech. The consonant vocabulary may be limited, and the child omits those sounds he has not learnt to articulate, substitutes those he can use, or transposes the order of the sounds he uses, and there is a failure to achieve the accurate reproduction of the sound sequences he is attempting to imitate.

Articulation in Articulatory Apraxia

Articulation is a learned neuromuscular skill associated with neurological maturation although acquired at a time in infancy before conscious imitation is involved to any great extent. When there is a failure of such development, varying defects of articulation occur. Some of these children are able to imitate a consonant sound such as [k] or [s] accurately in isolation when they are unable to use it in speech. In others even such imitation is not possible on auditory stimulus alone but can be accomplished if the child also watches the therapist making the sound and perhaps uses a mirror to watch the movements of his own tongue and lips. Imitation is helped by visual stimulus when the auditory stimulus alone is insufficient. This has been appreciated clinically by the therapist who uses a mirror during treatment.

Again, these children may be able to imitate accurately a simple syllable or isolated word but have insufficient ability to reproduce a multi-syllable word or a long sequence of sounds in a phrase or sentence. This may account for the evidence frequently given by the mother that at first the child spoke 'clearly', at a time when speech was probably limited to a few simple words. The ability to imitate normal articulation in long sequences of sounds being inadequate, the intelligibility of speech deteriorated as use of language progressed. How far the speed at which parents speak to their children influences their difficulty is not known. It is a possible factor, and children with some degree of apraxia for articulation may be helped if the speed of conversational speech is reduced.

Although some children are found to be consistent in their use of consonants and substitutions, others use them more readily in the final, initial or medial positions in words, but in many their use is erratic or may vary during treatment. Consonants may be used normally in some words but not in others, there may be mispronunciation of whole words such as 'enbelofe' for 'envelope', or perseveration of sounds as 'kak' or 'tat' for 'cat'. Frequently consonant sounds are transposed with reversal of the order in which they are used in words as 'breakufs' for 'breakfast', or 'bilikces (bailiksəs)' for 'bicycle'. Vowels and diphthongs are often normal, but may be affected in severe cases, especially diphthongs.

When the child is older and learns to read, the association between the visual appreciation of a letter and word, and its normal articulation, may be established, in which case the child learns to read with normal articulation. This may then assist a rapid and spontaneous improvement in the articulation of conversational speech. If, however, the faulty patterns of articulation remain unchanged, the child then learns to read using the same defects of articulation as he uses when speaking, and in writing, words may be spelled as they are spoken or read.

It is a striking fact that many of these children spontaneously gain assistance from watching the speaker's lips, so much so that one is reminded forcibly of the partially deaf child, and audiometric assessment of the hearing is essential. This also occurs in the adult patient who has lost his former ability to articulate normally following a cerebral vascular lesion. Consonant substitutions similar to those found in children then occur and there may also be mispronunciation of words. The adult differs from the child, however, in previously having had normal speech and is usually aware of his defective articulation. In this respect also he differs from the child with a developmental apraxia who is not aware that his speech differs from that of others.

The ability to imitate the sounds of speech includes, therefore, various mental processes. It is primarily dependent on the integrity of hearing and perception, and on the absence of any interference with the actual movements of those muscles used for speech as in dysarthria. Where there is some failure of organic origin to imitate accurately the sound sequences of speech not due to a perceptive hearing defect nor dysarthria, resulting in inadequate control and direction for the movements of articulation, we have used the term articulatory apraxia.

This condition has been particularly studied in 12 children. Of these, five were girls and seven were boys, and they were observed for periods ranging from one to seven years. The age range at the time of referral was four to ten years, apart from one adult, who was referred at the age of 28 years, having had unintelligible articulation since speech developed. The range of intelligence in these patients tended to be higher than in the children with developmental dysarthria, and on performance tests ranged from 105 to 130, the mean intelligence quotient being 114. Details concerning these 12 children are given in the following table (Fig. 65).

Articulatory Apraxia and other Conditions

Family tendency

There was a history of speech disorder in parents, siblings and close relations in six of the 12 families. In one family the grandfather had had a stammer. He had four sons; one had a stammer which he outgrew in early adult life, two were 'slow to speak' and in adult life 'did not always pronounce words properly'. They were unintelligible in childhood, but the details are not known. The remaining son, who was the second child in the family, had normal speech, but was the father of the child L. L. referred for speech therapy. She had begun to speak at 11 months, but had always been unintelligible except to her mother, who also had difficulty in understanding what she said at times. Some defective articulation persisted in speech until six and a half years, when she left the district, but articulation was normal when repeating stories phrase by phrase.

E. W. had a twin brother, whose speech development was normal. An elder and a younger sister also had normal speech, and a baby brother, age two, is developing speech normally. The mother had seven brothers, six of whom had normal speech. She herself did not speak well until she was seven years of age. She remembers that no one understood what she said, and her brother, now a squadron-leader in the Royal Air Force, did not speak at all until he was four years and had unintelligible speech until nearly eight years of age.

Position in family

Only two of the 12 children were first born (see Fig. 65), six were second children and four were third or fourth children.

Emotional disturbance

The majority of these children seen by us with an articulatory dyspraxia, as described, showed little evidence of emotional disturbance, and in other respects developed normally and happily in spite of their speech disability. There were, in some, intermittent emotional difficulties apparently not related to speech; or growing awareness of the inability of others to understand their speech produced, as time continued, a reticence and hesitation which was lacking in earlier years. Children with good intelligence who are unable to communicate easily with others after the age of four inevitably became aware of their disability, but clinical experience usually demonstrated that improvement in speech was associated with a decrease in anxiety and with growth of self-confidence. Such a change might be noticeable within a few weeks of the commencement of therapy when the child perhaps felt that the problem was understood, and correction of speech at home ceased. One six and a half year old girl had ceased to speak because not even her mother could understand her. After attending for therapy for four weeks her mother reported that she was talking again although speech was, of course, still unintelligible.

We could find no grounds for believing that psychogenic factors played any important part in this group of disorders,

	Sex	Position in family	Age period of observ. Years	Development of speech	
				Words	Phrases
B.A.	M	1	5½ to 7½	10/12	14/12
J.B.	M	2	4½ to 7	2	4
M.B.	F	3	28 to 29	?	about 2
M.C.	M	2	4½ to 8½	18/12	2
G.C.	M	3	4 to 5½	1	18/12
L.L.	F	2	4 4/12 to 5½	11/12	4
A.Mc.	M	4	10 to 17	'early'	'early'
J.N.	F	1	5 3/12 to 7½	18/12	2
R.P.	M	2	4 2/12 to 7½	18/12	2
F.S.	M	3	6 to 10	2	4
E.W.	F	2 Has a twin brother	5 3/12 to 10	2	4+
P.W.	F	2	4 2/12 to 7	3	4

FIG. 65

Details concerning 12 children with developmental articulatory apraxia.

Articulation defects	Assoc. language disorders	Family History	General Remarks
Erratic, e.g. [θ (th)]=[f] or [p] [k]=[t] initial position, but=[k] in final position.	Dyslexia & dysgraphia.	+	Speech was normal at 7½ years.
[j (y)], [v] [s] [ʃ (sh)] [θ (th)] =[w] [k]=[t] [g]=[d] [f]=[p] [tʃ (ch)] =[t] [dʒ (j)] =[d].	Some delay in the development of language. No dyslexia.	+	Speech normal at 7 years.
[p] [b] [t] [d] and [w] were the only consonants used. Consistent throughout.	No dyslexia. Spelling disability. She spelt as she spoke.	−	Some improvement, but she ceased to attend before speech was normal.
Plosives used normally, but all fricatives defective.	Dyslexia. Reading age at 8½=6½.	−	Some difficulty in the use of consonants persisted to 8½ years.
Many substitutions, omits final sounds, transposes sounds.	Nil.	+	[s] not quite normal at 5½ years.
All consonants defective except [p] [b] [t] [d] [l] [w]. Omits final sounds and transposes sounds and syllables.	Some delay in the use of sentences.	+	Speech almost normal at 5½ years.
[p] [b] [t] [d] only. Omits medial and final sounds. Erratic use of consonants in speech.	Stammer.	−	Speech adequate, but with some persisting lack of easy control of movements for articulation at 17 yrs.
[p] [b] [t] [d] [l] [w] only consonants used. Substitutions used consistently.	Nil.	+	
[p] [b] [l] [w] only sounds used. Mostly consistent, but many consonants omitted in speech.	Nil.	−	
[p] [b] [w] [j (y)] only. Most consonants omitted with use of glottal stop.	Dyslexia. Reading age at 9=6 yrs. at 10 =9 yrs.	−	Slow improvement. Consonants rarely defective at 8½, but not used easily. Normal at 10 yrs.
Few defective consonants in simple words, but had great difficulty in their use in speech.	Some delay in speech development.	+	Articulation better in reading than in speech, which is still unintelligible at 10 yrs.
	Some delay in speech development.		

FIG. 65 (*continued*)

and we considered that, as in developmental dysarthria, there was an organic cause for the speech disability.

Appearance and movements of lips, tongue and palate

In these children there was no limitation of movement of the lips, tongue or palate, and such movements appeared normal when carried out voluntarily on request. For articulation, however, the movements were awkward and misdirected and the child was unable to imitate the sounds of speech correctly in isolation, in simple syllables, or in the long sequence of sounds in conversational speech, according to the severity of the disability.

Associated disorders of language

Seven of these 12 children were using phrases or sentences by two years of age, whilst in five there was some delay in the first use of words; and phrases were not attempted before four years. The mean age for the first use of words in these 12 children was 19 to 20 months and for phrases 33 months, which is somewhat later than the average, but still within the normal range. In a few of these children there was an associated difficulty in the use of words and sentence construction, or developmental dysphasia, which continued into school and later life. In three there was a dyslexia, and in one, where unintelligible speech persisted into adult life, a spelling disability. One child had a stammer between the ages of 10 and 14 years which resolved spontaneously as articulation improved.

Prognosis

In many of these children there is a natural tendency towards spontaneous improvement, and if normal or at least intelligible articulation is established by four years of age, therapy may not be required. If not, speech therapy between the ages of four and five years may assist in the improvement of articulation so that speech may be intelligible when the child enters school. When learning to read, some children again are able to substitute normal for defective articulation and later use it spontaneously in speech. Where, however, there is a more severe disability, the defective articulation may persist in reading and in speech. As the child grows older, spontaneous improvement becomes more difficult, and faulty patterns of articulation may then persist into adult life. In some of these there may be only minimal signs, as when there is persistent defective articulation of only one consonant sound, but in a few speech may remain unintelligible.

Persisting familial articulatory apraxia

In one family of eight there were four men and four women, their ages ranging from 57 to 72 years when they were first seen. The parents were said to have had normal speech, but three of the men and one woman had unintelligible articulation and another woman had a less severe defect of articulation and spoke slowly and with obvious care. Two women and one man had normal speech. They had all been educated in the normal school, could read and write and had no difficulty in the use of figures and calculations as used in everyday life. The three men with unintelligible speech worked as miners in the pit. The woman with a less severe defect managed the home for these three brothers who had not married.

In their early life the parents had sought help and advice. Tonsils and adenoids had been removed, lingual fraenums cut and even the uvula excised. These children grew up together, but the actual consonant substitutions were not identical, and although the first and second, sixth and eighth had such a severe defect of articulation, the third had a much less severe defect, and the fourth, fifth and seventh children had normal speech. Direct imitation has probably not been the chief factor, therefore, in the defective development of articulation in this family.

Clinical Notes of Patients with Articulatory Dyspraxia

F. S. was referred at six years. He was the fourth child and was born prematurely, weighing three pounds. His behaviour during the first few weeks is not fully known, but at one stage 'he was not expected to live'. He did not dribble excessively, and there was no apparent difficulty in swallowing. He was walking at the age of 15 months and has always been a good runner. He did not begin to use words in any quantity until two years. When first seen he was a friendly active boy with no abnormality in the nervous system apart from defective speech. This was fluent, but intelligible only to his parents. The tongue, lips and palate were normal in appearance and movement, and he could sing accurately in tune but still with defective articulation. Although at first progress was rapid and he was thought to have a simple dyslalia, the subsequent slowing down and failure to respond further to treatment suggested a more complex speech disorder. He had difficulty in imitating and using consonant sounds, and was helped considerably by watching the therapist's lips. When imitation of consonants was possible in isolation and in single words, he still had great difficulty in incorporating consonants correctly into speech. Two and a half years later articulation was still defective, and with increasing awareness of this he became more cautious, often repeating words silently before speaking. He had difficulty in repeating phrases of a story and would change words, as in verbal paraphasia, or consonants, and often transpose them. For example, he pronounced 'Nelson' as 'Lenson', and 'stars' as 'sarts'. At nine years of age speech was usually intelligible. He also had some dyslexia, and at that time his reading age was only six and a half years. He had ceased to attend for speech therapy but returned for help with reading, and at ten years his reading age was nine years. Articulation in spontaneous speech was then usually normal. His intelligence quotient on the Wechsler Bellevue Scale at eight years was 113. On the verbal scale it was 108, and on the performance scale 121.

N. B. was not referred for speech therapy until she was 28 years. She had lived in the country, had first been taken to her own doctor at three years of age, and at five had been seen in hospital by a neurologist who suggested treatment as an in-patient because speech was not intelligible. She refused to stay in hospital, however, and was taken home again. The age of onset of speech is not known, but she was said to have been speaking at two years of age. School work was adequate, and she subsequently worked in a tweed factory and kept house for her father. The articulation of consonants was limited to [p] [b] [t] [d] [j (y)] and [w] and she substituted these for the remaining consonant sounds with some omissions. She could read fluently, but with the same unintelligible articulation. She could write, but tended to spell words as she pronounced them. Attendance for therapy was only possible for eight months. There was some improvement in intelligibility and in articulation when reading, but little in spontaneous speech.

Acquired articulatory apraxia

E. G. was referred at six and a half years. He was a twin who had a severe anoxic cerebral birth damage. At three he was found to have some right hemiparesis, more marked in the leg than in the arm. He had begun to have fits at the age of two, but these were well controlled. He used single words at 11 months and sentences early in his second year. Articulation was always intelligible, although at five years he had what was considered to be a slight dyslalia. At six years he had an illness which was thought to have been chicken-pox encephalitis. After this illness, whilst still in hospital, the mother stated that the boy was still talking in sentences but she 'could not understand a thing'. Later he tried to talk to her using only single words and gestures. Six months later he was beginning to use sentences again. He had then no apparent difficulty in moving the lips, tongue or palate except during speech, but articulation was usually unintelligible. Before his illness he had been right handed in spite of the slight right hemiparesis, but subsequently he used his left hand for a cup, spoon and knife, and for doing jig-saws and the posting box. He still, however, maintained the use of the right hand for writing and for using scissors and a hammer. He was also found to be right eyed and right footed, and there was no familial history of left-handedness. He had some difficulty with visual perception, and for some time was unable to identify or match plastic letters or shapes. Drawing was also very poor.

Improvement was rapid at first, but progress was not well maintained. It is probable that there was also some deterioration in the general level of intelligence. One had the impression that at first the child was to some extent aware of a change in himself and was anxious to gain what he had lost. Later he became somewhat apathetic, as though he had accepted himself as he then was. He then showed much less interest in speech therapy, although slow progress was maintained.

REFERENCES

Bastian, H. C. (1897). Some Problems in Connection with Aphasia and Other Speech Defects. *Lancet*, **1,** 933.

Brain, W. Russell (1952). *Diseases of the Nervous System.* Oxford Med. Publications.

Critchley, J. Macdonald (1952). Articulatory Defects in Aphasia. *J. Laryng.*, **60**, 1, and *Speech*, **17,** 4. Semon Lecture.

Darley, F. L. (1967). Lacunae and Research approaches to them.

Brain Mechanisms Underlying Speech and Language. New York and London, Grune & Stratton.

Geschwind, N. P. (1965). Disconnection Syndromes in Animals and Man. *Brain*, **88,** 237–294, 585–644.

Gubbay, S. S., Ellis, E., Walton, J. N., and Court, S. D. M. (1965). A Study of apraxia and agnosia defects in 21 children. *Brain*, **88,** 295–312.

Head, Henry (1926). *Aphasia and Kindred Disorders of Speech.* Camb. Univ. Press.

Illingworth, R. S. (1963). The Clumsy Child: minimal cerebral dysfunction. *Little Club Clinics in Developmental Medicine*, No. 10, p. 26.

Nathan, P. W. (1947). Facial Apraxia and Apraxic Dysarthria. *Brain*, **70,** 4, 449.

Orton, S. (1937). *Reading, Writing and Speech Problems in Children.* New York, Noton.

Schuell, H. (1954). Clinical Observations on Aphasia. *Neurology*, Minneapolis, **4,** 3.

Wilson, Kinnier S. (1921). An Introduction to the Study of Aphasia. *Lancet*, **2,** 1143.

Walton, J. N., Ellis, E., and Court, S. D. M. (1962). Clumsy Children: a study of developmental apraxia and agnosia. *Brain*, **85,** 603–612.

XIV. Dyslalia

ROBERTS (1967) investigated the various meanings attributed to the term 'dyslalia' such as—oral inaccuracy; phonetic defects; general dyslalia, also known as delayed speech; an acute form of lisping and lalling; a language disorder; a functional articulatory problem; articulation errors often emotional in origin; due to structural abnormalities of the articulatory organs or impaired hearing; functional and organic defects of articulation, and speech difficult of perception, to mention only a few definitions of this much abused term.

Here, it is suggested that the term should not be used where there is evidence of articulatory apraxia or any degree of dysarthria. Nor should it be used where there is an anatomical basis for the articulatory defect or a defect of hearing. In dyslalia there is no abnormality in the movements of the lips, tongue or palate. The defect is largely one of phonemic substitution, but speech is fluent even if unintelligible, and the development of speech is not delayed. During treatment these are the children who respond readily, and early spontaneous resolution of the abnormal phonological system is also common.

As described in Chapter III, many children have transient difficulties in the integration of their phonemic usage into normal linguistic sequences in early life. We have thought that the term dyslalia could be used to include such defects for which there may be more than one cause. We shall consider here:

1. Persistence of faulty habits of articulation.
2. Imitation of faulty patterns of articulation.
3. The influence of defects of vision on articulation.
4. Mental defect.
5. Environmental and psychogenic factors.

1. Persistence of Faulty Habits of Articulation

During the early development of speech the rapid development of language may be associated with a partial failure of accurate imitation for the consonants of speech. The defect may be attributable to slow maturation for the function of articulation which is yet within the normal range, but faulty patterns of articulation, once acquired, may tend to persist in some children when there remains no underlying dysfunction. The child's linguistic syntactical competence may have outstripped his phonological ability. Thus abnormal phonemic usage becomes stabilised through repeated usage, although the child's phonemic system for decoding is normal.

2. Imitation of Faulty Patterns of Articulation

The term dyslalia would also include those defects of articulation which are due to imitation of the defective speech of another child or adult, or even the speech of a partially deaf member of the family or one with cleft palate speech. Such defects of articulation cannot be attributed to any defect in the child's ability to imitate the speech of others, yet articulation is defective.

T. L., aged two years nine months, had adequate movement of the soft palate for blowing and for most consonant sounds, but [t] and [d] were nasopharyngeal plosives, and [s] [ʃ (sh)] [tʃ (ch)] and [dʒ (j)] were articulated as nasopharyngeal fricative sounds. When first seen it was thought that regular speech therapy might not be necessary, but the [*θ* and ð (th)] sounds were not being used, and these were taught. He rapidly incorporated them normally into spontaneous speech, and it was hoped that this would influence the use of the other fricative consonants. However, when seen a year later, these remained as before. Speech therapy was then commenced because he had been corrected at home and one day had remarked to his father, 'I haven't got a nice voice father', and also because his younger sister, aged two years, was imitating his speech exactly. In nine months T. L.'s speech was normal, but he had considerable difficulty in spite of a high intelligence, and was considered to be a case of articulatory dyspraxia. By this time the sister's speech was also normal without therapy or correction, her defect being dyslalia.

3. The Influence of Defects of Vision on Articulation

A blind child may have a persisting defect of articulation because the visual assistance used unconsciously by the normal child may be lacking. One child in our experience used a normal sounding [f] and [v], but articulated them with apposition of the lower teeth and upper lip. In some partially sighted children the temporary period of defective articulation may be prolonged, and where there is any degree of dyspraxia for the imitation of consonant sounds through hearing, these children with limited vision are at a disadvantage, and defective use of consonant sounds may persist.

4. Mental Defect

Dyslalia may occur when there is a general defect of mental development. There may then be an abnormal prolongation of the period of defective articulation found in many normal children at an earlier stage of speech development. Although, as previously described (Chapter VII), many mentally retarded children imitate and reproduce the sounds of speech accurately, in others a dyslalia may persist, frequently associated with delay in the development and use of language which is proportional to the general level of mental and motor development.

5. Environmental and Psychogenic Factors in Dyslalia

The home surroundings of the child may be such that use of speech is limited and the general standard of articulation low. It provides little need or encouragement for the use of speech and the continual development of the neuromuscular skills involved. Change in the environment of the child may improve his emotional state and response to others, the need to communicate then becomes more urgent, and speech may subsequently enter a phase of more rapid development. This does not, however, exclude the possibility that such improvement in speech might have occurred had the environmental conditions remained unchanged. Speech is a social function, and happiness and a sense of security must encourage its development and use.

Where speech has developed and subsequently there is failure to use it normally, there may be an underlying disorder of personal emotional development, and it should then be recognised and treated as such. It may not then be a true disorder of speech, and speech therapy may be contra-indicated.

Where there is a true reversion to speech of a more infantile level, the disability is a functional one with failure to use rather than to develop normal speech. It should not be confused, however, with the periods of relapsing articulation experienced by many children with disorders of speech of organic origin during their progress towards the use of stable, normal articulation. Such a relapse is possible under emotional stress in the execution of almost any learned muscular skill, and does not indicate a true regression.

Again, an older child may imitate the speech of a younger member of the family, using this as a means to regain attention which has been unwisely and entirely directed by the parents or other relatives to a younger child. It may then be an intelligent attempt to adjust his environment more favourably, and may not indicate a regression to either a more infantile pattern of behaviour or of articulation. It should always be borne in mind that under the most difficult of environmental conditions many children develop and maintain normal use of speech. For want of a term to describe the defective articulation associated with these conditions we have for the present used the term dyslalia, indicating a defect in the use of the phonetic sounds of speech which is not the result of an organic failure for the neurological development of speech.

In cases of dyslalia a family history is rarely found. Speech develops early and consonant sounds are used with fluency although there may be many substitutions of one sound for another whilst other associated difficulties such as dyslexia are unlikely to occur. However, dyslexia may also be associated with emotional disturbance, rather than the result of a true organic disability.

THE DIFFERENTIAL DIAGNOSIS

Where dysarthria is part of an obvious or persisting minimal cerebral palsy, its recognition is determined on physical examination, but the differential diagnosis between isolated dysarthria and articulatory dyspraxia and between the latter and dyslalia may be less clear, especially when the condition is not severe. In isolated developmental dysarthria the characteristic appearances and defective movements of the muscles used in articulation are similar to those associated with cerebral palsy. In children with an articulatory dyspraxia these movements are apparently normal except when used for articulation. The specific clumsiness evident then appears to depend on a disturbance of function arising at a higher level of the nervous system than is involved in cases where neuromuscular function is visibly abnormal for all movements. The differentiation of articulatory dyspraxia from dyslalia may be less clear and may be decided only by the rate of spontaneous improvement or the response to treatment, when the greater difficulties experienced by the child with dyspraxia will assist the diagnosis. A careful case history may also suggest the possibility of a neurogenic rather than a functional basis for the disorder of speech.

When general mental deficiency and hearing loss can be excluded, the following summary may be found useful in assisting the differential diagnosis between isolated developmental dysarthria, articulatory dyspraxia and dyslalia.

	Isolated developmental dysarthria.
Family history.	Often positive.
Movements of tongue, lips and palate.	Movements of one or more muscle groups obviously affected. There may be excessive dribbling, or sucking, swallowing or chewing difficulties. Movements are limited, slow and clumsy.
Development of speech.	May occur at the normal time, but there is usually some delay which may be developmental aphasia or anarthria.
Articulation.	May be normal in isolation, in single words or syllables or at a slow speed in speech according to the degree of dysarthria. Consonants often omitted. Substitutions may be consistent and determined by the group of muscles chiefly affected. Consonant combinations often defective.
Vowels and diphthongs.	Usually normal, but sometimes defective, particularly diphthongs.
Ability to imitate the sounds of speech.	Normal on auditory stimulus alone within, the limits of muscular movement.
Phonation.	There may be inco-ordination, of phonation and articulation, or of both with respiration.
Rate of speech.	Increased rate, anxiety or excitement causes deterioration in muscle movements and articulation. Such relapses persist so long as neuromuscular control is inadequate.
Associated disabilities.	Aphasia, which may be persistent, Dyslexia, Spelling disability or Dysgraphia may occur in association with this condition.
Lateral dominance.	Left-sidedness is found more commonly than in the normal population, or there may be left-handedness in association with a preferred right eye.

THE DIFFERENTIAL

Articulatory dyspraxia	Dyslalia.
Often positive.	Infrequent.
No spasticity, normal movements of tongue, etc., except for articulation. These movements are not well directed and may appear awkward and clumsy during speech.	No obvious difficulties in the movements of the muscles for speech.
Often a little retarded, but usually within the normal range.	Normal age for speech development. Fluent.
The imitation and use of single sounds, syllables or words is better than their use in long sequences. Use of consonants and substitutions often erratic. There may be faulty pronunciation of whole words, transposition of sounds, reversals and perseveration.	Consonant substitutions usually consistent, sounds rarely omitted except in mental deficiency.
Usually normal, but are affected in some severe cases.	Normal.
Auditory stimulus may be insufficient. Imitation is assisted by visual stimulus and may be normal when the child is watching the therapist's movements. Seeing the word in print helps the older child.	Normal.
Usually normal.	Normal.
Speech can be rapid without deterioration in muscle movements, but use of consonants may deteriorate with stress. Periods of relapse occur until new habits of articulation are fully stabilised.	Normal speed, but some relapsing articulation occurs until normal articulation is stabilised.
Aphasia is rare, but there may be verbal paraphasia, or difficulties in the use of words, rather than a severe delay in the onset of speech. Dyslexia, especially if visual discrimination and visual memory for printed symbols is not well developed. Spelling disability. Dysgraphia.	Rare.
Cross laterality occurs more frequently than in the normal population—usually right-handedness in association with a preferred left eye.	The majority right sided, the proportion of left-sidedness and cross laterality being similar to that in the normal population.

Diagnosis—Summary

The Case History

The following points may assist the diagnosis:

1. *A family history of speech disorder*

This is common in developmental dysarthria and articulatory apraxia, but rare in dyslalia.

2. *Information concerning pregnancy, delivery and the onset of respiration*

Illness of the mother during the first three months of pregnancy, prematurity, abnormal delivery, or neonatal anoxia may suggest a neurogenic basis for the articulatory disorder.

3. *Infancy*

Information as to sucking or swallowing difficulties in early life may indicate some abnormality or inco-ordination of such developmental behaviour, and again the possibility of a developmental dysarthria.

4. *Motor development*

The age at which the child passed the various milestones in motor development, including toilet control, will be a guide as to the possibility of some degree of general motor disability, mental defect, or a combination of both. It should be noted if hand, foot and eye preference has been established. Scribbling with a crayon, drawing or writing, throwing and kicking a ball, and the eye test as described in Chapter XXI will give some indication as to whether the child is ambidextrous, right or left sided or cross-lateral.

5. *The age of speech development*

The age when words and phrases were first used and the age at which intelligible speech was established should be ascertained where possible. In dyslalia speech develops around the normal age. There may be some delay associated with articulatory apraxia, but except when there has also been a developmental aphasia speech develops within the normal age range. In some children with developmental dysarthria there may be considerable delay or an associated developmental aphasia.

6. *Personal development*

Are the child's interests appropriate to his age? Play interests, ability to amuse himself, interest in books and everyday life, such information contributes towards a fuller knowledge of the child and his mental development.

7. *Social behaviour*

What are his relations with other children? Does he share in their games on an equal basis, and is he accepted and liked by the group? The extent of his urge to be independent may also be a guide to true assessment.

Speech Assessment in Defective Articulation

If the child has been able to play freely with toys under discreet observation by the therapist whilst the case history was being taken, some information concerning his movements and play interest will already have been obtained. A first assessment must always be provisional and subject to modification in a young child whose reactions will be influenced by the strangeness of his surroundings. If the child feels that attention is being directed towards his mother rather than to himself, and that the therapist and his mother have established a friendly relationship whilst he has been apparently ignored, some conversational speech and a desire to take part in the relationship is often spontaneously forthcoming.

Language

The child's ability to use language should be compared with what is appropriate for his age level. In the older child any reading, spelling or writing difficulties should be assessed, and attempts to draw may demonstrate any failure of visual or spatial perception (see also p. 44).

Movements of tongue and lips

Movements of the tongue, lips and lower jaw should be watched during speech, and if there is any nasality, palatal movements should be examined. The ability to protrude the tongue, move it from side to side and elevate the tip towards the nose should be noted, and also lip movements on request, but some children are too shy to permit a definite opinion, and movements may appear clumsy when this is in reality due to reluctance on the part of the child to co-operate fully. It is also important to observe these movements during the assessment of articulation.

Articulation

Before the therapist can begin to treat the child's defective phonological system, or decide whether or not treatment is necessary, an assessment of the child's phonological and phonemic ability is required.

There are many lengthy articulation tests, devised to assess the ability to use the phonetic sounds of speech in words, initially, medially and finally. However, these do not necessarily give a true indication of the child's ability or disability.

The ability to use certain phonetic sounds can vary under varying circumstances. It can vary according to its context and can be influenced by other sounds in sequence with it. For example, /ki:/ may be used normally when /ka:/ is not, the tongue position for the vowel sound modifying the articulation of /k/. The use of a phoneme can vary according to circumstances, such as whether the sound is produced in isolation, in a word, in a short phrase or in conversational speech. It may also vary if used spontaneously in naming an object or picture, or when repeating the same word after the therapist. If spontaneous improvement is occurring at the time of the assessment it is probable that there will be many temporary inconsistencies and variations in phonemic usage. Where improvement is occurring rapidly the results of a lengthy test obtained one day may be markedly changed a week, or a month later, depending on the rate of such spontaneous improvement. Psychological and physiological factors, such as boredom and fatigue also complicate the outcome of the test procedures. Winitz (1970) also describes the variables which affect the results of articulation tests and discusses sources of error which may contribute to the unreliability of such tests.

Following the initial assessment, there should be continuing evaluation during treatment based on the child's response and reactions. Tests which show the child's reactions to simple tests under varying circumstances have been found most useful to the clinician, and provide an initial assessment which can be modified, if necessary. The tests described are simple, and useful for children from approximately three years of age, but should be modified to some extent according to the age and intelligence of the child.

The speech is assessed according to:

I. Level of intelligibility in conversational speech.
II. Phonological ability under varying conditions.
III. Imitative ability (including auditory discrimination, short-term memory and control of oral movements.

I. Level of intelligibility

1. Is the child easily intelligible to (*a*) the therapist; (*b*) the mother; (*c*) other children?
2. If not, does he use mime, gesture or other means to assist communication?
3. What are his emotional reactions? Is he frustrated when not understood? Or is speech inhibited, perhaps indicating excessive correction at home?
4. Are there any circumstances under which speech is more intelligible? For example, when using single words? Does intelligibility deteriorate in longer sentences?

II. Phonological ability under varying linguistic conditions

1. Assessed in single words. The child is asked to repeat after the therapist a short series of words which should be familiar even to the young child, and which consist mainly of one consonant and one vowel or diphthong, for example, pie, boy, tie, door, car, go, fire, see, shoe, chair, jam, letter, water, you (or yellow, yes), red (or road, read). Phoneme clusters, or blends, may also be tested if there is no severe difficulty, spoon, stop, slide, smile, snail, swim, school.

   Use of the initial consonant is noted.
2. The child is next asked to repeat simple phrases and phoneme sequences.

Pay Paul for the paper.
It is tea-time.
A cup of coffee.
Four bonfires.
Shine your shoes.
A jar of jam.
A long letter.
A big boy.
To-day is Monday.

A good game.
Sing a song.
A lot of cheeping chicks.
Round and round in a ring.
Also, Spin a top; Stir the soup.
Swing up to the sky; A fly on the wall; Higher still they climb.

The use of individual phonemes is noted and of phoneme clusters as they are used in the phrases repeated. It is also noted whether voiced or voiceless consonants give greater difficulty, whether sounds are used in medial and final positions; whether plosive or fricative consonants present greater difficulty.

Careful assessment concerning the distinctive features used by the child will give some guide as to the severity of the condition. A child who can already use a distinctive feature, such as continuant (or fricative) in some phonemic sequences will have less difficulty in acquiring other phonemes with the same distinctive feature than one who cannot use this feature in any circumstances. For a full assessment the distinctive features, described by Jackson, Halle and Ernst,* as used by

* For a full description of the articulatory correlates of the distinctive features as discussed in this article, see 'On the Bases of Phonology' by Morris Halle in *The Structure of Language*, J. Foder and J. Katz (eds.) Prentice-Hall, Inc. June 1965. The following is a brief outline. *Grave* phonemes are articulated with a primary narrowing located at the periphery of the oral cavity (i.e. at the lips or in the velar region). *Nongrave* phonemes are produced with the primary narrowing in the central (i.e. dental-alveolar-palatal) region. [p], [m], [k], and [ŋ] are grave; [θ], [ʃ], [t], and [d] are nongrave. *Diffuse* phonemes are produced with a constriction in the front part of the vocal tract (i.e. alveolar ridge, forward). *Nondiffuse* phonemes have narrowings in the posterior part of the vocal tract, from behind the alveolar ridge, backward. [p], [d], and [s] are diffuse; [ʃ], [k], and [dʒ] are nondiffuse. *Strident* consonants are produced by directing the air stream at an angle across a sharp edge, or parallel over a rough surface, causing turbulence. *Nonstrident* consonants occur when one or several of these features are missing. [s], [tʃ], and [dʒ] are strident; [b], [θ], and [g] are nonstrident. *Voiced* phonemes are produced with vibration of the vocal folds. *Voiceless* phonemes are produced without vocal vibration. [v], [z], and [ʒ] are voiced; [t], [ʃ], and [k] are voiceless. *Nasal* phonemes are produced with the velum lowered. *Nonnasal* phonemes are produced with a raised velum and naso-pharyngeal closure. Only [m], [n], and [ŋ] are nasal, all other phonemes are non-nasal. *Continuant* phonemes are produced with a vocal tract which is narrowed but just short of full occlusion. *Interrupted* phonemes are produced when the vocal tract is effectively closed at some point of contact before release. [ð[, [ʒ], and [f] are continuant; [t], [d], and [g] are interrupted.

the child, will be an indication as to prognosis and whether or not spontaneous improvement is probable. A short description of these distinctive features is given in the footnote.

3. The child may then be asked to say a rhyme (if he knows one), and it is noted whether or not he is able to use the phonemes he was able to use in (1) and/or (2). Is he using them consistently in all positions in words, or is there deterioration in these longer linguistic sequences?

4. He is then asked to repeat a story, phrase by phrase, after the therapist, and again phonemic ability is noted in these longer sequences.

5. Phonological competence is next observed in conversational speech (if the child can be persuaded to talk freely whilst playing with toys, or with other children). A recording of the speech may be made and analysed later, if necessary.

III. Imitative ability

This is observed throughout the above tests. Does the child try to watch the therapist's oral movements? If so, does he imitate more accurately?

Does he attempt to use his fingers to guide his oral movements?

Was there any clumsiness or inaccuracy of movements of lips or tongue?

Was memory adequate for repetition of phrases of varying length?

Did phonemic ability deteriorate with phrases of increasing length?

Such tests are not standardised and cannot be used to compare the standard of one child's speech with that of another. Their value lies in the information they provide for prognosis and diagnosis. Such an assessment provides a clinical basis for initial treatment, and can be modified, if necessary, as treatment proceeds.

Hearing

If any doubt has arisen during the examination as to the child's ability to understand speech, a hearing assessment is necessary in order to arrive at a differential diagnosis between a partial hearing loss, receptive dysphasia, and mental deficiency.

Physical examination

If this has not been carried out before referral to the speech therapist, arrangements should be made for a full examination by a paediatrician or neurologist.

REFERENCES

Roberts, D. (1967). The Term Dyslalia: Its Uses and Values. *J. of Aust. Coll. of Sp. Therapists*, **17**, 2, 44.

Winitz, H. (1970). *Articulatory Acquisition and Behaviour*. New York, Appleton, Century Crofts.

XV. General Principles for the Treatment of Defective Articulation

SPEECH therapy aims to help each child to obtain speech which is useful for the purpose of communication, which is appropriate for his age, development and environment, and which does not attract undue attention as the result of any abnormality. It is not usually concerned with dialectal variations, nor does it attempt to develop the aesthetic use of speech as in reciting, or in association with dramatic art. Again it does not attempt merely to teach the correct pronunciation of words. It aims rather to ascertain any basic cause for the abnormal development of speech and to stimulate and encourage the development and use of those neurophysiological processes which are essential for the use of speech. The alteration of an abnormal phonological system may be more correctly described as the reorganisation of a function with the formation of a new functional system. In attempting this, the therapist must consider the patient as a whole, and in relation to his environment, and not merely his use, or mal-use, of articulate speech. Success is indicated not by ability to use phonemes normally in controlled, conscious speech but by the carry-over into conversational speech with normal linguistic competence. Knowledge of the phonemes of a language does not necessarily give one the ability to speak the language. What is required is the ability to speak without conscious effort whilst producing the sound patterns characteristic of the language of the community. Whilst knowledge of the phonemic structure of a language may be useful, even an essential basis for an adult acquiring a new language, it is doubtful if too much awareness of individual phonemes does not hinder rather than help the child in changing defective patterns of articulation.

There are many variations within the range of what may be considered normal speech, and in the level to which the individual's neuromuscular skills can be developed, but the majority are able to achieve what is the essential articulatory skill for speech, with or without assistance. Where the speech disability is so severe that this is not possible, the aim must always be the development of articulation which is as intelligible and as useful as is possible.

The treatment of defective articulation is based on the physiological processes involved in speaking and in motor learning, and an understanding of the neurophysiological basis of motor learning provides information as to a rationale for treatment. Abnormal neuromuscular patterns of articulation have been acquired, and if not changed either spontaneously by the child or with assistance, may become stabilised and persist throughout life. Therapy consists in the development of normal or improved movements for speech and the substitution of normal phonemic patterns of articulation for those that are defective.

Whatever the basic cause of the speech disorder, whether it is due to a structural condition of the lips, tongue, palate or larynx, or to a delay in the neurological maturation for the reproduction of articulation, the child's speech ability is the result of several contributing factors such as intelligence, environment, acuity of hearing, the potential ability to think clearly, and to formulate and express such thoughts with adequate phonological and linguistic sequences.

The more intelligent child may be able to compensate to a greater extent for a similar disability. An intelligent partially deaf child may be educable in the normal school, whereas a less intelligent child with a similar hearing loss may need education in a special school for the partially deaf. The child with a severe dysarthria as the result of cerebral trauma may have no articulatory apraxia, and may therefore achieve slow, laboured but intelligible articulation, whereas the child with a cleft palate and also some degree of apraxia for articulation may develop or retain faulty habits of articulation despite an excellent surgical result. Always the total sum of the factors involved must be recognised and considered in assessing the child's disability, the prognosis, and in planning treatment. Each child presents an individual problem, and treatment for defective articulation must be varied and designed to meet the level of intelligence, the stage of language development and any neurological or structural condition which may influence articulation.

Treatment should involve as little correction of actual speech as possible. The young child feels annoyed and frustrated if his conversational attempts are interrupted for the correction of a word he has pronounced incorrectly. Unaware that he is expressing his thoughts through articulation which may be unintelligible, he resents the interruption in his flow of speech and thought. He is not normally aware of the sounds he uses, nor even that speech consists of words, until he begins to read. Even should no non-fluency develop, the child may hesitate to speak for fear of using a sound which he has been told is incorrect. For this reason it has been suggested that therapy should make no direct approach to speech whatever, and that some form of self-expression through play therapy may be all that is necessary. The establishing of a friendly relationship between therapist and patient is always helpful, and indeed essential, and spontaneous improvement may gradually occur during such treatment. We have seen how, in the majority of children with defects of articulation such as dyslalia, or stammering during the early stages of speech development, there is gradual progress towards normal speech without any direct form of treatment. Play therapy has been found useful in such children who are too young for and may never need direct speech therapy. However, reassurance of the mother without some form of treatment may be insufficient to allay her anxiety, and positive help may be required. Ferrie (1952) stated that 'because no direct therapy has been given (the mother) continues to force speech upon her child, and so by her misdirected efforts at correction only increases the difficulty'.

Play therapy may be especially useful with young children who are late in developing expressive speech, as in developmental aphasia, and may be all that is possible with some more backward children where intelligent co-operation may never be gained. Observation of children's play also leads to a fuller understanding of the personality and difficulties of each child, and thereby may assist diagnosis of the speech or hearing defect.

Where the child has a more severe disorder of articulation, such as developmental dysarthria or articulatory apraxia, play therapy will generally be insufficient in itself, and a more direct approach to speech therapy will also be necessary.

Treatment for defective articulation must involve the physiological processes of motor learning, requiring, as it does, the neuromuscular skill for the initiation and control of the complex movements which make audible the phonological sounds in the correct phonemic sequences of any linguistic system. Only thus does spoken language become intelligible to others. In this way articulation is comparable to the expression of musical thought through the controlled and learned movements of the fingers on the keyboard of the piano, or of language through the typist's fingers on the keys of the typewriter. It is therefore dependent upon habit. The child learns through the performance of the action, and repeated sensorimotor experience would seem to be more important than reason in the actual process of acquiring or changing motor skills and co-ordinations.

Articulation requires the co-ordination of the muscles not only of the mouth, but also of those involved in respiration, and phonation, in addition to the oral movements and adjustments required for the differentiation of the phonetic sounds used in speech. Lenneberg (1967) pointed out that this includes muscles of the thoracic and abdominal walls, the neck, face pharynx and oral cavity, which means that over 100 muscles must be centrally controlled and used with great rapidity and variations of movement at the speed required for conversational speech. It is therefore essential that *automatic sequences*, or neurophysiological patterns develop, as voluntary, conscious control is impossible for the complexity and speed of the movements required. It is for this reason that children who are taught only to produce sounds, and use them in words with conscious control, fail to change easily their abnormal phonological patterns in syntactic and linguistic sequences in conversational speech.

It has been previously described how, during the process of acquiring articulate speech, muscle movements made by the child produce sounds, and he then experiences sensory feedback through multiple internal circuit loops (pp. 12–21). The receptor processes involved are (1) auditory feedback through the auditory system and (2) the surface receptors, with tactile, proprioceptive and kinaesthetic feedback for the contacts and movements produced. Thus the feedback loops complete the circuit, and sensorimotor activity becomes self-reinforcing (see also p. 14). When the child reproduces a sound which he hears made by another, external to himself, the sound which he utters is again reinforced through his own feedback experience, and identified with the sounds he hears as made by others. In this way he is learning through experience, and approximating his phonemic patterning towards the normal. If a child is unable to modify his own phoneme imitations towards the expected normal standards, then defective articulatory patterns will be used and increasingly stabilised. In this way the child develops two phonological systems, one which he hears and through which he understands the speech of others, and another his defective phonological system which he uses in speech.

Normally, we are unaware of the existence of these various sensory feedback processes, although they continue to monitor speech subconsciously. Their existence becomes more evident when an unaccustomed error occurs in one's own speech. Their importance may also be experienced when they are temporarily suspended, as in conditions of extreme noise, when one cannot hear oneself speak, or after a dental anaesthetic, when we cannot adequately monitor speech through a temporary failure of tactile and proprioceptive feedback.

Walking and articulate speech are two motor skills which we normally acquire so early in life that their development is mainly dependent upon direct imitation at a subconscious level. The muscle movements and co-ordinations are controlled below the level of conscious thought, and, once they have become established at the automatic level, attempts to bring any such activity into the foreground of consciousness may result in some degree of inco-ordination. This is an important consideration in planning therapy procedures.

Many have considered, and have investigated the possibility, that a limitation of auditory discrimination, or a tactile or proprioceptive deficiency, could be the cause of the faulty development of articulation.

Auditory discrimination. Tests for consonant discrimination and recognition, in older children and adults with normal articulation, indicates a considerable variation and range of normality, and it is apparent that some individuals who have normal articulation for all the phonological elements of speech, experience varying degrees of difficulty for the discrimination of speech sounds in certain prescribed tests, when hearing for pure tones is normal, and comprehension for spoken language is adequate. Such tests usually require conscious intellectual processes which may play little or no part in the spontaneous subconscious discrimination and developing use of articulation in infancy. Even the student of phonetics has been known to experience difficulty in reproducing an unfamiliar phonetic sound and yet be able to distinguish, recognise it, and write the correct symbol in phonetic dictation.

It may be suggested that slow maturation for the process of perception and sound discrimination may account for the development of faulty articulation in early childhood, which then persists due to habit when the causative factor is no longer operative. At an age when the tests would be valid, the child is too young to give a reliable response in such an unnatural situation. Training in auditory discrimination naturally produces an improved response, but this could result from increased attention, concentration and a learned ability to carry out the tests, and not necessarily from improvement in the neurophysiological processes of perception. Interest, auditory attention and other conditions relating to environment must also affect the results of such tests and of training for auditory discrimination.

Locke and Goldstein (1971) have studied the relationship between phoneme production and phoneme perception and state that it has never been determined whether discrimination tasks are appropriate in assessing children's phoneme perception. They think there is reason to believe that their use may be inappropriate. They, and others, have found that children's error rates are considerably greater on discrimination tests than they are on articulation tests (Kamil and Rudegeair, 1969) and that many children with normal articulation miss items on discrimination tests. They also found that recognition tests appeared to be a more sensitive index than discrimination tests in detecting perceptual errors in phonetic contexts produced incorrectly. However, they state, that neither test demonstrated a close relationship between misarticulation and misperception in children. Boothroyd (1968) studied the influence of the acoustical properties of sounds, probability of occurrence, and contextual factors, such as the influence of adjacent sounds, phoneme probabilities, and a vocabulary factor. His findings indicated that a score based upon the percentage of recognised phonemes is a more valid measure of the ability to make phonemic classifications from intrinsic acoustical clues than a score based on the percentage of recognised words.

Weiner (1967) distinguished between self-discrimination (SD) and 'other' discrimination (OD). The former required the child to monitor his own speech to discriminate between paired stimulii presented, whilst other discrimination requires the child to discriminate between paired stimulii produced by another speaker. Aungst and Frick (1964) and Woolf and Pilberg (1971) also report that the results of such tests have indicated that a judgement of 'right' or 'wrong', as the child listens to his own production of a word (that is SD) is the most difficult; that it is less difficult for him to respond correctly giving a 'same' or 'different' response to a word spoken by himself and also by another, but easy for him to give an accurate 'same' or 'different' response when the two words are spoken by another (OD). Winitz (1970) has given much attention to this subject and now questions the assumption that defective auditory discrimination is the main cause of defective articulation.

Fry (1968) suggests that children appear to possess *two* phonological systems, a normal one for perception, and an abnormal one for production. Whilst these two systems do not appear to be necessarily entirely independent, their limited correspondence would seem to question the value of the time spent on the testing and training of auditory discrimination and phoneme perception in treatment when it is divorced from simultaneous motor experience.

Surface receptor discrimination. Other sensory processes, tactile, kinaesthetic and proprioceptive, are also involved in the development and maintenance of speech. However, although they play an essential part, the accurate assessment of their relative significance in the appreciation of articulate sounds, or in sensorimotor control for the reproduction of phonemes in speech, is also difficult. Ringel *et al.* (1965) and others have carried out tests for tactile perception of the tongue, lips and palate, using two-point discrimination, and of texture discrimination (1967). They also designed tests for oral kinaesthesia which required intact central nervous relay networks for normal function. They found that significant differences existed for tactile discrimination between the various oral and extra oral structures, such as the lips, tongue and palate. Tests for oral stereognosis, or the ability to recognise the form of objects, have also been devised (Ringel *et al.*, 1968), using small plastic geometric shapes which can be placed in the mouth for testing discrimination of shape. Such tests, carried out on 22 university students with normal articulation, were compared with those on 27 students who had defective articulation. The age range was from 18 to 25 years. Their findings support the view that persons with articulation defects experience greater difficulty than those with normal articulation in tests of oral discrimination.

Fawcus (1971) reports on techniques he has devised to assess the efficiency of the lingual sensorimotor system and to explore the relationship between performance in these tests and differing types of articulatory dysfunction. He describes difficulties such as the maintenance of the subject's head in one position, the employment of transducers and connecting wires in the mouth, and the difficulty which many individuals encounter when attempting to articulate with foreign objects in the mouth, all of which tend to invalidate the findings. He has used a device which will transmit information regarding pressure changes in the mouth during speech with no more interference than may normally be incurred in wearing a dental plate. This will be used to investigate the relationship between feedback and articulatory performance, but no results are presented as yet.

It is probable that the indefinite and sometimes contradictory findings in such testing is due to the selection of individuals with defective articulation. As has been described (p. 207) this is not a simple group. Some children may have a severe defect and signs indicative of articulatory dyspraxia or minimal dysarthria, whilst others may have defects related to agnosia. Others may have less severe defects where there is little or no residual underlying sensorimotor disability at the time of testing. Were the selection of individuals based on a more accurate diagnosis of the underlying condition, it is possible that, in some types of defective articulation, sensory defects might prove to be significant.

Present day trends in thinking are therefore tending to place a decreasing emphasis on auditory training and discrimination during therapy.

To summarise the processes involved in the development of articulation in speech: The infant's utterance of sounds are at first *reflex*, then *spontaneous* and finally, *imitative*. By this means sensorimotor experience is acquired and the motor skill developed. Vocalising and babbling develop the co-ordinations of breath with vocal tone and oral sounds, and it matters little what sounds are uttered, as all provide exercise for the development, control and co-ordination of the essential skills for eventual phonological competence. The child is not taught to imitate. How does he know what movements to make? He cannot see himself and the oral movements he is making. Environmental reinforcement may encourage him to continue, but does not account for the fact that such imitative behaviour is universal in children, regardless of environment and reinforcement.

During these developmental stages the child reproduces and associates both the sounds he himself makes, that is self imitation, and the sounds he hears from others (see p. 13). Thus vocalising and babbling reinforce the sensory feedback processes, auditory, tactile and kinaesthetic, at the same time as the motor skill is developing. Increasing discrimination for phonemic sequences is associated with increasing mobility, selectivity, control and co-ordination of the motor activity for articulation. This is the basis for all such development, continuing until the child's speech approaches that of his environment through maturation and learning.

Learning, in its psychological aspects, involves the acquisition of new goals through direct information, imitation, and the association of new goals with existing ones, stimulated through reinforcement of the required behaviour. Through such learning, behaviour can be shaped within the limits of anatomical and neurological potential, to approximate to the required response, or extinction of a non-required response by withdrawal of reinforcement. Learning also occurs through, and is reinforced by experience.

This developing skill is probably innate in an organism biologically predisposed to the production of oral language (Lenneberg, 1967; Geschwind, 1965). A child exposed to a particular language system will systematically and rapidly acquire its phonological and grammatical rules. These rules are not explicitly presented to the child by his environment which, in general, is not consciously aware of them (Chomsky, 1965). In further support of this view, it has been demonstrated that, regardless of their culture, most children appropriately use the basic structure of their language by three and a half years of age (McNeill, 1966; Morley, see p. 44) and most acquire adequate control of the phonology by about four and a half years at the latest. However, speech patterns are essential, and environmental stimulation and reinforcement helpful, to the child's acquisition of any particular language system, in all its linguistic, social and psycholinguistic aspects. The child learns *what* to produce from his environment, but the environment does not usually teach him *how* to produce it; this he does for himself with very little effort in the process of acquiring an entire language system (Morley and Fox, 1969).

As linguistic performance develops, the child does not necessarily select the phonological sounds he requires from his repertoire of babbling sounds, but rather uses his acquired sensorimotor skills to imitate directly the phonemic sequences he hears. Thus he may not always use correctly the phonological elements he used in babbling. Through the development of sensorimotor skills, he has at his disposal the phonological ability required to imitate a linguistic sequence, and this he does normally or not according to the length and complexity of the sequence and his underlying ability.

Changing a child's phonemic patterns, when it is necessary to do so and however it is done, must produce at least some temporary difficulties and selfconsciousness, and if the child is expected to consciously discriminate between sounds, and to change phonemic sequences in his conversational speech, it is demanding much. If the therapist has attempted to change one phoneme for another, say /t/ for /k/ in his own conversational speech for a period of five minutes he can appreciate a little of what is being asked of the child. It matters little that one is substituting a faulty sound. This is how it appears to the child.

This difficulty must be due to the fact that speech does not consist of a series of phonetic sounds, but of integrated phonemic and linguistic sequences and patterns, established through usage. The child has increasingly stabilised his own sensorimotor feedback circuit for such sequences, and accepted his defective articulation as normal. However, if he hears a recording of his own speech, or hears it repeated by others through the external feedback circuit, he is at once aware that it differs from what he normally hears used by others.

Resistance to change. Due to the way in which a child develops his phonological system, as described, through learning, maturation and sensorimotor experience, he equates his own phonological patterning with that of others. Being unaware that his speech differs from that which he hears, unless corrected or not understood, he can make little or no attempt to change his defective phonemic patterns without help. He will resist change when required to incorporate what are to him incorrect phoneme sequences into his own linguistic system. The use of newly acquired phonemes in speech is therefore difficult until such time as the new sensorimotor associations are fully developed at the automatic level, at first independently of linguistic context, until they can be accepted by the child in both their motor and sensory aspects. Only when such resistance to change is fully overcome, will the child begin to incorporate, without conscious thought, his new phonological ability into his linguistic system.

Correction of a child's speech should, therefore, not be undertaken lightly, especially if there is any possibility that speech may improve spontaneously. Spontaneous improvement can be assessed if the child is seen at intervals of one month for a period of three months. At each visit the speech is assessed as previously described, when it becomes obvious if the disability is static, or there is any tendency towards improvement in phonemic usage without treatment.

Reasons for treatment. However, there are several reasons which indicate that direct therapy should not be delayed. Firstly, if the phonological ability is inadequate for the child's needs to communicate with others. The more intelligent the child, and the greater his linguistic ability, apart from intelligibility, the greater the need for therapy to obviate the frustration that he will experience.

Secondly, entrance to school may be questioned, or progress retarded in school, if unintelligible speech persists. It is useful if the child is at least intelligible when he enters school and broadens his social contacts outside the home circle.

Thirdly, if the parents are anxious, and unable to avoid correcting the child's speech to the point of exasperation by the mother, and inhibition of speech on the part of the child, something should be done without further delay. The child will be reassured that his problem is understood and help available, and the mother's anxiety relieved by the fact that her child is receiving treatment, and by guidance in understanding how to help her child in a useful way, and so provide an outlet for her problem.

Treatment. It is suggested, therefore, that therapy should follow these normal developmental processes, as described, training sensorimotor skills and using maturation and learning. Therapy will therefore be dependent upon the change of movement patterns associated with phonological changes, rather than the introduction of individual sounds into linguistic sequences in conversational speech, at least in the early stages of treatment.

Because the present state of our knowledge makes us uncertain as to the exact point of breakdown in the sensorimotor circuit, the method of treatment to be described aims to develop normal phonological patterning with no isolated approach to either the motor or sensory processes involved. The motor, transmitting, integrating and sensory functions are simultaneously involved, and thereby auditory discrimination in association with other sensory processes and with motor patterning, is directly improved.

Prognosis. Progress will be slow in the treatment of children with a severe developmental dysarthria or articulatory dyspraxia. The ability to increase the range, ease and speed of the movements of articulation will vary according to the severity of the brain damage or the extent of the delay in maturation, as will also the child's ability to imitate consonant sounds normally in isolation, in single words, phrases, or in conversational speech. Sometimes articulation may be almost normal when speech is slow, but there may be failure to maintain it at conversational speed or under stress.

Where faulty phonemic patterns have become stabilised in older children, improvement in articulation may be hindered when there has been progress or recovery in the underlying potential neuromuscular ability. One child, aged 11 years, was referred for speech therapy following an illness diagnosed as bulbar poliomyelitis. The soft palate had been affected, and nine months after recovery from her illness speech was of cleft palate type, almost unintelligible, and with incompetent use of the nasopharyngeal sphincter. Following referral for speech therapy, progress was rapid during the first month, suggesting that the child had failed to make use of what physical improvement had occurred. At this stage a slight nasal leak of air persisted, and this was only slowly eradicated during the following six months. It seems possible, therefore, that the patient's ear may become accustomed to the abnormal phonemic patterns arising at a time when there is an organic dysfunction, and that if this condition persists for a sufficiently long period the ability to regain normal articulation spontaneously may be lost, even when the organic basis for the dysfunction may have resolved completely.

Many therapists develop their own methods of treatment through experience, and such methods may be more successful in their hands than any other. The method of treatment to be described here was developed from an appreciation of the processes underlying the normal development of articulation as described, and has sometimes been described as 'Babbling'. However, apart from the pleasure associated with the utterance of sounds, it does not correspond to the spontaneous babbling of infancy. It is based on and follows normal development of phonemic patterns, being the growth, elaboration and integration with developing language of the various phonological elements to ensure that language is intelligible to others. It is related to normal linguistic development in that it requires first, the development of the use of the simplest phonological element—the phonetic sound; secondly, the association of this sound with other sounds in phonemic sequences, and thirdly, its gradual introduction into linguistic sequences of increasing length.

Principles of treatment will first be described for those articulatory disorders of speech where there is no associated general motor disability causing dysarthria. In children with generalised spasticity or involuntary movements, the treatment as outlined requires certain modifications which will be subsequently described.

In describing this method of treatment one is describing nothing new, but merely utilising the normal and natural processes of speech development in both its physiological and linguistic aspects, as has been outlined previously. It is based upon the psychological factors involved in learning, and maturation of the neurophysiological skills which are basic to the normal acquisition and usage of the phonological elements in their linguistic contexts.

Aims of treatment

(1) To establish a normal relationship between the child's phonological system for reception of speech, usually normal, and his defective system for production.

(2) To establish the normal *movements* for articulation of the phonetic elements which are defective or absent from the child's phonological system.

Various processes are involved in motor learning: (*a*) inhibition of faulty movements; (*b*) facilitation of correct movements; (*c*) association of these movements into phonemic units and sequences and sensorimotor associations; and (*d*) stabilisation of these new patterns of movement through adequate experience and practice. Active movement is essential for the origin and maintenance of normal sensorimotor co-ordinations.

(3) To give the child sufficient sensorimotor experience until the new phonemic patterns are (*a*) acceptable to the child, and (*b*) can be used at an appropriate speed, automatically, and without conscious thought and control.

(4) To prevent any disruption of the normal rhythm and fluency of the child's speech, whether this be intelligible to others or not. There should be no correction at home or during therapy of the defective articulation as the child uses it in his conversational speech. He will accept it in other circumstances (to be described, p. 328).

Once the child has gained adequate control of the normal phonetic sounds, and normal phoneme sequences are fully established during treatment, the majority of children will themselves gradually incorporate them into their own speech, naturally, with the minimum of guidance, and in all normal linguistic sequences, usually quite unaware that they are doing so. Thus the phonological system becomes increasingly normal and speech intelligible to others.

Four steps in treatment

Therapy is arranged in four steps as follows:

1. Correct movement for and imitation of the simplest linguistic elements of speech; that is the correct movement for the production of a phonetic sound in isolation, based on inhibition of the faulty movements and facilitation of the correct one.
2. The second step requires the introduction of this new sound into the simplest phonetic sequences, that is the syllable, consisting of one consonant and one vowel—CV. This involves the building up of associations between one sound and another in sequences. Physiologically, the syllable is the morphological unit of speech, and articulatory movements are auxiliary movements in the syllable. Therefore, if the child can use articulatory movements automatically in syllables he will be able to combine these syllables in words, phrases and sentences. Van Riper also describes how the phonetic stabilisation of a new sound is best begun through the use of what he describes as 'nonsense' syllables used for strengthening a new sound, and not associated with faulty linguistic patterns already acquired.

   Linguistically, the English structure is based on sounds organised into syllables (Gleason, 1955), one or more consonant sounds being associated with a vowel, V, either before the vowel, CV, or following the vowel, VC. Words then consist of one or more syllables. Whilst vocabulary changes with time, and is a transient feature of language, the basic structure of sound patterns remains constant.
3. The syllable is next incorporated into the simplest form of

phrase without meaning, that is the repetition of one consonant/vowel syllable in sequence, as CV CV CV, or [pɑ:pɑ:pɑ:]. In this way, through practice, the new sequential associations are stabilised until they are completely automatic.

4. At this stage the consonant/vowel sequences are varied in meaningful linguistic phrases, involving increasing associations and stabilisation of the newly acquired patterns of articulation as they are used in linguistic sequences.

Stage 1. Correct movement for each phonetic sound in isolation

When substituting a new consonant sound for a defective one the child is required to inhibit the old faulty sensorimotor pattern and substitute another. The difficulty in accomplishing this can be better appreciated if one considers substituting, for example, /t/ for /s/ in one's own speech, or developing the use of a consonant sound used in the language of another country of which one has no experience in one's own speech.

At first it may be necessary to obtain and practise the sound in isolation. In so doing it is helpful if the defective muscular movement is restrained, as, for example, by holding the lower lip away from the upper incisor teeth with the fingers whilst the child attempts to substitute a tongue movement for the articulation of [*θ* (th)], when formerly [f] was used. Similarly, the tip of the tongue may be prevented from touching the alveolus by restraining its upward movement with a finger, spatula or spoon handle whilst attempting the movement of the tongue required for [k], when [t] has previously been substituted. Closing the nostrils by finger pressure will inhibit nasal escape of air when there is inadequate use of the nasopharyngeal sphincter until control is acquired and whilst the child experiences the normal articulation of a consonant sound. Pressure of the cheeks against the lateral teeth by the child's or therapist's fingers will prevent lateral escape of air as on a lateral [s] until the child has so adjusted the position of the tongue tip that the air stream can be directed between the central incisor teeth for the normal articulation of [s].

The therapist assists the child in every possible way, by guiding the tongue or lips, using a spatula, a teaspoon, a finger, or the child's finger, etc. and visual guidance, either direct imitation of the therapist or using a mirror, until the required sound, perhaps through a series of approximations, is achieved. The child then experiences the sound as a new phonetic unit and can accept it more readily because it is divorced from his normal linguistic usage and familiar conversational speech.

If the consonant is a plosive it will be associated with a simple voiced or unvoiced vowel sound such as /ə/ or /ʌ/. If it is a fricative (continuant) it should be sustained as C-------, thus allowing time for the child to fully experience both the motor and sensory aspects of the sound he is producing. This training by direct imitation is continued intermittently so as to maintain the child's interest until he reproduces the required sound normally, automatically and without hesitation, on direct stimulation by the therapist. Through such imitation he develops the correct association between what he hears from the therapist and the sound he makes himself. Although operant conditioning, as such, is not used, nevertheless the child is of course told when the sound he is making is good (faulty attempts being ignored), and encouragement being given for improvement and approach towards the normal, as well as for complete success.

Each phenome to be corrected should be introduced as a 'new' (to the child) phonetic sound, and practised as an isolated sound for possibly half a minute several times a day, for perhaps a week. This is not done as a lesson but at odd moments, preferably at home with the mother, during play or even in the bath!

In severe cases of dysarthria associated with cerebral palsy, inhibition may be used in a wider sphere to restrain abnormal movements of the whole body, or parts of the body, as the result of abnormal reflex activity.

Facilitation

As described, the development of a new articulatory movement is facilitated by inhibition of the old defective one, and the child may then be able to imitate the normal movements required for articulation of a sound, at least in isolation, on auditory stimulus alone. Watching the therapist's tongue and lip movements, or his own in a mirror, may also facilitate normal articulatory movements. All therapists develop various devices for facilitating the movements required for articulation, but the following are suggestions based on clinical experience. These are related to the order of development of new consonant sounds, the use of associated articulatory positions, of similarities and of contrasts.

The order of development of consonant sounds. Use should always be made, in the first place, of what the child is able to do. It is therefore useful initially to practise simple multi-syllable drills on consonant sounds the child can use normally. These may be /p/ /b/ /t/ or /d/. Lip and tongue-tip movements and control are improved thereby, and the child gains confidence and pleasure in doing what is well within his power.

New sounds should always be learnt and practised in the order which the individual child finds most easy. This must be found by testing, and is extremely variable. The practice of some sounds may facilitate the use of others. For example, the practice of [t] or [θ (th)], if normal, may help the control of the tongue tip and render it less difficult to obtain [s].

Associated positions for articulation. If a consonant sound is made too far back in the mouth, a sound more forward than the one required should first be practised. For example, when [s] is produced by a fricative sound in the position of the plosive sound [k], or is pharyngeal, the practice of [θ (th)] or of [f] is useful in first giving the sensation of a fricative sound further forward in the mouth. Such over-correction may assist the production of [s]. This may be obtained approximately at first, or even temporarily, as an interdental lisp.

The consonants [k] and [g] are sometimes acquired more easily in conjunction with a vowel sound requiring a similar position of the tongue such as [i: (ee)], and children who can imitate [ki:] may have greater difficulty in obtaining [kɑ:] and continue to say [tɑ:].

Again, a child who can use [s] normally when associated with [p] in *spoon* may substitute [f] for [s] when it is associated with [w] as in *swim*, and say *fwim*. Whilst such faulty associations must be broken down, this principle may also be applied to help the child to acquire new consonant sounds.

Similarities. Most children have more difficulty in using fricative rather than plosive consonants, although this is not always so. It is most useful then to obtain one fricative sound, or even a sibilant soft whistle through the teeth or lips. Whichever fricative sound can be obtained most easily should first be developed. Other fricative consonants can later be obtained by changing the position at which the sound is produced on the outgoing air stream, once it has been acquired and controlled for one such sound.

Voiceless consonants are frequently more defective, and may be more difficult to obtain, than the voiced consonants. This is commonly so in articulatory apraxia, whilst in the child with a cleft palate the reverse is often found, as a result of faulty neuromuscular co-ordinations between phonation and the use of the nasopharyngeal sphincter. Again, treatment should be so arranged that one voiced or voiceless consonant should first be acquired. As neuromuscular control improves with the practice of what the child finds possible, he is eventually able to obtain the sounds which at one time were too difficult.

Contrasts. Some children may be helped by the practice of contrasting sounds such as [t] and [k], if [t] has been substituted for [k]. The child is thereby helped to appreciate the difference between the old and the new sensori-motor patterns as said by himself. He can usually readily hear the difference when the sounds are articulated by the therapist, and the only ear training which is probably of value is that which ensues as the child hears *himself* repeating the sounds, and associates them correctly with those he hears said by others.

Some children may have a temporary difficulty in retaining a consonant sound already in use. For example, if [t] has been substituted for [k] and the child develops the use of [k], he may lose the sound [t] and substitute [k] for [t]. *Cat*, which was formerly *tat*, will then be *kak*, and *tea* will become *kee*. If the child then practises the two sounds alternately, contrasting them in such exercises as [tə:kə:tə:kə:tə:kə:], he will more readily appreciate the difference between them and retain both sounds.

Auditory training. Although training in auditory discrimination is not used in isolation, it occurs naturally throughout. The child is continually associating the new motor and sensory patterns through his own internal feedback loops, and simultaneously comparing and associating the new sounds he is making with those used by the therapist through an external feedback circuit.

Where there is a severe dysarthria or articulatory apraxia it may be necessary to facilitate the actual movement required, assisting the movements of lips or tongue by the fingers or with a spatula until the child experiences the actual sensorimotor patterns of normal articulation. Again such children may be helped, as is the blind or deaf child, by feeling with his fingers the movements of the therapist's tongue or lips.

Stage 2. Association—Sounds in simplest phonemic clusters, that is phonetic sequences in simple syllables

A newly developed isolated consonant sound will not be used in speech until it has been associated with vowel or other consonant sounds, as in simple syllables. Speech is a sequence of syllables rather than of isolated sounds, and the ability to use such sounds in association with others may not develop spontaneously.

Again, there must be development of the child's association between his changing auditory and kinaesthetic sensations involving repeated experience, and a gradual growth of association between the new articulatory patterns as now being attempted by the child with those he hears used by others.

Once the required movement has been achieved, and the correct sound produced, the building up of such normal associations and co-ordinations begins. Therefore, when a phonetic sound can be produced easily as described in (1) it is incorporated into the simplest *non-meaningful* sequence, the phoneme cluster or syllable, consisting of one consonant and one vowel, as CV, (or C-----V if C is continuant). The same consonant is then used with changing vowels, as CV_1, CV_2, CV_3, CV_4, CV_5 (*e.g.* kɑː, kei, kiː, kou, kuː). At first each syllable is repeated after the therapist. No more effort must be used than is normally used in uttering such a syllable. If there is difficulty in joining the consonant to the vowel a slight break between the consonant and vowel may help at first. It should not be emphasised, and the two sounds should be smoothly joined as soon as possible.

Again each syllable is repeated in turn after the therapist allowing exposure time for adequate sensorimotor experience.

At the same time the ability to imitate is trained by allowing the child to associate what he is saying with what the therapist has said.

It is important that in these initial stages these phoneme clusters should be disassociated from meaningful linguistic sequences, as in words and sentences, where the child has acquired defective patterning. The correct sounds are acquired with greater ease as *new* syllables, as the child is not then required, at this stage of therapy, to inhibit his established faulty linguistic associations in an attempt to replace them by new ones. For example, a child may have greater difficulty with the syllables Kɑː and kiː than with kouː as the first two may represent familiar objects, car and key, in which words he may have already substituted [t] as 'tar' and 'tea' (taː and tiː), and these patterns have become established and associated with meaning.

However, the vowel sounds and diphthongs used with the consonants should be those which occur frequently in the child's speech, such as [ɑː], [eiː], [iː], [ouː], [uː]. Many of these, with a consonant actually form either words of one syllable, or the initial syllable of a word, but, at this stage, it is best to discourage association with meaning.

Where the sound [s] has not been used and [t] has been substituted, the child may have difficulty in using the newly acquired [s] in syllables such as [siː]. He formerly said [tiː], and although he may now begin by using [s] he is unable to disassociate his former articulatory pattern and often uses [stiː]. The use of [t], being formerly associated with the vowel sound, is retained in addition to [s]. Practice of syllables using [st] as in [stɑː stiː stoː] and so forth deliberately, often contributes towards the child's appreciation of the difference between [siː] and [stiː] as said by himself, also contrasting the sounds in the syllables as [stɑː sɑː stiː siː stoː soː] and so forth.

Stage 3. Phonetic sequences of increasing length, without meaning

The syllable, once established, is next incorporated into the simplest form of phrase, that is the repetition of the CV syllable in sequences as CV CV CV, or CV × 3 (*e.g.* kɑː kɑː kɑː), with varying inflexion, intonation and rhythm as in normal speech.

The child should now be able to repeat the 3-syllable phrase after the therapist, perhaps slowly at first, but lightly and easily. As in (2), other vowels are used as $CV_1 \times 3$, $CV_2 \times 3$, etc. When automatic control of these 'phrases' is adequate, the speed is gradually increased until it at least equals that required for conversational speech. Until he can use the elements of speech automatically he cannot use them without conscious direction in speech.

If the child omits final consonants in his speech, he may require similar practice using consonants in the final position in syllables, as VC, or VC---- if C is a continuant, then V_1C, V_2C, etc. It is seldom necessary to practise these syllables rapidly; it is usually sufficient for the child to experience a consonant in the final position relative to a vowel. Consonants in the medial position occur in the three-syllable 'phrases' that is the $CV \times 3$ 'phrase'.

Similar treatment is also used for consonant blends at stages (2) and (3) as CC_1V, or C-----C_1V) as s----pɑ:, if the initial consonant is [s]. It is, of course, presumed that the child can already use the consonants separately as in (1) and (2) and (3), before proceeding to attempt blends.

Children enjoy the practice of these basic sounds and articulatory movements, and there should be no attempt to incorporate them into speech until their speed and ease are adequate.

The practice of isolated words involving meaning is entirely ignored at this stage in the treatment of a young child, and no correction of the pronunciation of words is permitted either at home or at the clinic. It is easier at first to obtain normal articulation of consonant sounds as described in simple exercises than in familiar words where the faulty articulatory pattern must be inhibited before a new pattern can be substituted.

If the right approach is used and the child's co-operation is obtained, he will achieve pleasure and satisfaction in the accomplishment of what is well within his capacity. The exercises are so simple that they can be carried out successfully by the mother each day in the home for a few minutes only, the length of time varying according to the age of the child and the stage reached in treatment. They are used as a form of vocal play and not taught as a lesson, and such practice not only assists but is probably essential for the acquisition of the associations which must be developed before the new articulatory patterns can be easily introduced into speech.

Exercises for movements of the tongue or lips are not generally used. The development of normal co-ordinations for speech involves a total pattern of response, associated with pleasure in the utterance of sounds, and not the development of individual muscles or isolated muscle groups. Articulation also requires very fine rapid movements, and these are probably best developed in exercises, which are accomplished with less effort and self-consciousness than when attention is directed towards unnecessarily exaggerated movements of the tongue and lips. Exercises may be needed for control of the muscles used in obtaining nasopharyngeal closure and for their co-ordination with articulation, or stretching exercises for the tongue may be useful when there is a short fraenum.

Again, in the child with a severe dysarthria or apraxia, associated with more widespread brain damage, the basic movements and co-ordinations of the lips, tongue or palate may need to be developed before exercises for articulation are attempted.

Stage 4. The incorporation of phonemic patterns into meaningful linguistic sequences

When at least four consonants can be used easily in 'phrases', as described in (3), the child can proceed directly to the introduction of these syllables into meaningful linguistic sequences, that is phrases involving the use of varying consonants and vowels. This is done through the repetition of meaningful phrases (not single words) of a story. (It should be noted that no attempt is made to teach the child to repeat lists of single words.) This procedure is begun before the child has full control of all normal phonology in order to maintain interest, and to accustom him to such repetition.

The child is not expected to incorporate into these linguistic sequences those phonemes which he cannot yet use, as described in (3), that is automatically at the speed of speech. Faulty articulation of phonemes should only be corrected in rhymes and stories when these are adequately controlled at stage (3), otherwise all errors are ignored until such time as the therapist knows that the required level of sensorimotor competence has been achieved, and the correct phoneme can be used and integrated into sequences with little or no loss of fluency.

As the child progresses, the length of the phrase to be imitated is increased from approximately two to four words or more, depending upon the number of syllables in each word. At times, it may be necessary to isolate a 3- or 4-syllable word, as perhaps 'elephant'. The number of syllables presented to the child is more important than the number of words, but meaning and suitable context are important within the child's ability at any one time.

When correction of any phoneme is necessary it should be done by reducing the length of the phrase, presenting the word with the defective phoneme in isolation but still as part of a phrase, or perhaps placing it *first* in a phrase, always, so far as is possible, maintaining the context. The skill of the therapist lies in presenting these phoneme sequences to the child so that he is given the greatest assistance with the minimum of conscious effort on his part. Rhythm, and suitable intonation must be used as the interest and meaning of the story require, and the child should be encouraged to look at pictures rather than attend too consciously and seriously to the phonemes and words he is using. Direct repetition is maintained at the automatic level, previously achieved in the earlier stages, so far as is possible. The faulty word may be repeated in isolation two or three times, but if a correct response is not available the faulty articulation should be accepted and further practice given on the incorrect phonological element as at the earlier stages.

The child who feels justly annoyed when his spontaneous speech is interrupted for the correction of defects of articulation will accept such correction much more readily when repeating rhymes or stories. Very simple rhymes are used, and an attempt is made to incorporate a new consonant sound into one or two words only. Little is lost if defective articulation of other words continues for the time being. Short sentences may be used, especially with meaning and personal significance for the child, but most children enjoy the rhythm of simple rhymes. More difficult rhymes should not be used. They can be of great value to the child with poor articulation and no true organic speech disability, who requires speech training only. Many of these rhymes include words which are much too difficult for the child with a real disorder of speech.

Stage 4. Stabilisation—Practice for the stabilisation of new phonemic sequences

In any learned motor skill, practice is essential until control can be relegated to the automatic level. In the procedures described there should be daily practice at each stage. This may vary from one minute or less several times a day, to five or ten minutes twice a day, or longer periods for older children and adults, according to the needs and possibilities of the individual.

Everyday experience proves that the performance of any action is rendered easier by repetition, and articulation is no exception. At first a sequence of actions may be slow and consciously directed, as in the young child endeavouring to fasten a button, tie a shoe lace or slowly repeat articulatory syllables, but repeated attempts renders the activity more and more automatic until it is performed rapidly and easily without conscious thought.

This, then, is the aim in the practice of the developing patterns of articulation, and in order that they may be incorporated easily into speech they must be included in sound sequences and their associations intensified and stabilised until they can be recalled at will when necessary and eventually without conscious thought. The level of consciousness at which this is achieved varies with the age and reactions of each patient. Some become aware of the difference between the old and the new, and may then consciously discard one and substitute the other. In young children especially, the change often occurs at a lower level of consciousness, and the child is unaware that it is taking place.

At all stages of treatment practice is continuous until the phonological patterns are so well established that they are used without conscious thought, automatically, and in the same way integrated into linguistic usage in phrases of increasing length. Use is made of the fact that the neurological functions which initially serve in the planning of an activity become unnecessary to its execution. Expression of thought through language is never, however, automatic, except in a few specific exclamations.

Individual adaptation. All treatment must be adapted to the needs and progress of the individual child based upon the treatment as outlined. For example, where a child can use four consonants such as [p], [b], [t] and [d] before treatment begins, he may be given these four consonants in simple sequences, as at stage (3), during the first treatment period, and for practice at home the following week. He gains confidence because he can do this easily, and a pattern is established for further therapy.

When attempting to use a new consonant in isolation, the therapist should test various phonetic sounds, not yet in use, and choose to work next with the one the particular child can produce most easily at any stage of treatment. As articulatory skill develops, and with increasing sensorimotor experience, the sounds which at one time were more difficult for the child, will be acquired more easily.

Reinforcement in the form of encouragement, pleasure at the child's improvement, if not success, and a star in his work notebook for work well done, is useful. The therapist shows pleasure in the child's progress, but not displeasure at his mistakes. Responsibility for obtaining what is required from the child is dependent upon the skill of the therapist, and also for obtaining the child's willing and happy co-operation.

Most children under the age of seven or eight years can, by easy stages, be led towards the use of normal articulation in the way described, whilst correction of, and interference with spontaneous speech is avoided. If the procedures, as outlined, are followed, it is usual for normal articulation of phonemes to be gradually incorporated by the child into his conversational speech, whilst he is unaware that any change is occurring. Improving articulation may be noticed within a few weeks, but it is usual for this to be more apparent within two to three months after correct phonemes can be used freely, without conscious control and on direct imitation in repeated reading and in rhymes, as at stage (4).

When sounds are being used easily in stories and in rhymes, exercises at stages (1), (2) and (3) are only continued if any particular consonant, or consonant blend, is not being used consistently with ease. The use of normal articulation in conversational speech, therefore, lags behind ability to use it in rhymes and stories, and again when conversational speech can be normal it is to be expected that there will be relapse at times into the use of the former defective patterns of articulation. This is especially so during moments of stress and excitement, the normal patterns of articulation in speech being insufficiently stabilised.

Although the ease with which this process is achieved depends to a great extent on the age of the patient, other factors are related. The defective patterns of articulation are so firmly established in the speech of some young children that they are difficult to eradicate, whilst the improvement in the speech of others may be apparent after two or three months, or even after a few weeks. Much depends on the severity of the underlying basic condition.

A Typical Treatment Period

This may include treatment at all four stages, according to the stage reached in the acquisition of the various consonant sounds.

For example, after running through the exercises the child has been practising at home at stages (2) and (3) and noting what is still required, the next step will be the selection of a new consonant sound. This is practised at stage (1) and perhaps stage (2). Exercises already easy at stage (2) are then practised at stage (3). Practice is then given at stage (4) in rhymes and reading. Treatment will possibly, therefore, include all four stages, according to the stage reached in the acquisition of the various consonant sounds.

Once all phonemes can be used at stage (4), regular attendance at the clinic may be unnecessary, the mother continuing with story repetition and rhymes at home until full stabilisation is realised. During this period the child may return to the clinic perhaps once a month for two or three months, depending on progress, after which a final interval of three months may elapse. It is then quite usual to find that the child's speech is normal, equal to that of his environment and adequate for his needs.

However, one can only proceed at a rate which is dependent upon the maturation and development of the underlying neurophysiological functions, and for some children therapy may be required over periods of two or three years, and for some even longer.

Where the defect of articulation has persisted into school life, the child may also be helped by associating a symbol, plastic or written, with the sound he is attempting to make, and later he may associate a word, again built with plastic letters, written or printed, with the word he is saying. This method can only be used, however, when the appropriate stage of recognition for symbols and reading readiness has developed.

With older children and adults, whether the difficulty is developmental or acquired, the same procedures are followed (with, of course, appropriate modifications) for the establishment of normal articulatory patterns, based on sensorimotor experience, until they become automatic. Phoneme acquisition at stages (1) to (4) may proceed much more quickly than with the young children, but more time will be required before the faulty use of phonemes in linguistic sequence, as in conversational speech, can be modified.

Treatment can include combined repetition after the therapist and reading, using auditory and visual clues simultaneously; then repeating using auditory clues alone; followed by reading aloud with no auditory stimulation from the therapist, using visual clues alone; and repeating learned rhymes or poems, where both visual and auditory stimulus patterns are eliminated. Such treatment helps the individual to gain the use of normal articulation in conversational speech, or to regain useful speech, in the acquired condition.

This procedure has the advantage of naturally and effectively assisting or rehabilitating the individuals articulatory ability. Especially with the young child, the therapist has the responsibility for helping the child to acquire the necessary sensorimotor competence and linguistic patterning, but the child should be allowed to gradually incorporate this competency into his own linguistic performance. He can do this best.

Age for Treatment

Defective articulation is normally noticed early, and if the child is not intelligible by the age of three or four years the mother becomes worried and seeks advice.

The child, unaware that his speech differs from that of others, also becomes anxious when he realises at the age of three and a half to four years of age that his attempts to speak are not understood. His anxiety is often increased when repeated correction of his speech by others causes loss of self-confidence and even inhibition of speech itself, with consequent frustration. He may use intelligent gesture, amounting in some to excellent mime, and so make known his wants, but lack of ability to express adequately the increasing variety of ideas in a rapidly growing mind is the inevitable result of such a speech disability.

In general we have found it useful and advisable to wait until the child is about four years of age before commencing regular treatment. By so doing we allow time for as much natural and spontaneous improvement as may occur, and in some children therapy is then unnecessary. At this age there is also time and the possibility of achieving useful and intelligible, if not normal, speech before the child goes to school at the age of five years. He is often more co-operative and interested at this age, perhaps as the result of experiencing the frustration associated with his speech disability, whilst new habits of articulation are more rapidly and easily incorporated into spontaneous conversational speech than at a later age.

If speech therapy is postponed beyond this stage, the child may be subjected to misguided and repeated correction of his speech at home, may have to endure teasing by other children because his speech is 'different', or may be refused admission to certain types of school.

Again, it is stressed, that should there be any possibility of continuing spontaneous improvement, the child should be observed over a period of from three to six months before treatment is commenced. A simple assessment, as previously described (p. 301) of the child's level of articulation at a visit once a month will indicate whether or not any improvement is occurring. If so, observation should be continued and there may be no need for treatment. The mother's anxiety will also be allayed, and there should be no stressful correction of the child's speech at home during this period of observation.

Self-consciousness

R.W. was referred at the age of seven years. She had an older sister aged eight years and a younger one aged 16 months.

Speech was a little late in developing, but she used words by two years and phrases by three and a half years. Articulation was defective and speech unintelligible except to those in close association with her. She was referred by a doctor, who stated that 'the mother was quite unable to give a clear account of the difficulty or to imitate it, although it is clear that whatever the primary difficulty there is now a marked element of anxiety and self-consciousness. Apparently the child at times completely refuses to attempt to speak, and will pour with sweat at these times, and this behaviour is more marked at school than at home. In fact, she proved quite friendly in the clinic after a while and co-operated quite well'.

When seen by the speech therapist it was found that she was beginning to read and that she did so with normal articulation. Speech, however, was so unintelligible that she refused to go a message. Recently a shopkeeper had been unable to understand that she wanted 'a dozen eggs'.

Because this disorder of articulation had persisted so long there was a marked state of anxiety which was concerned only with situations requiring speech and did not extend to other aspects of school, play or home life.

Such emotional reactions are only too frequent and should be avoided if possible by the commencement of speech therapy at an earlier age.

Speech therapy must always be designed to meet the needs of the individual child, and although some group work may be possible, and advisable, at times, we have found individual treatment more useful, especially if carried out in the presence of, and with the full understanding and co-operation of, the mother.

Speech Therapy and the Mother

Many of these children show more emotional attachment to, and dependence on, the mother than is usual for their age. As the child (once a biological part of his mother) grows, his desire for independence gradually increases, and he asserts himself in ways which are sometimes described as behaviour problems rather than accepted as the only way he has of expressing his progress towards maturity. The adult must respect the child's desire for independence, but in many children with unintelligible speech there is delay in developing this desire for a separate independent existence, which is perhaps not unnatural if the mother is the only one who can understand his speech or interpret what he says to others.

It has been found that the desire for independence in these children often develops gradually and naturally during treatment, and with improvement in the use of intelligible speech. Until this occurs it may be unwise to attempt to force the separation of the child from his mother.

There must also be recognition of the justifiable anxiety which the mother feels for her child, which is probably the reason for her attendance with the child at the speech therapy clinic. This anxiety may have originated in her own mind, as she noticed her child's development in comparsion with that of the children of her neighbours or relatives, or it may have been implanted there by the remarks of others and their doubts as to the child's intelligence. The mother's anxiety may then have been transmitted to the child through repeated correction of mispronounced words, which may have served only to impress on the child that there is 'something wrong' concerning his speech.

As full an explanation as is possible, suited to her understanding, must be given to the mother concerning the difficulty which her child is experiencing. Where possible she must be reassured as to the true level of her child's development. It must be explained that children with speech defects are not necessarily defective in a general sense, a fear which may be very persistent in her mind, despite the fact that she may state that, apart from his speech, development and behaviour have not differed from that of her other children.

Again, the mother must be reassured as to the future outlook where speech is concerned, but she must also realise that the child has a real difficulty and is not being stupid, obstinate nor lazy.

Her desire to help the child by correction of his speech must be guided into channels which will be more fruitful and less irksome to the child than the usual home correction, thus taking part in his treatment rather than hindering his progress. In many hospitals mothers are admitted to nurse their own children under the guidance of the nursing staff. The late Sir James Spence (1947*a*) once said, 'It is an advantage to the child, it is an advantage to the mother, for to have undergone this experience and to have felt that she has been responsible for her own child's recovery establishes a relationship with her child and confidence in herself which bodes well for the future'. It seems also important that the mother should share in the treatment of her own child when speech is defective (see also Miller, 1948). We have always arranged for the mother to be present during treatment. In this way she acquires insight into and understanding of the speech difficulties experienced by her child, and she learns, more unconsciously than by direction, how to carry out regular simple treatment at home. It is essential that the mother should fully appreciate not only *what* she should do, but *how* she should do it. It is most successful when the mother observes the treatment by the therapist. She remains in the room, somewhat apart and behind her child. Thus she observes how the therapist handles her child's difficulties.

Through friendly contact with the mother the therapist is also helped to see the child in relation to his family background and so maintains a realistic understanding of the amount and type of treatment which can best be carried out in the home between visits to the out-patient clinic. Spence (1947*b*) has also said, 'The family exists first, to ensure growth and physical health; second, to give the right scope for emotional experience; third, to preserve the art of motherhood; and fourth, to teach behaviour.' We cannot presume to separate the young child from his family, nor should we seek as speech therapists to change the lives of the child or his family, but rather than treat the child alone, while the mother is excluded from the room, we should maintain contact with her, so that through the mother-child-therapist relationship the child may be helped by a more complete understanding of his problems to which each contributes.

Some consider that the mother is not the best person to handle her child's problem. However, the young child spends the greater part of his early life with his mother, and the success of treatment may depend upon her understanding, and the relationship between mother and child. Experienced and wise paediatricians have found that the mother can be guided to nurse her physically sick child when in hospital, that this increases her confidence, and is helpful to the mother-child relationship. Similarly, the mother can help with the treatment of her child's defective articulation.

If at any stage of treatment the child wishes to come alone, either because he is gaining independence or to avoid any self-consciousness, the mother remains outside the room. She has by this time seen and appreciated the way the therapist works, and after treatment the child is asked to invite the mother into the room to show her how he has carried out his exercises. It is not enough to show her the book with exercises written therein. In this way the therapist is enabled to understand each child's needs as fully as possible and to plan the treatment which will be most useful.

Whilst the therapist may see the child only once a week, the mother is in daily contact with him. If her understanding and co-operation can be gained, improvement in speech can be assisted through treatment carried out naturally and regularly for a few minutes each day, the length of time depending on the age of the child. A set 'speech lesson' should always be avoided.

In the treatment of the older child who is at school, attendance with the mother may not be possible nor desirable. Contact with the school and the teachers, however, is most useful, so that not only does the therapist gain understanding of the child's environment but the teachers are also interested to know of any way in which they may assist by further understanding of the child's problem.*

The method of treatment described has been found useful in the majority of children with defective articulation. It can be adapted for the treatment of children with a developmental dysarthria, as in children with cerebral palsy or minimal

* Useful information—Advice to Mothers—Talking is Child's Play, Parts 1 and 2. (General suggestions for the prevention of speech disorders and how the mother can encourage speech development.)
The role of the Health Visitor. (A guide to normal speech development.)

Prepared by four parents who are also speech therapists, one other speech therapist, and a nurse who is a Health Visitor for Kent County Education Authority. Obtainable from The College of Speech Therapists, 47, St. John's Wood High Street, London, N.W.8.

cerebral dysfunction. In children with a persisting underlying dyspraxia progress will be much slower, and some disability may persist throughout life. This may not interfere with general intelligibility but may show itself in certain difficulties with especially long words, unfamiliar words and so forth. Where the defective articulation is associated with a cleft palate, exercises for control and co-ordination of the oral and naso-pharyngeal airways during speech may also be required. The adaptation of the basic principles for treatment will be described in the following chapters.

ADDITIONAL SUGGESTIONS FOR THE USE OF THE GENERAL PRINCIPLES IN THE TREATMENT OF DEVELOPMENTAL DYSARTHRIA WHEN ASSOCIATED WITH A SEVERE GENERAL MOTOR DISABILITY

Treatment for children with isolated dysarthria or dysarthria associated with minimal cerebral palsy may follow the principles of treatment already described, always bearing in mind that the aim in the treatment of these disorders is, firstly, ease of movement, and secondly, the increase in speed of articulatory movements up to that required for conversational speech.

Where the dysarthria is associated with a general motor disability, as in cerebral palsy, treatment may fail if it does not take into account the general condition. In many of these children attempts to speak produce a general increase in spasticity or of involuntary movements of the head and neck, of the limbs or throughout the body. Abnormalities of muscle tone, of posture and of movements then interfere with the easy rapid movements of the lips and tongue for articulation and with the normal co-ordinations of respiration with phonation and articulation.

Speech Therapy in Cerebral Palsy

Various methods of speech therapy have been described, some based on the practice and improvement of the reflex actions of sucking, chewing and swallowing, and others on muscle training and the improved mobility and control of the muscles used for articulation by means of tongue, lip and jaw exercises. These aim to increase both the extent and speed of movement. Much further research is needed into this aspect of speech therapy before any definite rules for treatment can be laid down. With limited personal experience, the following suggestions indicate the lines along which treatment has tentatively been developing.

Lencione (1965), describing how it is known that a defect in one area may often cause defects in other areas, suggests that, by the same token, the improvement of a handicap in one area may even improve handicaps in other areas. This could ultimately lead to the child having increasingly meaningful activities and accomplishments.

As previously described (Chapter XIII), Bobath (1955) believes that spasticity and athetosis result from the absence of the normal inhibition of unwanted mass reflex movements due to brain damage. Such inhibition is the basis of co-ordinated muscle movements and of motor skills, including articulation which then develops on a background of normal muscle tone. When the muscle tone is abnormal, normal movements are impossible, whether of the jaw, tongue and lips or of the whole body. Bobath (1955) has stated:

> We think that the motor disorders of patients with lesions of the central nervous system are due to:
>
> 1. The released and disordered activity of lower centres of the central nervous system with abnormal strength and distribution of muscle tone.
> 2. The absence of normal development of automatic motor activity.
> 3. Inadequate inhibitory control with failure to develop skilled and independent movements.

Treatment has been designed to inhibit the abnormal reflex activity resulting in a general condition of more normal muscle tone. The development of automatic movements and skilled movements may then occur on this background of more normal tone throughout the body.

As the speech disorder in these children is the result of inadequate neuromuscular movement and control of the muscle groups used for speech, it seems reasonable to suppose that speech therapy should follow similar lines to that used by physiotherapists in treating the general motor disability.

The dysarthria in children with cerebral palsy is not isolated but is closely associated with the general condition, and may be due to widespread interference with the whole of the motor activity required for speech. The development of more normal movements for speech may therefore require, firstly, the positioning of the child so that more normal muscle tone is experienced through the inhibition of abnormal reflex activity, secondly, the improvement of respiratory movements, thirdly, the more normal co-ordination of such movements with voicing and phonation and, fourthly, their co-ordination with the muscle movements required for articulation.

Normal and abnormal patterns of respiration, phonation and articulation have already been described (Chapter XII), and before treatment is begun there should be a careful analysis of the motor activity, and that associated with speech, in each individual child. Certain postural reflex patterns of activity may be demonstrated in children with cerebral palsy. These reflex reactions occur in response to changes in position of the head and neck in relation to the body. Two such reflexes are the tonic neck reflex and the tonic labyrinthine reflex. The tonic neck reflex (T.N.R.) may be symmetrical or asymmetrical.

Asymmetrical T.N.R.

If the child is in supine and the head is turned or bent over to one side, there will be extension of the limbs on the side to which the head is turned, with simultaneous flexion of the limbs on the opposite side. In less severe cases this may be demonstrated only as an increase of extensor tone in the muscles of one side without obvious movement, and with increase of flexor tone in the muscles of the other side.

Symmetrical T.N.R.

If the child is lying face downwards in the prone position, raising the head will cause increase of extensor tone in the arms, with flexion of the legs. The arms therefore become extended and the legs bent. Lowering the head will produce the opposite reaction with flexion of the arms and extension of the legs. Where there is no obvious movement of the limbs, changes of muscle tone may be felt on testing the resistance to passive extension or flexion.

The tonic labyrinthine reflex

This reflex produces changes of muscle tone in all four limbs simultaneously. The child lying on his back in the supine position will experience an increase of extensor tone with extension of the limbs and spine, whilst the reverse occurs in the prone position, with an increase of flexor tone and flexion of the spine and limbs.

Due to lack of cortical control and inhibition in the child with cerebral palsy, these reflexes may persist and cause abnormal postures, and movements. The reflexes described may act together, and it may not be possible to differentiate between them, the child's movements being the resultant of a combination of reflex activity.

As the child attempts the normal movements of infancy, rolling over, getting on to all fours, crawling and so forth, such reflex activity prevents or hinders him. For example, if the child wishes to turn over on to his right side he first turns his head in that direction. The right side of the body, arm and leg may then extend due to the influence of the tonic neck reflex, and it is then impossible for him to turn on to that side against the resistance of the extended arm and leg.

During treatment by reflex inhibition the therapist places the child in certain positions which inhibit such tonic reflex activity, and by so doing enables the child to experience the sensation of muscle tone which is nearer to that which is normal, and subsequently the movements of turning and other righting reflexes are experienced.

Analysis of Postures and Movements associated with Speech

A careful analysis must first be made of abnormal reactions occurring during speech when the child is in various postures. There may be abnormal increase and distribution of muscle tone causing movements of the limbs, head or neck during speech, or abnormal muscle tone may only be detected if the limbs or head and neck are gently flexed and extended whilst the child is using voice or speech. The child should be examined on a wide couch, or on a rug on the floor, and should be undressed so that abnormal respiratory movements may be observed during speech and at rest.

Observations should be carried out with the child in the following postures:

(1) lying flat on his back in supine; (2) lying face down in prone; (3) in side lying; (4) when sitting; and (5) when standing.

The following motor patterns should be observed in these various postures:

1. *Respiratory movements*
   (*a*) When the child is at rest.
   (*b*) When voicing.
   (*c*) When speaking.

2. *Movements of the jaw*
   (*a*) Opening and closing the mouth.
   (*b*) Chewing.

3. *Movements of the tongue*
   (*a*) Protrusion.
   (*b*) Elevation of the tip.
   (*c*) Lateral movements.

4. *Facial muscles*
   (*a*) Movements of the lips.
   (*b*) Opening and closing of the eyes.

Speech, however, requires a co-ordinated motor pattern involving movements of all these muscle groups and should be studied as a total response during (1) phonation and (2) speech.

Phonation

Movements and abnormal distribution of muscle tone should be observed whilst the child is phonating in the various postures described. Abnormal movements should be noted concerning:

1. Respiratory movements.
2. Movements of the head on the cervical spine.
3. Movements of the mandible on the skull.

4. Movements of the tongue and floor of the mouth.
5. Abnormal muscle tone in the neck and facial muscles.
6. Other movements or abnormal increase in muscle tone in the limbs or trunk.

Speech

These six observations should then be repeated whilst the child is speaking. In many, a generalised increase of muscle tone or of involuntary movements can be observed just before the onset of speech when the child is preparing to speak.

Articulation. It should be noted how far the disability is limited to abnormalities of muscle tone or of movements affecting mainly the speed and ease of speech, and how far there is in addition a difficulty in imitating the sounds of speech as in articulatory apraxia.

Language. Is there full use of words and sentences, even if these are unintelligible at times, or is there also some degree of developmental aphasia?

Lencione (1968) stresses that adequate, complete and continuous diagnosis is an essential part of therapy. A period of diagnostic therapy in which revaluations are made should be an important part in all speech therapy.

TREATMENT

Treatment requires that abnormalities of movement or of posture, resulting from abnormal reflex activity, should be inhibited, and that more normal movements of the muscles used in speech should then be allowed to develop or be facilitated.

Inhibition

The use of reflex inhibition has been fully described by Bobath (1955) and reflex inhibiting postures which may be used for speech therapy by Marland (1953).

The aim of such treatment is to normalise so far as is possible the muscle tone of the trunk and limbs, and also of the muscles of the jaw, neck, tongue, lips and pharynx. When this has been achieved, normal movements are encouraged on this background of normal muscle tone. The patient then experiences more normal sensations of movement, until, with repeated experience, the reactions become increasingly automatic and can be maintained by the patient unassisted.

Positions must therefore be found which lessen abnormal and unwanted activity throughout the body and facilitate normal movements and co-ordination, especially of those required for speech.

Marland has suggested the following reflex inhibiting postures:

1. Supine with flexed abducted knees; shoulders and arms flexed.
2. Kneel sitting with trunk forward on couch; head down between extended arms; dorsal spine extended.
3. Sitting with legs down over side of couch; hips well flexed, spine extended; extended arms raised to therapist's shoulders; head up (and central) but not back.

It is probable that no actual speech therapy should be attempted until the child can be placed in at least one reflex inhibiting posture with the achievement of some reduction in spasticity.

From the findings already described it is apparent that the greatest difficulty in articulation is experienced when the muscles of the tongue, the floor of the mouth and the ventral muscles of the neck are severely involved, and change of posture may not be clearly associated with any marked improvement in the condition of these muscles during speech. There is, however, a habit factor which cannot be ignored and involves the set of the child's compensatory muscular patterns preparatory to and for speech.

It has been found that the position of maximum ease for speech varied from child to child, but in general, speech was facilitated when in supine or in side lying positions with flexed arms and legs, the head being in a position which was in normal relation to the cervical spine, and the mandible then in normal position in relation to the head.

Speech tends to deteriorate in the prone position, which is that tending to increase in flexor tone, and in sitting and standing, where there is increased extensor tone. In certain positions, as in lying with legs outstretched and standing, associated with increase of extensor tone, the ability to protrude the tongue may be increased; but there is then increased spasticity in the muscles of the tongue, and rapid movements, involving the intrinsic muscles of the tongue, are not then possible.

Treatment, therefore, aims to find reflex inhibiting postures which will decrease the general spasticity associated with speech and particularly of those muscles involved in speech, and which will maintain the head in normal relation to the cervical spine, so that the mandible may move in normal relation to the head and assist the movements of the tongue on the floor of the mouth. Better positions of the head and jaw will also assist phonation, as this can only be normal when the muscle tone in the larynx, neck and shoulders is also normal.

These improved relative positions may first be obtained with the child in supine, or in side lying, with flexed arms and legs, but should later be obtained, and maintained so far as is possible in sitting and in standing.

Each treatment should include the facilitation and development of more normal breathing movements, phonation and articulatory movements.

Respiration

There may be excessive expansion of the lower rib margins with indrawing of the abdominal wall and little diaphragm movement. More normal respiratory movements may be induced if the abnormal thoracic expansion is inhibited by lateral pressure of the therapist's hands, when diaphragm movement may increase spontaneously. With improvement in respiratory movements phonation may also improve.

Phonation

This may be facilitated by vibration with the hands over the lower thorax, diaphragm or abdominal wall whilst the child is in a reflex inhibiting posture, or it may be found that under such conditions the child voices spontaneously.

Articulation

Movements of the mandible may be facilitated during the repetition of such sounds as [b-b-b]. Movements of the lips may be facilitated by the therapist, so that the child experiences a more normal sensation of movement against a background of improved muscle tone, and previous effort and abnormal co-ordinations are avoided.

Treatment for articulatory movements will also require the development of selectivity and of the inhibition of unwanted movements. Isolated movements of the tongue or lips must be encouraged without more widespread movements involving the neck, head and jaw.

Language. Lencione (1968) describes conditions which will produce language development. She also describes the attention which should be given to the modification of atypical breathing patterns, co-ordination of respiration with phonation and the development of chewing, sucking and swallowing reflexes to form a background for the movements which are necessary for complex articulatory activity.

She also states that, clinically, an understanding of the child's development, and the stages of linguistic development already achieved, as well as those stages which have been omitted, provides one way of assessing the problems of the impact of cerebral palsy on language and articulation.

Treatment should follow the normal developmental sequence through vocal play to babbling or assisted babbling and finally speech, but only as the child progresses and arrives at a state of readiness for each stage of speech development. In the older child faulty patterns of compensation must be inhibited whilst more normal patterns of speech are experienced and practised until they can be maintained.

Each treatment should be limited to two or three new sensations of movement or co-ordination, and should be practised daily at home by the mother under the guidance of the therapist in order to develop more automatic reactions which can be maintained during speech. The child thus develops new motor skills through repeated experience of the new sensations associated with speech until they are fully stabilised.

In many children, however, normal speech may not be possible and the aim must necessarily be to achieve speech which is useful for communication, the final result being determined by the extent of the underlying disability.

Where athetosis is the predominating condition, attempts to

speak are usually associated with an increase of the involuntary movements, in spite of exercises for relaxation. In many of these patients there may also be some degree of spasticity, especially in the tongue and facial muscles, or those of the neck and floor of the mouth.

Reflex inhibiting postures will assist the child to experience speech without such involuntary movements, but the extent to which the child may eventually maintain such control himself is uncertain.

This is by no means a full account of this method of treatment, but it may indicate some of the possibilities to be explored and also discourage the practice of exercises for lips, tongue or articulation when it is found that these cause increased abnormality of muscle tone and of spasticity or involuntary movements.

As it is improbable that many of these children will obtain normal physical movements, so speech may never achieve normality. Again, we do not know how far physiotherapy based on reflex inhibition in the very young child may contribute towards a general alleviation of the condition and how far spontaneous improvement in the use of speech may be associated with such improvement in the child's general physical state. Whenever possible, the speech therapist should work in conjunction with the physiotherapist so that both may contribute what is possible towards improvement in the child's general physical activity and in those specialised movements and co-ordinations required for speech.

ADDITIONAL SUGGESTIONS FOR THE USE OF THE GENERAL PRINCIPLES OF TREATMENT FOR ARTICULATORY DYSPRAXIA

In the child with articulatory dyspraxia movements of the muscles used for articulation are apparently normal except for speech, and there is no abnormality of muscle tone. Respiratory movements are normal, but there may be inco-ordination between respiration and phonation, or between phonation and articulation, and the articulatory dyspraxia may be associated with apraxia of the facial muscles, tongue or palate, and perhaps with other forms of apraxia, especially in children with more extensive signs of brain damage.

The disability varies in extent from inability to imitate the articulation of a single isolated consonant or syllable to inability to use the phonetic sounds of speech normally in the long sequences of conversational speech. Treatment will therefore depend on what the child can do.

If the articulatory dyspraxia is uncomplicated, treatment as previously described under general principles may be all that is required. The simple babble exercises develop a store of automatic sensori-motor patterns of articulation upon which the use of sounds in speech is based. Their incorporation into speech, may, however, require months or even years of practice before they can be used normally in word sequences.

The aim of treatment is to stimulate and, if possible, increase the rate of development of the neurological processes by means of which we normally imitate the sounds of speech. At the same time the faulty motor patterns of articulation already acquired are changed, so avoiding their gradual stabilisation, until the child's articulatory skill is adequate for his needs.

Visual stimulation

Children with articulatory apraxia have difficulty in directing the movements of articulation through auditory control alone, and they are helped if they can watch the therapist's movements for articulation and also their own in a mirror. Some children find it easier if at first they rely on visual imitation of movement alone and are unable to hear the sound they themselves are making. Later they must associate the articulatory movement with the sound they are producing before auditory control can be achieved.

Reading

Many of these children have difficulty in learning to read. If they have good visual appreciation for the printed symbols and good visual memory, they may learn to understand printed language but yet read aloud with the same patterns of defective articulation as used in speech.

Other children, where visual ability is less well developed, fail entirely in their attempts to learn to read.

If the articulatory dyspraxia is less severe and persistent, a child may learn to read using normal articulation when spontaneous speech may still be defective or even unintelligible. The slow articulation of words during the early stages of learning to read may assist the association between normal articulation and the visual impression of the printed symbols of speech. Ability to read with normal articulation may then be extended to the spontaneous improvement of articulation in conversational speech.

In the child who is over six years of age the association between consonant sounds and their symbols, in plastic letters or print, should be used to help to establish normal sensori-motor patterns more firmly, and the therapist may use the ability to read with normal articulation, when developed, to assist the use and stabilisation of normal articulation in speech.

It must be remembered that these children have a basic organic disability which may not respond readily to treatment.

Clinically it has been found that improvement may be very slow until a stage is reached when progress becomes much more rapid. Whether this is the result of neurological maturation it is not possible to say, nor is it possible to forecast when this stage will be reached in any individual child.

In the meantime patient and persistent treatment is required.

REFERENCES

Aungst, L. F., and Frick, J. V. (1964). Auditory discriminative ability and consistency of articulation of /r/. *J. Speech Hear. Dis.*, **29**, 76.

Boothroyd, A. (1965). Statistical Theory and the Speech Discrimination Score. *J. Acoust. Soc. Am.* **43** (2), 362.

Bobath, B. (1955). The Treatment of Motor Disorders of Pyramidal and Extrapyramidal Origin by Reflex Inhibition and by Facilitation of Movement. *Physiotherapy*, **41**, 146.

Chomsky, N. (1965). *Aspects of Theory and Syntax.* Cambridge, Mass., M.I.T. Press.

Fawcus, R. (1971). The Psychological and Physiological Aspects of Articulatory Performance. *Brit. J. Dis. Commun. II*, **2**, 99.

Ferrie, M. W. (1955). The Place of Play Therapy in the Treatment of Defects of Speech in Young Children. *College of Speech Tharapists Conference Report*, p. 3.

Fry, D. (1966). The Development of the Phonological System in the Normal and Deaf Children. In *The Genesis of Language*. Eds. F. Smith and G. A. Miller. Cambridge, Mass., M.I.T. Press.

Fry, D. (1968). The Phonemic System in Children's Speech. *Brit. J. Dis. Commun. III*, **1**, 13.

Geschwind, N. P. (1965). Disconnection Syndrome in Animals and Man. *Brain*, **88**, 237–295 and 585–644.

Gleason, H. A. (1955 and 1958). *An Introduction to Descriptive Linguistics*. New York, Henry Holt.

Gubbay, S. S., Ellis, E., Walton, J. N., and Court, S. D. M. (1965). A Study of apraxia and agnosia defects in 21 children. *Brain*, **88**, 295–312.

Halle, M. (1965). On the Bases of Phonology in *The Structure of Language*. Eds. J. Foder and J. Katz. New York, Prentice Hall.

Illingworth, R. S. (1963). The Clumsy Child: Minimal Cerebral Dysfunction. *Little Club Clinics in Developmental Medicine*, No. 10, p. 26.

Lencione, R. (1965). *Speech and Language Problems in Cerebral Palsy*. Ed. W. Cruickshank. Syracuse Univ. Press.

Lencione, R. (1968). A Rationale for Speech and Language Evaluation in Cerebral Palsy. *Brit. J. Dis. Commun. III*, **2**, 161.

Lenneberg, E. H. (1967). *Biological Foundations of Language*. New York, John Wiley and Son.

Locke, J. L., and Goldstein, J. I. (1971). Children's Identification and Discrimination of phonemes. *Brit. J. Dis. Commun. VI*, **2**, 107.

McNeill, D. (1966). Developmental Psycholinguistics. In *The Genesis of Language*. Eds. F. Smith and G. A. Miller. Cambridge, Mass., M.I.T. Press.

Marland, P. (1953). Speech Therapy for Cerebral Palsy Based on Reflex Inhibition. *Speech*, **17**, No. 2, 65.

Miller, F. J. W. (1948). Home Nursing of Premature Babies. *Lancet*, **2**, 703.

Morley, M. E., and Fox, J. (1969). Disorders of Articulation: Theory and Therapy. *Brit. J. Dis. Commun. IV*, **2**, 151.

Orton, S. (1937). *Reading, Writing and Speech Problems in Children*. New York, Noton.

Paine, R. S. (1966). *Develop. Med. Child. Neurol.*, **4**, 21.

Ringel, R. L., and Ewanowski, S. J. (1965). Oral Perception: I. Two-point Discrimination. *J. Speech and Hear. Res*. Vol. 8, **4**, 389.

Ringel, R. L., Saxman, J. H., and Brooks, A. R. (1967). Oral Perception: II. Mandibular Kinaesthesia. *J. Speech and Hear. Res*. Vol. 10, **3**, 637.

Ringel, R. L., and Fletcher, H. M. (1967). Oral Perception: III. Texture Discrimination. *J. Speech and Hear. Res*. Vol. 10, **3**, 642.

Ringel, R. L., Burk, K. W., and Scott, C. M. (1968). Tactile Perception: Form Discrimination in the Mouth. *Brit. J. Dis. Commun. III*, **2**, 150.

Spence, J. C. (1947). The Care of Children in Hospital. *Brit. med. J.*, **1**, 125. Charles West Lecture.

Spence, J. C. (1947). *The Purpose of the Family*, 2nd ed. London, Epworth Press.

Vygotsky, L. S. (1934, trs. 1962). *Thought and Language*. Ed. and Trans. E. Haufman and G. Vakar. Cambridge, Mass., M.I.T. Press.

Walton, J. N., Ellis, E., and Court, S. D. M. (1962). Clumsy Children: a study of developmental apraxia and agnosia. *Brain*, **85**, 603–612.

Weiner, P. (1967). Auditory Discrimination and Articulation. *J. Speech and Hear. Dis.*, **32**, 19.

Winitz, H. (1970). *Articulatory Acquisition and Behaviour*. New York, Appleton, Century Crofts.

Woolf, G., and Pilberg, M. S. (1971). A comparison of three tests of auditory discrimination and their relationship to performance on a deep test of articulation. *J. Commun. Dis.*, **4**, 239.

XVI. Defects of Speech due to a Partial Hearing Loss

In addition to the children with delayed speech development due to a severe hearing defect already described, others are frequently referred for speech therapy with varying degrees of defective articulation when it has not been realised that the basic cause is a partial hearing loss. This may be for all frequencies or only for the higher frequencies of sound; it may be congenital or acquired after the development of speech, and it may be a conductive or a perceptive hearing loss.

Perceptive Hearing Loss

Where there is failure of cochlear response, with distorted appreciation of the consonant sounds of speech, increase in the volume of sound reaching the ear may fail to provide better discrimination and understanding for speech. There are many varying gradients and degrees of such hearing loss affecting comprehension for speech, and its imitation and use is therefore dependent on the extent of the hearing defect and the child's intelligence and ability to compensate for it.

High Frequency Hearing Loss

If the loss of hearing is chiefly or only for the higher frequencies of sound, with useful hearing up to perhaps 4000 c.p.s., there may have been little or no delay in the onset of speech, and the hearing loss may not have interfered to any noticeable extent with the child's social adequacy and apparent hearing for speech. Many children compensate for their inadequate hearing by lip reading spontaneously acquired, and the true nature of their disability and the cause of their defective articulation may not have been understood.

Where there is a more severe hearing defect of this type, affecting hearing for most consonant sounds and comprehension for speech to a greater extent, articulation may be unintelligible. In school there is resulting failure to make progress, yet hearing for voice and the sounds of everyday life is apparently normal, and a diagnosis of mental deficiency may even have been made.

As previously described (Chapter VIII), the vowel sounds of speech require appreciation of the frequency range from approximately 120 to 3000 c.p.s., the fundamental tone of the male voice being an octave lower than that of the female voice. The voiced consonants also have a fundamental tone in this range, but for their discrimination and imitation, and for that of the voiceless consonants such as [f] [θ (th)] [ʃ (sh)] and [s] there must be adequate hearing for the frequencies of sound between 1000 and 3000 c.p.s., and true appreciation of the sounds [s] and [θ (th)] may require useful hearing up to 4000 or even 6000 c.p.s. If there is a hearing defect for these frequencies of sound, either congenital or acquired in early life, there will be defects of articulation. Hearing for the consonant sounds will be distorted, and the child will imitate only what he hears.

Partial Hearing Loss for all Frequencies

A partial hearing loss of inner ear type affecting all frequencies of sound over the speech range may cause some delay in the onset of speech. The child is less aware of the use of speech around him than is the child with good hearing for the low frequencies and inadequate hearing for only the higher frequencies of sound. These children will again develop lip reading spontaneously if intelligence is normal, but articulation will be defective.

In a few children the hearing loss may be greater for the lower frequencies of sound than for the higher, or the greatest loss may occur in the middle range. Hearing for the high-frequency sounds such as [s] and [θ (th)] may then be adequate, and normal use of these sounds in speech may lead to a wrong diagnosis in the absence of audiometric assessment.

Transmission Hearing Loss

If the partial hearing loss is due to a conductive failure, as in conditions affecting the middle ear, the lower frequencies of sound are chiefly affected and there may be little or no failure of hearing for the range of frequencies required for appreciation of the consonant sounds of speech. Increase in the volume of sound, as by raising the voice, may then be all that is required to ensure that the sounds penetrate to the inner ear, and, in the absence of any defect there, will be appreciated normally. Such a hearing loss in young children is frequently intermittent and associated with colds or other infections of the nasal airway and middle ear. Speech is therefore heard normally in the intervals between such periods of reduced hearing. When hearing is subnormal, consonant sounds are heard without distortion if the voice is raised, and normal articulation usually develops and is maintained.

Congenital Hearing Loss

Many children with defective hearing have never at any time heard the sounds of speech normally, as the result of some partial failure of development, generally due to causes unknown.

In other children an illness early in life, and before speech has developed, will cause as severe a handicap as the hearing defect which is congenital.

Acquired Hearing Loss

The effect which such a hearing loss has upon acquired speech will depend on the age of the child when it occurs and also on its severity. Where speech was fully developed before the onset of an illness such as meningitis, it may or may not be maintained, depending on the extent to which speech had become stabilised. In children under seven years of age normal speech rarely persists and, in the child of four years or under, it may be entirely lost. If the child is over ten years of age, on the other hand, it is probable that normal use of expressive speech, and perhaps articulation, will persist in spite of a severe loss in comprehension for speech through the auditory pathways.

The potentialities of each child must therefore be assessed individually and will vary according to the age at which the hearing loss occurred, its type, degree, the response to amplification, together with the intelligence and ability to compensate for his disability, and to some extent on the help which he receives from his family at home. It must also be recognised that some of these children may have in addition some failure of neurological development for speech, resulting in dysarthria or articulatory dyspraxia which may then be responsible for some of the variations in articulatory defects in children with similar degrees of hearing loss.

In addition, therefore, to those children who are referred to the speech therapist with delayed development of speech associated with a severe hearing deficiency, children are also referred with defective articulation when the hearing loss is less severe. The effect of a severe hearing loss on the development of speech has already been described (Chapter VIII) in 110 children. Ninety-five children have also been referred to one hospital speech therapy department during the last four years with partial hearing loss of varying extent.

Speech and Partial Hearing Loss in 95 Children

These children were referred for three different reasons.

Forty-one were referred for speech therapy because articulation was defective, the hearing loss being unsuspected.

Sixteen had an acquired partial hearing loss subsequent to the development of speech, and instruction in lip reading was requested.

Thirty-eight were referred to the department for assessment of hearing, tests of response to speech with or without a hearing aid, for auditory training and for supervision in the use of a hearing aid.

Referred for speech therapy with defective articulation

Forty-one children who were referred for treatment because their articulation was defective were subsequently found to have a partial hearing loss. Obvious signs indicating such a hearing defect were: difficulty in the understanding of simple speech, associated with defective articulation of certain consonants, especially [s] [θ (th)] and [f], and unusual attention directed to the speaker's face, resulting in improved comprehension for speech (Figs. 66, 67 and 68).

PARTIAL HEARING LOSS IN CHILDREN REFERRED WITH DEFECTIVE ARTICULATION

(Figures 61 and 62)

Right = O Left = X Air = —— Bone = ----

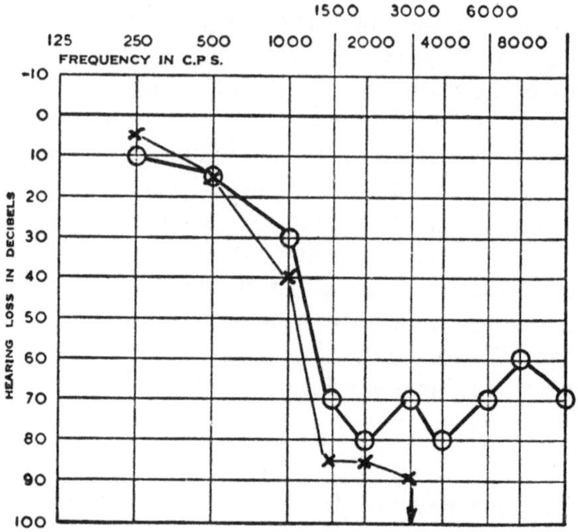

FIG. 66

D. P. was referred at three years of age because his general practitioner thought he was 'very backward in speech'. His birth weight was five pounds, and he thrived well. He walked at 15 months, and speech development was not later than that of his brother. At three years of age his mother was worried because he did not 'speak clearly', but she did not think that he was deaf. He attended for speech therapy at four years of age, and at first the hearing loss was not suspected. His mother was not convinced that he was partially deaf until he was five and a half years old. When hearing aids became available under the National Health Service he was nine years of age, and he found one useful in school. His intelligence quotient on the Wechsler Bellevue scale for children was 104, and at ten years of age he was eighth in his class where there were 54 children. His voice lacked variety of intonation and some defective articulation persisted in conversational speech although he was easily intelligible. The degree of hearing loss is shown by the audiogram.

Referred for lip reading instruction

Sixteen children were referred with a partial hearing loss and normal speech which had been acquired before the illness which was responsible for the hearing loss. Where the hearing loss affects mainly the higher frequencies of sound, a hearing

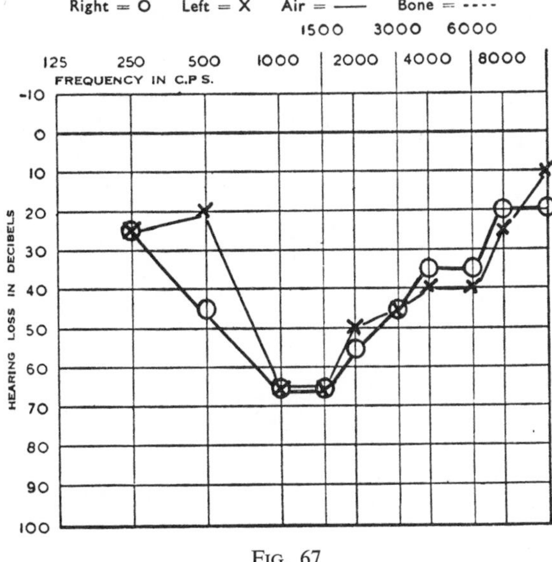

FIG. 67

R. C. was referred at five years ten months. His parents had never thought that he might be partially deaf. His birth weight was five pounds two ounces and he had been 'blue' in the first few days of life. He had walked at 14 months and used first words between two and three years. He had had no serious illness. By the age of four years he was using many more words, and at the time of referral had adequate use of language. He could repeat many nursery rhymes, but speech was unintelligible even in the home because of defective articulation, and he used gesture to explain his meaning. He also had violent temper tantrums when not understood. Play was normal, and he was interested in books and pictures, and his intelligence quotient on the Drever Collins performance scale was 106. Audiometric assessment proved a marked hearing loss for the frequencies of sound between 1000 and 4000 c.p.s. of inner ear type. A hearing aid was very useful in this case and he was able to continue his education in the normal school.

aid may be of little assistance. Hearing for the lower frequencies and perhaps for voice may be almost normal, and before the higher frequencies can be amplified sufficiently to be appreciated similar amplification of the lower frequencies may render them unbearably loud. The result may be comparable to one with normal hearing attempting to understand speech in a noisy factory. Other complex factors such as recruitment and noise intolerance may also limit the usefulness of a hearing aid. Lip reading is then of the utmost use, and, although it has many

AUDIOGRAMS OF A CHILD SHOWING VARIATIONS

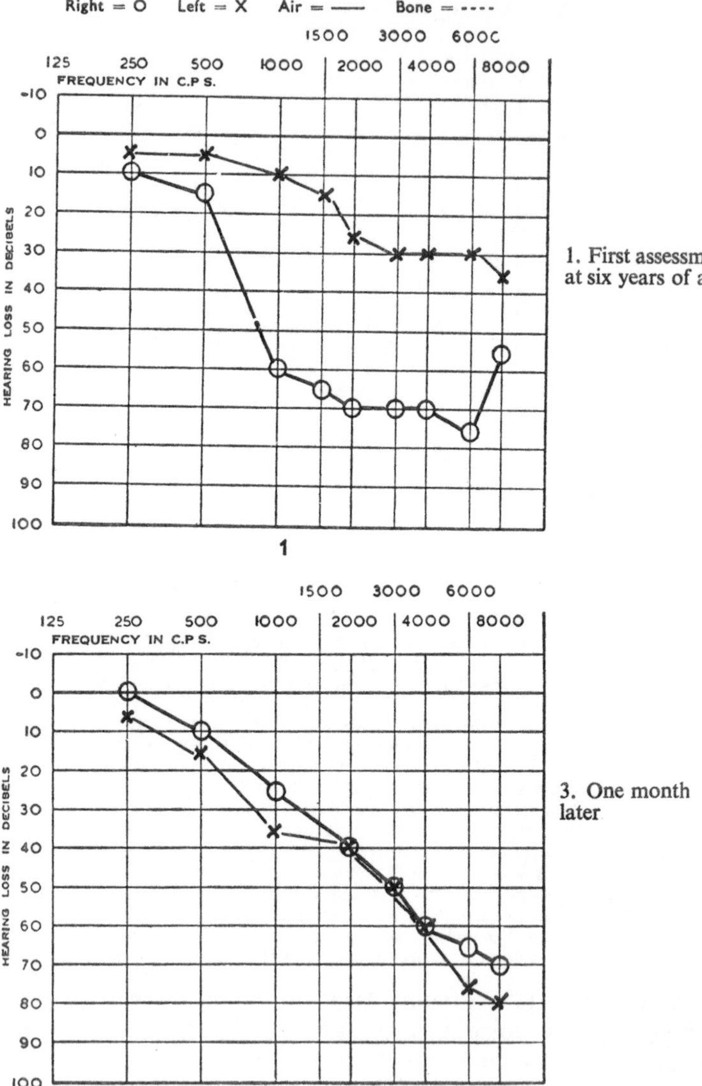

1. First assessment at six years of age

3. One month later

FIG. 68

Referred with defective articulation and an unsuspected hearing loss.

N. S. was an only child who was first seen at the age of 6 years. There was no family history of deafness or defective speech. Born normally at term she sat up at 6 months, walked at 17 months and could feed herself by 18 months. She had had a severe attack of measles at one year. She made no attempt to speak before two years, but after this speech developed slowly with silent intervals, and she could say 'Mummy' and 'Daddy' and a few other words by 3 years. She always responded to household sounds, and her mother did not think she was deaf. She liked books and stories, but from 4 years of age her mother noticed that the child turned round to watch her face when she was reading to her. She played naturally, alone and with other children. At 5 years tonsils

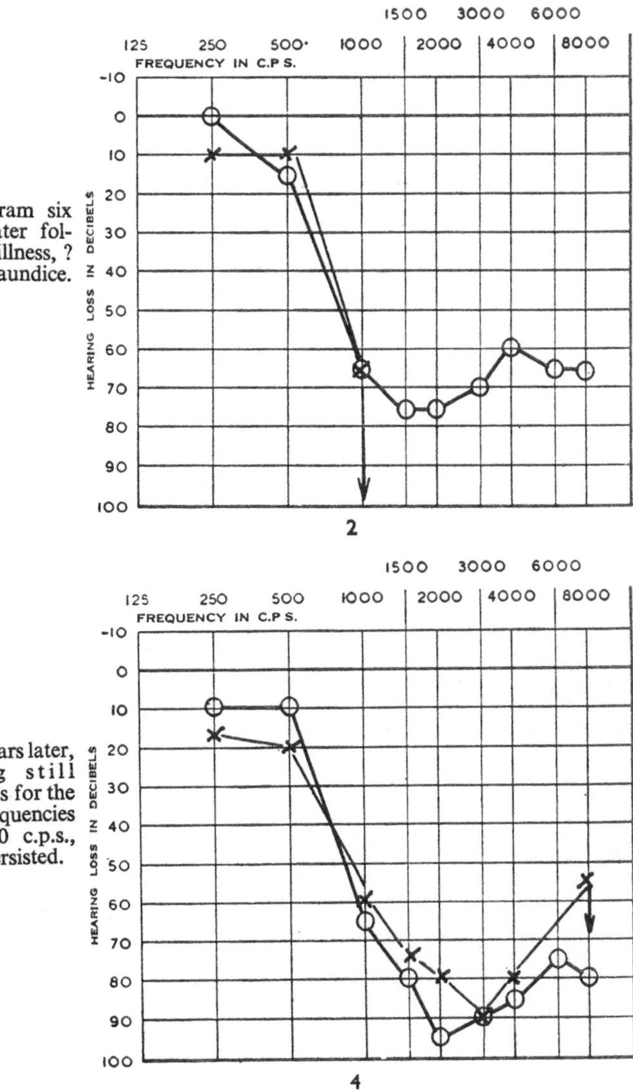

2. Audiogram six months later following an illness, ? infective jaundice.

4. Four years later, showing still further loss for the higher frequencies above 500 c.p.s., which persisted.

FIG. 68 (*continued*)

and adenoids were removed to improve her speech, which was fluent but unintelligible. There had been no history of tonsilitis, otitis or nasal obstruction.

At six years speech was still unintelligible, but she talked freely. She was unable to understand what was said if she could not see the speaker's face, although always aware when someone was speaking. Audiometric assessment showed defective reception especially for the higher frequencies required for the appreciation of the consonant sounds of speech. Her hearing was also found to vary from time to time, with a general progressive loss. She was reading well at 7½ years after having had special assistance by the speech therapist, and was able, though not without difficulty, to maintain her place in the normal school. Articulation gradually improved and was almost normal in reading, but there was greater difficulty in using consonants correctly in spontaneous speech.

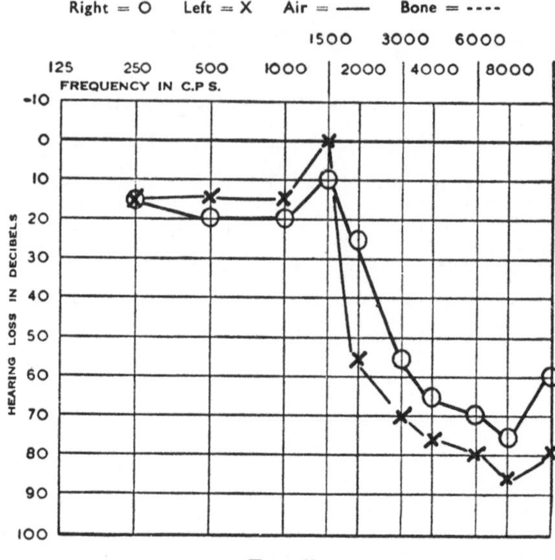

FIG. 69

C. C. The hearing loss in this case was congenital. Articulation was defective, but with the help of a hearing aid he was able to maintain progress in the normal school.

C. C. This boy was first seen at two and a half years of age. He was using words, but only a few phrases, and articulation was defective. Development had been normal in other respects, and he had walked at one year. He was referred with a diagnosis of a severe hearing defect. He was seen at intervals, but persistently refused to co-operate with any form of hearing test. Speech continued to develop, and at four years he had useful conversational speech apart from defective use of the consonants [t], [d], [s], [f], [th], and [ch].

Between the ages of three and five and a half years management was difficult as he had temper tantrums when he failed to make others understand his speech. His own comprehension for speech was good with the aid of lip reading.

At five years he was using language freely, but was still not intelligible to his teacher at school, although he could articulate all consonant sounds normally with care. Because of his pronounced aversion to audiometric testing a reliable assessment of his hearing was not possible until he was seven years of age.

At first it was impossible to prove that a hearing aid was useful, but at eight years he commenced to use one. As hearing for speech with the aid must have differed considerably from that to which he was accustomed it was some time before he gained any benefit from it. He liked to use it, however, and although it could not give him a normal hearing response, it was eventually proved that it was useful and may have improved his hearing for the frequencies between 2000 and 3000 c.p.s., and assisted consonant discrimination.

In spite of his handicap he continued to make good progress in the normal school, and at eight years nine months his reading age was eight years. His standard of work in other subjects, especially arithmetic, was equal to, or above that of his class. In this child high intelligence assisted compensation for a severe hearing disability.

limitations, may assist the child to maintain his place in society. In others lip reading may be useful to supplement the use of a hearing aid (Fig. 69).

Referred with a suspected hearing loss for assessment

Thirty-eight children of varying ages were referred to the speech therapy department for assessment of a suspected partial hearing loss, auditory training with or without a hearing aid, speech therapy for defective articulation, and encouragement of or lessons in lip reading. These children were seen at regular intervals to ensure that adequate use was being made of the hearing aid, and the mother was given guidance as to how she could best help the child at home.

The Assessment of Hearing in the Partially Deaf Child

Accurate assessment of the child's residual hearing by audiometric response to pure tones, and especially of his appreciation for the sounds of speech, is even more important in the child with a partial hearing loss than in the severely deaf child. The response to speech must be ascertained, and again using amplification such as is obtained with a hearing aid. On the results of such tests will depend the management of the child in the home and the arrangements for his education.

Speech response

Before audiometric assessment is attempted, especially in the young child, an approximate estimate of the usefulness of his hearing for speech should be obtained. This is simply and most easily obtained by asking the child to carry out some action as 'shut the door', 'give this to Mother', to point to a named object or picture, or to carry out simple instructions with a group of toys. The volume of the voice may be varied, using a normal conversational voice, then a quiet or a loud voice, as is appropriate. The distance between the child and the speaker should also be varied, remembering that twice the distance reduces the volume or intensity of sound reaching the listener by one quarter.

Response to sounds

In the very young child who has not yet developed speech, response to varying sounds should be noted. The child carries out some action, such as dropping a marble into a box, or placing pegs in a peg-board, when he hears the sound. We have used sounds of varying pitch and intensity such as a bell, a whistle, a mouth organ and the squeak of a rubber mouse for this purpose, at varying distances. The response to the voiced and voiceless consonants of speech, such as [b] [d] [g], and [p] [t] [k] [s], and [ʃ (sh)], may also be tested in the same way, and vowel sounds in monosyllables such as 'boo', 'now', 'go' and so forth.

Audiometric assessment

This should next be attempted as described in Chapter VIII. The younger the child, the more tests will probably be required before a true and reliable result can be obtained. It may be necessary to test the hearing several days in succession, or on several occasions at weekly intervals, until similar findings suggest some degree of reliability. If the hearing loss is confirmed, the child must be referred for examination and the opinion of an otologist.

Response to a hearing aid

This may be tested using the sounds already described, (*a*) noises, (*b*) consonant sounds and (*c*) single syllables with vowel sounds, with varying degrees of amplification. Increase in the volume of sound should be used cautiously, as unpleasantly loud sounds may cause discomfort or frighten the child who may be unused to such noises.

Any improvement in the response to speech should also be assessed, but in this respect it must be remembered that where the hearing loss is congenital and speech has previously been heard with varying degrees of distortion, speech with amplification may be an unknown or at least an unfamiliar language. An improved response to speech may not be obtained, therefore, until the aid has been used consistently for a considerable period of time. On the other hand, the child who has had normal hearing for speech, and recently suffered a loss of hearing, may immediately obtain improved understanding for speech through the use of a hearing aid, depending, of course, on the extent and type of the hearing loss.

THE MANAGEMENT AND TREATMENT OF THE CHILD WITH PARTIAL HEARING

Education

Children with a partial loss of hearing may be divided into two main groups. These are, *firstly*, those whose disability is so slight that they are able to remain in the normal school. A seat near the front of the class may be desirable, and they may use lip reading to supplement their hearing.

In addition there are those children who have a more extensive hearing loss, but obtain adequate hearing for speech with a hearing aid.

All these children have normal language development, although there may be varying degrees of defective articulation. Comprehension for speech is, however, adequate with or without a hearing aid.

Secondly, there are children with inadequate hearing who are helped only partially or not at all by a hearing aid. They rely on lip reading, associated with what hearing they have for vowel sounds and voice. Many of these children struggle to maintain their place in the normal school. They face a severe handicap, often resulting in constant feelings of inferiority and anxiety. They may also have difficulty in learning to read. The hearing aid, if it helps at all, may fail to provide useful speech reception, and lip reading is only of use when the child can see the teacher's face. The older child is therefore at a disadvantage when taking notes from dictation, or when the teacher's face is turned away.

The partially deaf child should be taught as far as is possible through the auditory pathways and should not therefore be educated with children who are severely deaf and who are taught largely through the visual pathways. They may continue to attend a normal school and associate with hearing children, but should be taught in special classes by a trained teacher of the deaf. Hearing aids and classroom amplification can then be used to the best possible advantage, and the standard of educational achievement may be maintained at the normal level. Treatment of the defective articulation is then an important and integral part of their education in the hands of such trained teachers of the deaf.

If such special facilities are not available, it is important that the teacher in the normal school should fully understand the child's disability, and treatment for the defective articulation should then be undertaken by a speech therapist.

Always the teacher must be aware that part of the child's understanding for speech is dependent on intelligent anticipation or guessing, and resulting misunderstandings must be patiently explained. It may also be necessary for the teacher of a young child to have some understanding and supervision of the use of the hearing aid to ensure that it is being used to the best advantage in school.

If the child is dependent on lip reading, he should sit where he has the light behind him and a good view of the teacher's face. He must also have an adequate view of the blackboard, as he will be more dependent on what is written than is the child with full hearing.

Where the child has difficulty in learning to read, special help will be necessary, but once he can do so his ability to learn will be considerably increased, especially if he is given some guidance as to how he may supplement, by reading from a textbook, what he has missed in general class teaching.

Many partially deaf intelligent children have been given such understanding assistance by their teachers in the normal school that they have been able to maintain their place in class without undue strain, and have later been able to proceed to a higher school or university education and lead a normal life in society.

Speech Therapy

The work of the speech therapist will vary according to the educational facilities provided for the partially deaf children in the area where she works.

Treatment of defective articulation. She is concerned, firstly, with those children with defective articulation who are too young to go to a special school or class, or who are being educated in the normal school.

Lip reading instruction. Secondly, lip reading instruction may be required for those children who have an acquired hearing loss in association with normal speech, unless local arrangements provide such facilities under a teacher of the deaf.

In some children a hearing loss may develop gradually and be progressive. It may not be suspected at first, as speech may have developed normally before the onset of the hearing loss, and an older child may be considerably disturbed when such a disability is overtaking him and when his difficulty is not understood. This occurred in one boy, F. S. A hearing loss was first suspected at thirteen years and was confirmed by audiometric tests (Fig. 70 a, b and c). Six months later another test confirmed a further loss of hearing, and he attended for lip reading instruction. A further test five years later showed further severe deterioration in hearing, but normal articulation persisted and he was able to understand speech through lip reading.

The Pre-school Child with a Partial Hearing Loss

The treatment of the young partially deaf child requires guidance in lip reading and auditory training.

Auditory training

This has been described in connection with the severely deaf child (Chapter VIII), but is more important and often of greater value in the child with a less extensive hearing loss. It should begin as early as possible so that the auditory centres of the cortex receive stimulation at the time when a child is normally becoming aware of the meaning of sounds and of speech, and when the neurological mechanisms for executive speech are developing rapidly. Fry and Whetnall (1954) state that:

> The ability to recognise the meaning of sounds or of words is by far the most important factor in normal hearing. It is called auditory discrimination and has to be learnt by the auditory centres in the cortex. A sound is not learnt on once hearing it but only through frequent repetition; memories of sounds and associations with their meaning are acquired slowly. Auditory training is the

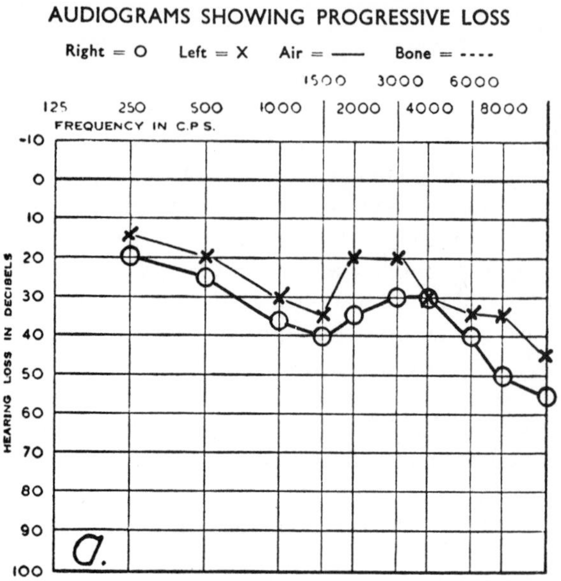

AUDIOGRAMS SHOWING PROGRESSIVE LOSS

Right = O Left = X Air = —— Bone = ----

(*a*) Audiogram at 13½ years.

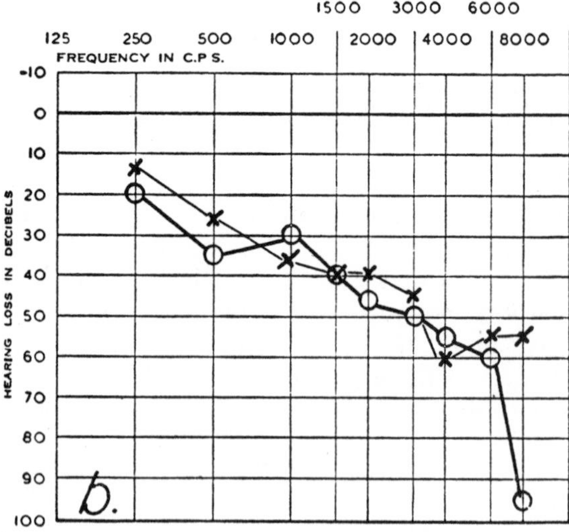

(*b*) Audiogram 7 months later.

FIG. 70 (*continued overleaf*)

F. S. Showing a progressive hearing loss for which there was no obvious cause. Speech was normal.

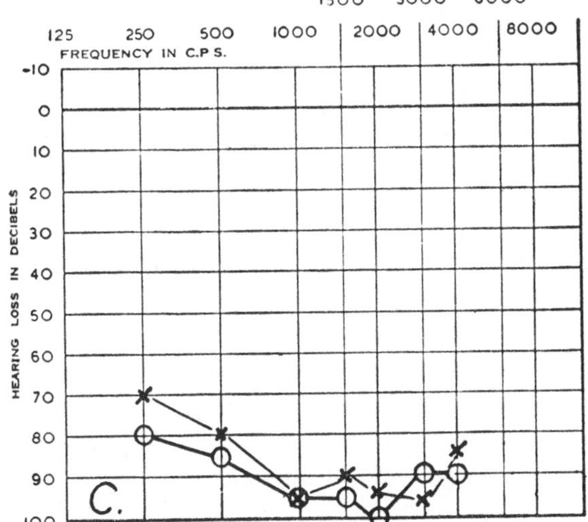

(*c*) Five years later, showing still further deterioration.

FIG. 70 (*continued*)

means by which the cortical areas are given additional practice in discrimination for both the background sounds of everyday life and speech patterns.

They believe that such auditory training should start early in life and consider that:

although the results (of auditory training) are quite good at two or three years, the ideal is to start as soon as possible after the birth of the child, so that listening opportunities can approximate as nearly as possible to those of the child with normal hearing.

This, of course, presupposes that the hearing loss is suspected. Although this may be so in the severely deaf child, a partial hearing loss is frequently not suspected until much later in life when speech fails to develop normally. A hearing aid may assist such auditory training, and should be provided even before accurate assessment of the hearing is possible if an improved response to noises and perhaps to vocal sounds is apparent.

The mother should be advised as to how she can give the child auditory stimulation in the daily life of the home, using an aid, or by speaking close to the child's ear, and in the training of appreciation and imitation of the sounds of speech. The child and the mother should be seen frequently in order to ensure that such training is being carried out to the best advantage at all stages of the child's development. If adequate understanding and some use of language has developed by five years of age, the child may then be able to attend a normal school, even if executive speech is limited and articulation is defective.

Lip reading

Many children with a congenital partial hearing loss develop lip reading spontaneously during the first few years of life. This is assisted when there is hearing for voice and the vowel sounds of speech. If such development is delayed, advice should be given to the mother as to how she can train the child to watch her facial movements during speech. It is important that these should not be exaggerated in any way but should be easy and natural. Further suggestions have already been described in connection with the treatment of the child who has a more severe hearing loss (Chapter VIII).

Maintenance of speech already acquired

Where a hearing loss is acquired after the development of speech, every attempt should be made to maintain communication through speech. The neuromuscular patterns of articulation and the formulative processes through which we speak may be insufficiently stabilised and fail to persist if the loss of hearing is severe and the child finds his world has become strange and silent. A hearing aid may be all that is necessary to restore useful appreciation of speech and maintain the normal channels of communication. If it is of little or no use lip reading instruction may be required to help the child to maintain adequate social contacts as it may not be acquired as easily or spontaneously as when the hearing loss has existed since infancy. The child has, however, the great advantage of having developed speech under conditions of normal hearing.

Treatment for the Older Child with a Partial Hearing Loss

Treatment for the older child involves treatment for defective articulation and instruction in lip reading. Speech is usually maintained without assistance when the hearing loss occurs at a later age, although there may be some deterioration in articulation.

Defective articulation

In these children defects of articulation are the direct result of the child's normal neurophysiological processes by which he imitates the sounds of speech, but with a partial hearing loss he hears them with varying degrees of distortion and reproduces them as they are received. The improvement of articulation in children with a partial hearing loss is therefore not easy. If there is an improved hearing response to speech with a hearing aid, this will be helpful and improvement in the use of articulation may then be spontaneous, or speech therapy may be required in addition to help the child to substitute normal articulation for the defective use of speech sounds already acquired.

If a hearing aid fails to give improved appreciation of the sounds of speech, even after a period of constant listening, speech therapy must depend on the use of other sensory means to guide the child's articulatory movements. The use of tactile and kinaesthetic sensory impressions may be encouraged to compensate for the defective auditory sense, and the visual pathways must be used to a greater extent.

As found in the child with articulatory apraxia, the association of correct articulatory movements with the visual impressions of printed and written letters and words is also of great assistance in helping the child who has learnt or is ready to learn to read, to recall and stabilise articulatory patterns of movement.

The child can be helped not only by the kinaesthetic and tactile sensations of his own lips and tongue movements but also by feeling with his hand the air released on the articulation of consonant sounds by the therapist and by himself. He should also feel the vibration on phonation of vowel sounds and the voiced consonant sounds.

In other ways speech therapy may follow the general principle for the treatment of defects of articulation as already described (Chapter XV). Progress will be slow, as always such patients are attempting to speak as they are taught and not as they hear, and the visual, tactile and kinaesthetic sensory stimuli are a much less useful guide than the normal auditory control for speech. Articulation may eventually be normal when reading aloud, or with care, but in spontaneous conversational speech there may be frequent relapses into the use of articulation as it is heard by the child.

Voice and intonation

In some patients the normal use of voice may not be maintained. There may be difficulty in controlling the volume of the vocal tone, and the patient may either raise the voice or speak too quietly. In noisy surroundings, as in a train or restaurant, the voice may not be raised above the background noise, and it may then be the listener with normal hearing who must attempt to lip read. The patient may be helped to adjust his voice according to varying degrees of sensation in the larynx, and should also be guided by the apparent effect of his voice on those to whom he is speaking. If they are apparently straining to catch what he says, or withdrawing somewhat from too loud a voice, the patient must attempt to adjust the volume of vocal tone accordingly.

Intonation may cease to be variable and become monotonous, and again voice exercises may be necessary to regain or maintain intonation which is as near normal as is possible.

Lip reading

Instruction in lip reading involves first of all eye training, the child being encouraged to watch the speaker's face easily and yet carefully. Even when lip reading is well developed, however, it has its limitations. It cannot be used for appreciation of speech on the radio, nor when there is insufficient light. When the individual is aware of the subject of the conversation he may be able to anticipate some of the words which are not easily visible, but following a change of topic, or of speaker in a group, a sentence or more may be lost before the lip reader is once more able to follow the conversation. One service patient in the Royal Air Force described how he always placed himself, if possible with his back to the light and whenever he could started the topic of conversation. The lip reader will also develop ability to anticipate and to guess from the context, and in so doing may make extraordinary mistakes at times. With normal hearing, comprehension for speech is not dependent on the reception of all the sounds or words spoken. We do not appreciate this under ordinary circumstances until we fail to hear accurately an unfamiliar name of a place or person, perhaps as transmitted through the telephone. Fry and Kerridge (1939) described how 'the brain is ordinarily helped by context and custom to supply what the ear does not perceive, a process so easy that it is commonly unsuspected'. It is probable that the further development of such mental processes plays a considerable part in the understanding of speech through lip reading.

The approach to lip reading should be, as far as possible, at the automatic level. It is the appreciation of the meaning of words and sentences which is required, and not the identification of consonant and vowel sounds. These must be seen rather as part of a sequence of movements, just as with hearing we appreciate the meaning of what is said and not the individual sounds which are used in the articulation of the spoken words and sentences.

The methods used for the development of lip reading ability will depend on the age of the child. Following on from what has already been described for the pre-school child, use can be made of various games involving speech, the lip reading of rhymes and stories, assisted by pictures and sequences of pictures as found in children's 'comic' newspapers.

With older children and adults we have used three simultaneous lines of approach. These are: (1) eye training in watching and discriminating movements (this corresponds to auditory training which is spontaneous in the child with normal hearing); (2) conscious recognition, or the practice of recognising and associating lip movements with meaning; and (3) direct lip reading. This is used from the beginning with very simple material.

1. *Eye training*. The patient watches words where certain consonant sounds occur repeatedly. For example, a list of words is read using the bilabial consonants [p] [b] and [m]. The aim is to familiarise the patient with a certain movement repeated frequently. He is not asked to attempt to understand the words. Isolated words are difficult to lip read as there is no context to assist anticipation of meaning, and words such as 'bad', 'mat' and 'man' look alike to the individual depending

on lip reading, and are only to be distinguished in conversational speech by the context.

2. *Recognition and association.* A limited number of sentences, perhaps ten, are given, containing as many of the consonant sounds being practised in (1) as possible. The patient first watches for the particular articulatory movements just practised and then tries to understand and repeat the sentence. These sentences may be spoken slowly at first, but there must be no break in the continuity of the speech sounds, nor must there be any exaggeration of the lip or tongue movements. Eventually the patient is familiar with the sentences; they are then given in varying order and he is able to discriminate and recognise through lip reading which sentence is being spoken, and repeat it.

3. *Direct lip reading.* From the beginning the patient must be helped to lip read spontaneously, as any attempt to use conscious mental processes of discrimination is impossible at the speed of speech.

It is useful to begin with a list of words in groups, as for example numbers, days of the week, months of the year, the brands of cigarettes, makes of motor cars, names of footballers, contents of a greengrocer's shop, or anything which will interest the particular patient, and he is asked to repeat the words spoken. Here lip reading is facilitated by a recognised limitation of the context.

This process should be extended to the discrimination of nursery rhymes, the playing of games involving speech, and to the understanding of short stories or paragraphs.

A very short story may be read rather slowly at first, and the patient merely asked to find out, if he can, what it is about. The same story may be read two or three times, when there is generally increased understanding. The patient is then allowed to read the story himself, after which he again watches it read. As he progresses he is asked to repeat the story, phrase by phrase after the speaker, so building up verbal associations with visible lip movements.

As progress continues, conversation practice should be a part of each period of treatment.

Many people think lip reading will be difficult to learn, and care must be taken to develop confidence by ensuring that the exercises given are adapted to and well within the scope of the individual. He must be encouraged to relax and watch rather than to make strenuous efforts to understand, and be content at first with accepting what comes easily.

Patients must also be helped to feel that they can develop the use of their eyes to hear. In fact, many patients say after a few weeks that they think their hearing has improved. Closing their eyes proves to them that this impression is the result of the developing association of the visual impressions of speech with the previously established auditory patterns, and only in this way can lip reading be acquired easily, become a natural process and of assistance in the understanding of what others say.

REFERENCES

Fry, D. B., and Kerridge, P. M. T. (1939). Tests for Hearing and Speech by Deaf People. *Lancet*, **1,** 106.

Fry, D. B., and Whetnall, E. (1954). The Auditory Approach in the Training of Deaf Children. *Lancet*, **1,** 583.

XVII. Defects of Articulation and Structural Abnormalities

CERTAIN conditions which affect the growth and development of the mouth may hinder or prevent the use of normal articulation. Structural abnormalities in the pharynx or oral and nasal airways may interfere with the movements and adjustments of the tongue or lips, or prevent adequate control of the essential intra-oral air pressure for the articulation of the plosive and fricative consonant sounds of speech. In spite of adequate neurological development for speech, normal articulation may then be impossible.

The tongue is capable of so much compensatory adjustment that dental irregularities are rarely responsible for gross defects of articulation unless there is also some degree of associated dyspraxia or dysarthria which hinders such compensation. The child beginning to talk may have normal articulation in spite of incomplete dental equipment, and most children readily adjust their articulation when teeth are temporarily absent during the second dentition. There may be a transient lisp, but even this is not inevitable. Inability to control the outlet of air through the nasopharynx and nasal airways, as the result of an incompetent nasopharyngeal sphincter, causes a much more serious interference with the development and use of normal articulation.

The structural conditions which will be discussed in their relation to defects of articulation are (1) the incompetent nasopharyngeal sphincter, (2) macroglossia, (3) tongue tie, (4) dental abnormalities, and (5) tonsils and adenoids.

THE NASOPHARYNGEAL SPHINCTER OR VALVE

The expiratory air stream used for speech is normally controlled by three valves or sphincters in three positions, namely:

1. In the larynx at the level of the vocal folds, or ventricular bands.

2. In the nasopharynx, by the nasopharyngeal sphincter.
3. At the lips, by the orbicularis oris and other facial muscles.

Normal speech requires primarily the adaptation and co-ordination of the muscles concerned in the action of these three valves. The issuing air stream is modified and set into vibration at the level of the vocal folds for phonation, and thus forms a basis for the vowel sounds and voiced consonants. This air stream is also modified and its vibrations amplified as a result of resonance in the various resonating cavities in the chest and below the level of the larynx, and of the pharynx, mouth and nasal airways. Such resonance varies according to the individual shape and size of these cavities, and is also affected by the action and degree of tension in the muscles of the pharynx, oropharyngeal isthmus, tongue and lips. In addition the air stream is modified or interrupted at varying positions in the mouth through contacts between the tongue and the teeth, alveolus, or palate, for articulation.

Anatomy

The muscles concerned in the control of the nasopharyngeal sphincter are (*a*) palatal and (*b*) pharyngeal. The palatal muscles are arranged in pairs, one on each side. The tensor palati enters the upper surface of the palate after passing round the hamular processes, its tendons from either side meeting to form the palatal aponeurosis (Figs. 71 and 72). The levator palati, the palatopharyngeus and certain fibres of the superior constrictor from the pharynx also enter the upper surface of the palate from each side and are inserted into the palatal aponeurosis. The palato-glossus enters the palate and is attached to the lower surface (Fig. 71).

The pharyngeal muscles concerned are the superior constrictor, and, perhaps to a lesser extent, the salpingopharyngeus. Whillis (1930) found that some of the fibres of the superior constrictor passed round the lateral walls of the pharynx to be inserted into the palatal aponeurosis, thus acting synchronously with the levators and on contraction causing a sphincteric or valvular mechanism which, when closed, prevented the passage of air through the nasopharynx. It has been thought that the tensor palati acted in opposition to these muscles to cause

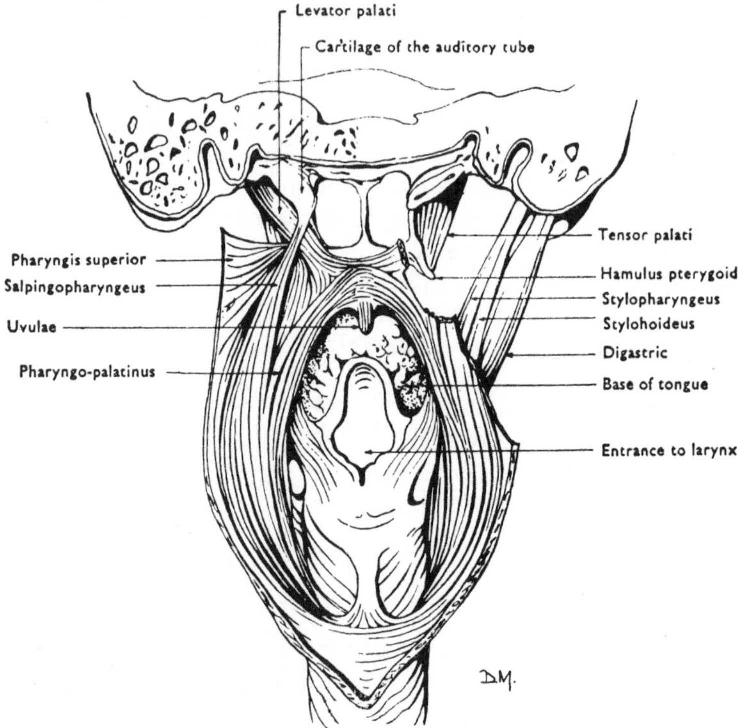

FIG. 71

Movements of the soft palate. Diagram showing the muscles concerned with the opening and closure of the nasopharyngeal airway.

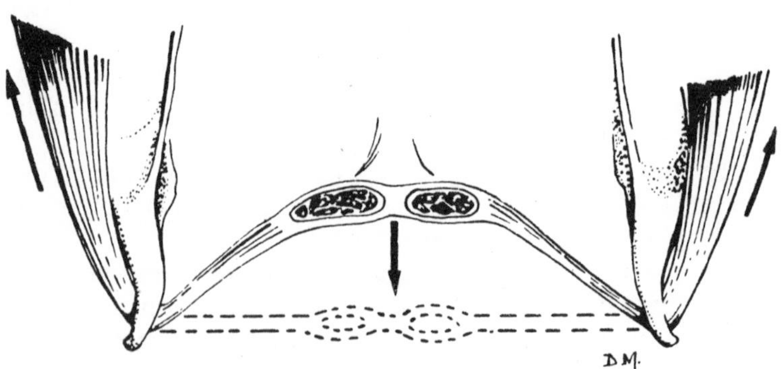

FIG. 72

The tensor palati and the hamular processes. This muscle lowers the soft palate and may be concerned chiefly with swallowing rather than with speech.

lowering of the palate and opening of the nasopharyngeal sphincter (Fig. 72).

Podvinec (1952) has suggested that each pair of these muscles forms a sling with its concavity upwards or downwards.

(*a*) With concavity upwards	Tensor palati, Levator palati, and Superior constrictor muscle slings.
(*b*) With concavity downwards	Palatoglossus, and Palatopharyngeus muscle slings.

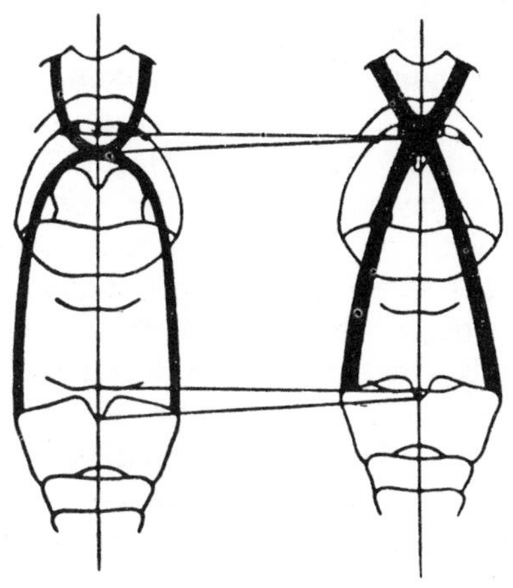

FIG. 73

Diagram representing the slings of the levator and palatopharyngeus muscles when relaxed and when contracted. (*Podvinec* (1952).)

He suggests that the movement of the soft palate results from the simultaneous contraction of two of these muscle slings, namely that of the levator and the palatopharyngeus and that of the superior constrictor acting with the levator, in assisting closure in the nasopharynx. The action of the muscle slings formed by the levatores and the palatopharyngeus are shown diagrammatically in Figure 73, firstly in a state of relaxation and secondly when simultaneously contracted. The sling of the palatoglossus is thought to oppose the lifting action of these muscles, acting as a depressor of the palate, and relaxing when the soft palate is raised. This action is also shown in the diagram (Figs. 74 and 75). Podvinec suggests that the decisive factor in raising the palate in order to obtain nasopharyngeal closure is the rèsultant component of force towards the posterior pharyngeal wall of the tensions in the two muscle slings of the levator and palatopharyngeus. This is shown in Figure 76, firstly when the soft palate is relaxed and rests on the tongue and secondly when raised into contact with the posterior pharyngeal wall.

Passavant, 1861, described a ridge which formed across the posterior pharyngeal wall during speech. It was later thought that this was assisted by the contraction of some of the fibres of the superior constrictor. More recently doubt has arisen as to the importance of this ridge for speech. Calnan (1955) believes that this ridge is not present in the normal, but is essentially related to effort in speech and particularly to closure during swallowing. It might therefore be possible that the ridge of Passavant as seen in patients with cleft palate represents hypertrophy of the muscles concerned in an attempt to compensate for an open nasopharynx. Ardran and Kemp (1952) have found through radiographic studies that the ridge of Passavant does take some part in speech in certain patients with normal nasopharyngeal closure and anatomy. However, whether the ridge of Passavant is present or not, it seems certain that adequate closure in the nasopharynx occurs and is essential for normal speech, and that it is associated with much bunching of the mucosa, and with firm closure occurring at various levels in the nasopharynx.

THE FUNCTION OF THE NASOPHARYNGEAL SPHINCTER, OR VALVE

Co-ordinated use of the muscles involved in the action of the three sphincters or valves controlling the respiratory air stream at the lips, in the larynx and in the nasopharynx is essential for normal speech, and the absence of such normal co-ordinations when the nasopharyngeal sphincter is incompetent is responsible for the various abnormalities of articulation which occur in cleft palate speech. Such co-ordinations normally develop at birth for the physiological processes involved in respiration, sucking and swallowing, whilst phonation occurs with the first cry. This usually has a nasal quality and may not be associated with closure of the nasopharyngeal sphincter during the first few days of life.

Podvinec (1952) believes that the innervation for speech may not be the same as that for swallowing and other physiological processes. He suggests that there is evidence to support the theory that the levator has a double innervation—from the facial nerve and from the pharyngeal branches of the vagus, and that during speech it is the facial nerve which takes the lead in co-ordinating movements of the palate and the facial muscles such as those of the tongue tip and lips. During swallowing the glossopharyngeus and the pharyngeal branches of the vagus are thought to ensure harmony of movements of the muscles of the pharynx and oesophagus. This theory might then account for the condition of those children who are able to obtain nasopharyngeal closure and co-ordination for swallowing but not for speech.

The function of nasopharyngeal closure will be described under varying conditions.

Respiration

Respiration may take place through the nose with the nasopharyngeal sphincter open, or through the mouth with the soft palate raised and the nasopharyngeal sphincter closed. It rarely occurs through both airways simultaneously, although this may be easily accomplished with conscious control.

Sucking

In the normal adult method of sucking, fluids are drawn into the mouth by the movements of the tongue, the lips sealing the opening into the mouth around the tube, straw, or cup margin. The dorsum of the tongue is at first elevated against the soft palate, which is somewhat depressed, closing the oropharyngeal isthmus. The nasopharyngeal sphincter is then partially open, or at least not firmly closed. The floor of the mouth, mandible and tongue are then lowered, and a negative pressure is thus set up in the mouth. The fluid is drawn up into the space so created, assisted by the action of the muscles of the lips and cheeks and movements of the tongue.

In sucking, when large quantitites of fluid are drawn up by inspiratory effort from the chest, the nasopharyngeal sphincter is normally closed, but may at times be open to allow air to be drawn simultaneously through the oral and nasal airways. This is the usual method employed by the child with incompetent nasopharyngeal closure.

In the infant the nasopharyngeal sphincter remains open during sucking as the child continues to breathe through the nose, alternately or simultaneously with sucking. The soft palate is depressed and the dorsum of the tongue raised, thus closing the oropharyngeal isthmus. The lips enclose the nipple and seal the entrance to the mouth whilst the nipple is then pressed between the tongue and the alveolus. This infantile method of sucking persists in the patient with the incompetent nasopharyngeal sphincter, and may not always be changed in the cleft palate patient following successful surgical repair.

Swallowing

Fluids are held in the mouth, resting in a depression upon the upper surface of the forepart of the tongue, which then directs the fluid to the back of the mouth and through the oropharyngeal isthmus. This has been fully described by Ardran and Kemp (1955). Whillis (Lucas and Whillis, 1950) states that during this voluntary stage of swallowing the nasopharyngeal sphincter is open and there is closure of the mouth by the lips or by the tongue against the alveolus. As the bolus reaches the pharynx it is directed into the oesophagus by the constrictors of the pharynx, the nasopharyngeal sphincter remaining open. The sensation of attempting to swallow with the nasopharyngeal sphincter closed can be experienced during a severe cold in the head, when the nasopharyngeal airways are occluded, or simply by attempting to swallow whilst the anterior nares are closed by finger pressure. Similar control of the nasopharyngeal sphincter is maintained during the swallowing of solids.

The presence of a nasopharyngeal sphincter is not therefore essential to life, but the infant with a cleft of the alveolus will first experience difficulty because he cannot adequately compress the nipple between the tongue and alveolus, and because the development of the necessary negative pressure in the mouth may be difficult, although not always impossible. Swallowing

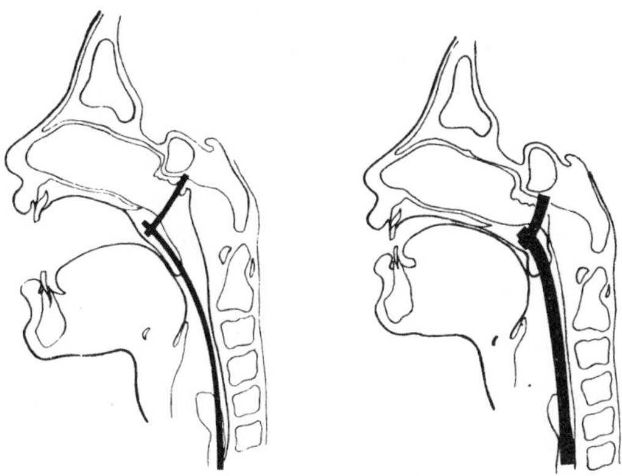

Fig. 74
Lateral view showing the effect of interaction of the levator and palatopharyngeus muscles on the movement of the soft palate. (*Podvinec* (1952).)

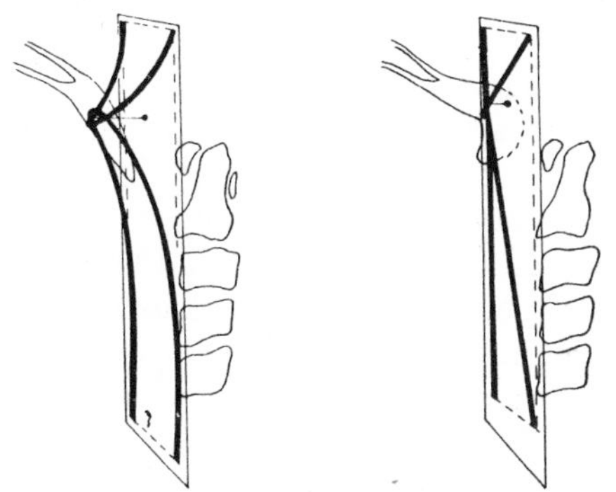

Fig. 75
Diagrammatic view of the muscle action in Fig. 74. (*Podvinec* (1952).)

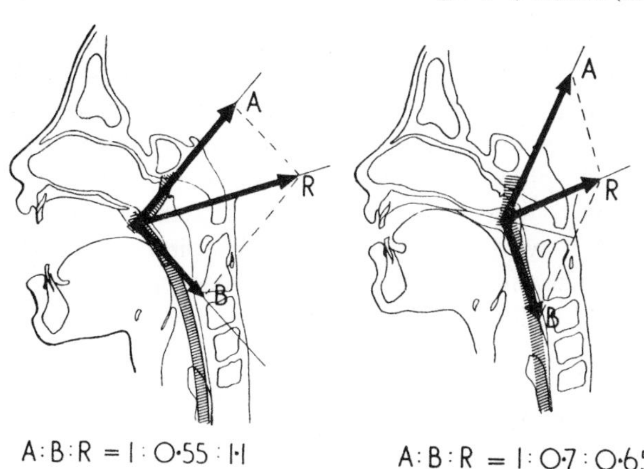

Fig. 76
Diagram illustrating the resultant force and its direction on the soft palate of the two forces occurring on contracture of the levator and palatopharyngeus muscles. (*Podvinec* (1952).)

is not markedly hindered apart from the difficulty of regurgitation of fluids and solids into the nasopharynx and nostrils. Most babies with cleft palates unconsciously adapt to their need to maintain life, but feeding with a spoon may be necessary until the lip and alveolus have been repaired in cases of complete unilateral or bilateral alveolar clefts.

Blowing

Blowing usually requires that the breath should be directed at or into some object, as when blowing out a flame or inflating a balloon. Although blowing may be sustained simultaneously through the mouth and nose, greater and more effective pressure is obtained if the nasopharyngeal airway is closed for the normal act of blowing through the mouth, and if the mouth is closed when blowing through the nose, as when clearing mucus from the nasal airways.

When the cheeks are distended with air, against the resistance of the muscles of the cheeks and closed lips, considerable pressure can be maintained in the mouth. The nasopharyngeal sphincter is closed, otherwise air would leak through the nasal passages and the maintenance of pressure be impossible. This air, held under pressure in the mouth, may be released at will either through the lips or through the nasopharyngeal sphincter.

If closure in the nasopharynx is not possible, air may still be held in the mouth under some degree of pressure if the oropharyngeal isthmus is closed by the depression of the palate and elevation of the dorsum of the tongue. This method is sometimes used by the child with an incompetent nasopharyngeal sphincter. Under such conditions the release of air through the mouth is not supported by the pressure of expiratory air from the lungs, which accompanies this action when the nasopharyngeal sphincter controls the outlet of air through the nasopharynx, and the oropharyngeal isthmus remains open. In the child with an incompetent nasopharyngeal sphincter, blowing is therefore ineffective rather than impossible, and can be assisted by closure of the nasal airways at the anterior nares.

Speech

The normal articulation of most consonant sounds requires a degree of air pressure in the mouth which cannot be maintained if air escapes through the nasopharynx and nostrils. Although much less oral pressure is required for vowel sounds, a balance between oral and nasal resonance which approaches normal must be achieved, and this may sound grossly distorted if the nasopharyngeal sphincter is incompetent or the pharyngeal dimensions are abnormal. The degree of nasopharyngeal closure for vowel sounds also depends on the adjacent consonant sounds, and vowels associated with the nasal resonants [m] [n] and [ŋ (ng)] may be partially nasalised. This occurs more commonly in French or some other languages than it does in standard English pronunciation, but in conversational speech complete closure, even apart from the nasal consonants, is not consistently maintained. The mucosa of the palate approximates to the posterior pharyngeal wall, from which position it can achieve extremely rapid movements, effecting adequate closure when required for the normal articulation of consonant sounds. This requires accurate timing and co-ordination of movements of the lips and tongue with palatal movements.

The position of the tongue for most vowel sounds offers little resistance to the passage of air through the mouth. The vowel [i: (ee)] being produced with the blade of the tongue raised towards the palate causes more resistance than a vowel sound such as [ɑ: (ah)], but very much less than is caused by the position of the articulatory organs for the plosive and fricative consonant sounds.

Similarly, the consonants [l] and [r], and the semi-vowels [j (y)] and [w], offer little resistance to the issuing air stream, and may approach normal even when the nasopharyngeal sphincter is incompetent. Some change of resonance may be obvious, but this may not interfere with the intelligibility of these sounds when used in speech.

The plosive consonants, however, require that air should be held under pressure in the mouth momentarily, and then released. This pressure can only be adequately obtained when there is simultaneous closure of the nasal and oral outlets, the latter occurring at the lips for the articulation of [p] and [b], by the tongue against the alveolus for [t] and [d], and by the dorsum of the tongue against the palate for [k] and [g]. The actual consonant sound is then produced by an explosive release of air through these positions of the articulatory muscles. For the corresponding nasal consonants [m] [n] and [ŋ (ng)] the position is maintained, the oral outlet remains closed and the sounds are produced through the nasopharyngeal sphincter and nasal airways. The sphincter is not completely relaxed, however, as for nasal breathing, and its nearly closed position may contribute to the resonance of these sounds forming a resonance node.

The fricative consonants used in speech also require considerable air pressure. They require that the air stream should pass through a small airway between the parts of the mouth used for their articulation. In the case of each of the fricative consonants [f] [v] [s] [z] [ʃ (sh)] [ʒ] and [θ and ð (th)] the airway must be sufficiently small for the issuing air to be set into vibration, producing a fricative sound. This may be voiceless or superimposed on a fundamental laryngeal tone as in the voiced consonants [v] [z] [ʒ] and [ð]. Because the aperture for the sounds must be small, sustained air pressure in the mouth is essential, and can only be adequately achieved if the nasopharyngeal airway is closed. The consonant [s] in particular requires the maintenance of good air pressure as far forward in the mouth as the alevolar ridge and incisor teeth. Because of the high pressure required for this sound there is a greater tendency for air to escape through the nasopharynx when closure is incomplete.

Inadequate Nasopharyngeal Closure

The nasopharyngeal sphincter may be incompetent for various reasons, as when it is incomplete in a cleft of the palate, or when function is inadequate for normal articulation as in paresis of the soft palate. In the latter case it is not a structural defect, but so far as speech is concerned the condition causes a similar functional disability. Conditions which may be associated with an incompetent nasopharyngeal sphincter are (1) a cleft palate, (2) a submucous cleft, (3) a short soft palate, or excessively large nasopharynx and (4) defects in the palate. It may also occur as the result of (5) paresis of the soft palate (6) operation for tonsils and adenoids or (7) inco-ordination in the use of the nasopharyngeal sphincter in the absence of any anatomical insufficiency or paresis.

1. *Cleft palate*

Where the two halves of the palate have failed to unite, wholly or in part, the child is unable to control the expiratory air stream and to vary its direction at will through the mouth or through the nose. Expiration occurs simultaneously through both airways, or through the nose if the mouth is closed, and the infant is unable to obtain the requisite air pressure for the plosive and fricative consonant sounds during the babbling stage of speech development. He may develop abnormal co-ordinations for the physiological processes of sucking and swallowing but is unable to accomplish many of the actions common in babies, such as blowing out his cheeks, making noises with his lips and tongue and blowing saliva bubbles, all of which contribute in the child with a normal palate to the developing control of the three sphincters used in speech, especially those of the lips and nasopharynx.

Abnormal patterns of co-ordination of the palatal and pharyngeal muscles develop, therefore, in infancy, with inability to acquire normal control of the respiratory and vocal air stream and adequate intra-oral air pressure.

Mal-development of the palate has usually been classified according to the severity of the defect, or the position at which failure of normal union ceased. There may therefore be post-alveolar clefts of any extent, varying from a cleft of the uvula to a complete cleft of the soft and hard palates. Where the alveolus is also divided, the cleft may be unilateral or bilateral. Pre-alveolar clefts of the lip may vary in extent, be unilateral or bilateral, and may be associated with clefts of the palate whilst the alveolus is or is not intact. There may also be clefts of the lip, with or without partial clefts of the alveolus, and no cleft of the palate.

There are, however, many variations of development. In some the palatal plates and tissues have developed well yet failed to unite, whilst in others there is minimal development of the palatal tissues, resulting in a wide cleft and little material with which to close it. Again there may be more development of tissue on one side than on the other, and the surgeon is faced with the problem of uniting two unequal halves, one of which may be considerably longer than the other. Each presents an individual problem due to many varying degrees of developmental failure of the lip, alveolus and palate.

Although the first essential for speech is the ability to achieve competent nasopharyngeal closure, resulting deformities of the maxilla and alveolus may affect articulation. A narrowing of the maxilla may impede movements of the tongue, or residual grooves in the surface of the alveolus may cause difficulty in controlling the frequency of vibration of the air stream for the consonant [s], for which no amount of adjustment on the part of the tongue may compensate satisfactorily. Faulty dentition with many irregularities will also contribute to the difficulties experienced by the cleft palate patient in the acquisition of normal speech, but the greatest difficulty is encountered when sufficient intra-oral air pressure for articulation is unobtainable.

The bifid uvula. This represents a minimal cleft of the soft palate and may not interfere with normal nasopharyngeal closure unless associated with incomplete development of the palate. The levatores are inserted into the palatal aponeurosis which is situated about half way between the anterior and posterior borders of the soft palate, and it is here where the movement occurs which is chiefly concerned with closure in the nasopharynx. Such closure is achieved by bunching of the mucosa, and may be adequate when there is no deficiency of tissue. If the bifid uvula is associated with a submucous cleft, it is more probable that the nasopharyngeal sphincter may be incompetent.

2. *The submucous cleft*

This condition occurs when the muscles of the two halves of the palate have failed to unite in the mid-line but the mucous membrane is intact and no cleft is apparent. Movement of the soft palate is not normal, however, and attempts to raise the palate whilst saying ‘ah’ produce a widening and flattening of the soft palate with limited upward and backward movement. The tissues in the mid-line may appear translucent, or a notch may be felt in the posterior border of the hard palate. Because the muscles on each side have failed to unite, the lifting action of the levatores is inadequate. When the mucous membrane of the palate is incised at operation, the two halves of the palate fall apart.

In such cases articulation will depend on the degree of developmental failure and the extent to which there may have been development or hypertrophy of various muscles to assist nasopharyngeal closure. This may be adequate for speech, accomplished only on sustained effort, or the sphincter may be incompetent.

J. P., aged seven years, had a submucous cleft of the palate. Vowel sounds were nasalised, and all consonant sounds were weak as sufficient oral air pressure could not be maintained. Speech was mostly unintelligible. Surgery was considered, but it was decided by the surgeon that it should be postponed until attempts had been made to improve the use of the nasopharyngeal sphincter and articulation by speech therapy. Exercises were given to develop the use of the nasopharyngeal sphincter and to improve the air direction, encouraging maximum outlet through the mouth to strengthen the articulation of consonant sounds. Speech improved and became intelligible, but tended to lapse at times of stress or when hurried, and normal closure in the nasopharynx with adequate oral pressure for articulation could not be maintained. Eventually the palate was repaired by the usual surgical procedures, with considerable immediate improvement in articulation, and finally normal speech was achieved and persisted.

3. *The short soft palate*

This may be a congenital condition, or the result of surgery which has failed to produce the possibility of normal control of the nasopharyngeal outlet. There is no cleft of the palate, but in both conditions the nasopharyngeal sphincter is incompetent, and escape of air through the nasal airways cannot be prevented or controlled as required for articulation.

Following surgery there may have been deficient growth of the palatal tissues, or there may have been such a limited development of palatal tissues before operation that the surgeon's aim could not be achieved. Again the dimensions of the nasopharynx may be abnormally large and nasopharyngeal closure inadequate.

In some of these children, closure of the nasopharyngeal sphincter may be possible on sustained effort, as in blowing, but be inadequate for the rapid movements required during speech.

4. *Defects in the palate*

There may be a fistula in the palate due to trauma, or as a result of a breakdown of the palatal tissues after operation. Such openings in the palate allow the air to leak into the nostrils, and adequate air pressure is unobtainable. This may occur when the nasopharyngeal sphincter is competent, and if the fistula is then near the alveolus it may be possible for the child to obtain normal articulation with adequate pressure for [k] and [g], but not for sounds such as [s] [t] or [d] which require sustained pressure further forward in the mouth.

5. *Paresis of the soft palate*

Here there is no anatomical or structural failure, but there is deficient function of the muscles concerned in the closure of the nasopharyngeal sphincter. This condition has already been described under developmental dysarthria (Chapter XII).

It is doubtful if operation is advisable in this condition. The difficulty is one of movement rather than of a structural abnormality, and surgical interference may even hinder rather than help the movement of the palatal and pharyngeal muscles.

6. *Following operation for removal of tonsils and adenoids*

After such operations there may be a temporary or more persistent incompetence of the nasopharyngeal sphincter, with defective articulation resembling cleft palate speech occurring in children who previously had normal speech. This usually responds readily to exercises for control of the nasopharyngeal sphincter. However, it may also result from scarring causing a permanent defect, or from a previously unsuspected palatal paresis or enlarged nasopharynx.

The need for removal of tonsils and adenoids in a child with a repaired cleft palate presents a greater problem than in other children. Many are more susceptible to infections of the nasal airways, the pharynx and middle ear, with the possibility of permanent damage to the conductive mechanisms of the middle ear. In some of these children the adenoid pad may have developed in compensation for the enlarged dimensions of the pharynx and may have assisted nasopharyngeal closure during speech. Its removal may then cause a more persistent or even permanent deterioration in speech with subsequent inability to regain nasopharyngeal closure and normal speech. Surgical treatment for removal of adenoids should be carried out only in these children after consultation between the plastic surgeon and the ear, nose and throat surgeon concerned, and after assessment of speech by a speech therapist. If it is thought that speech will be seriously affected, such removal of adenoids is only justified if it is essential for the maintenance of normal hearing.

7. *Inco-ordination in the use of the nasopharyngeal sphincter*

It is possible that a nasopharyngeal sphincter may be competent but not used in speech. This may occur following surgery, or even when there has been no cleft of the palate, and be the result of an articulatory dyspraxia. In a minor degree it occurs only on the consonant [s], or on a few other fricative sounds. A fricative sound made through the nasopharyngeal sphincter is substituted whilst the tongue or lips completely occlude the oral outlet. The defect may also extend to some plosive consonants, such as [t] and [d], when a nasopharyngeal plosive sound is substituted. The absence of any true organic abnormality is proved by the ability to articulate other consonants with adequate oral pressure.

T. L., aged three years, had normal articulation except for the consonants [s] [ʃ (sh)] [t] [d] [tʃ (ch)] and [dʒ (j)], for which fricative or plosive sounds were made through the nasopharyngeal sphincter. The consonants [*θ* and ð (th)] had not been attempted. Initial attempts to obtain normal articulation by indirect means such as blowing for breath direction and hissing sounds in isolation were tried, but failed to improve the articulation. The sound [th] was then taught, and this was rapidly and normally incorporated into spontaneous speech whilst the other defective sounds persisted for another year. More direct speech therapy was then attempted, and speech was normal within four months.

Such an apraxia for the control and co-ordination of the palatal and pharyngeal muscles required for articulation may also persist in the child or adult following successful surgery. In most patients normal co-ordinations for the reflex acts of sucking and swallowing are established soon after operation and are quickly followed by improved use of the nasopharyngeal sphincter for speech. However, if, as previously suggested, the innervation for palatal movements for swallowing differs from that for articulation, improved function for sucking and swallowing may not necessarily assist the palatal movements for articulation. Faulty patterns of co-ordination of these muscles for speech may then persist, and may hinder or prevent the development of normal articulation.

THE TREATMENT OF INCOMPETENT NASOPHARYNGEAL CLOSURE

Treatment for incompetent nasopharyngeal closure, especially as it occurs in cases of cleft palate, may require surgery, the fitting of an obturator, or speech therapy, or the combined efforts of a team consisting of a surgeon, orthodontist and speech therapist. The problems which may arise, and pre-surgical orthodontics have been discussed more fully in *Cleft Palate and Speech* (1969).

The Obturator

This was first designed and used many years ago as an alternative to surgery, in the first instance to cover the cleft in the palate. When the need for closure in the nasopharynx was first realised, obturators were fitted with an extension or bulb, which fitted into the nasopharynx and was designed to assist closure.

In modern times such prostheses have been modified. They are lighter in weight and in some the bulb is replaced by a broad extension into the pharynx around which the constrictors of the pharynx can contract. Speech may be considerably improved thereby, and they may offer a better prognosis than surgery carried out by those unskilled in the special techniques required for the treatment of cleft palate.

Where there is a residual fistula in the hard palate following surgery, a dental plate which covers the aperture and prevents the leakage of air pressure from the mouth is of the utmost value. Even a small aperture may prevent the normal development of speech, and such an appliance should be fitted as early in life as the dental surgeon considers possible in order to permit normal development of speech rather than the establishment of faulty patterns of articulation due to inadequate intra-oral air pressure. Especially is this important in those children where nasopharyngeal closure is adequate.

Where surgical failure has resulted in a short soft palate, a 'push back' operation may assist speech but leave a large aperture in the hard palate which will require a dental prosthesis to compensate for the partial absence of tissue in the region of the hard palate and which will assist in maintaining the more backward position of the soft palate.

SURGERY

The problem facing the cleft palate surgeon is not a simple one whichever of the various methods he uses for closure of the cleft, and in every case his technique must be modified and designed to meet the individual need. Where there is insufficient tissue for complete palatal closure, the production of a competent nasopharyngeal sphincter is of more importance for speech than a complete hard palate. An aperture or fistula remaining in the hard palate may later be covered by a dental plate, as previously described, but an obturator may not provide an adequate substitute for a mobile soft palate and effective physiological function.

The history and growth of cleft palate surgery has been described elsewhere (Morley, 1969). In the seventeenth century operations were carried out on the pharyngeal wall by Passavant and Rosenthal, and later Wardill (1937) and Hynes (1950) devised pharyngoplasty operations designed to narrow the excessive dimensions of the nasopharynx and to compensate for the inadequate soft palate.

Wardill combined such pharyngoplasty with a four-flap operation, whilst Hynes is now using his method of pharyngoplasty as a means of obtaining nasopharyngeal closure with as little surgical interference with the palate as possible. Other surgeons think that operations on the normal pharyngeal wall may hinder its mobility, and Braithwaite has obtained successful results during the last five years without incision of the muscles of the posterior pharyngeal wall.

Any surgery which is designed to improve the speech of the

patient must include the freeing of the muscles so that the palate may be sutured without tension, otherwise there may be interference with the mobility of the soft palate, breakdowns in the suture line and the formation of tension fistulas. There must be careful suture to minimise the formation of scar tissue, as the growth and development of the palate will be hindered by hard fibrosed tissues. Successful surgery will produce a mobile soft palate and the possibility of adequate nasopharyngeal closure.

The Age of Operation

This must be considered from at least two points of view, namely the age when the surgeon is able to operate most advantageously as regards the actual technique, and the best age for the subsequent development of normal speech.

Speech

From the point of view of normal speech development early operation is an advantage. The basic neuromuscular patterns of speech, including the co-ordination of the three sphincters controlling expiratory air, are laid down early in life from the time of the first cry. Consonant sounds make their appearance in the infant's vocal play from the fourth month, and in the child with a cleft palate these activities must necessarily be abnormal. If the use of language develops before operation, inability to use the nasopharyngeal sphincter will cause faulty neuromuscular patterns of co-ordination between the oral muscles of articulation and those of the soft palate and pharynx. These will become more and more firmly stabilised, and as time passes will become increasingly difficult to eradicate.

It has been found that when operation has been unavoidably postponed until the third or fourth year of life, although normal speech may eventually be acquired spontaneously, the child will pass through a variable period of time when articulation is defective. Other factors being equal, the younger the child when operation is performed, the shorter the period of defective articulation through which the child will pass.

However, other factors are concerned in the child's ability to develop normal speech spontaneously after operation. A partial or severe hearing loss or general mental defect will obviously interfere with the child's ability to develop normal patterns of articulation. Again, as previously described in connection with the speech of the children in 1000 families in Newcastle-upon-Tyne (Chapter IV), 31 per cent of these children had defective articulation at the age of three years ten months, whilst 11 per cent had such a severe defect that speech was not intelligible to any but those in the child's immediate environment. There was generally spontaneous improvement, so that at four years nine months, 11 per cent had defective articulation but only five per cent were unintelligible. In one per cent, speech was still unintelligible at six and a half years of age. In only one case in the series was there a child with a cleft palate, and he had normal speech following successful surgery at the age of one year.

It is important to remember, therefore, when assessing the post-operative development of speech in children with cleft palate, that allowance must be made for some who may have in addition a dyslalia, developmental dysarthria or articulatory dyspraxia, and who will have additional difficulty in obtaining normal speech.

Where operation has been postponed until adult life, or where secondary operation is required following failed operation in infancy, faulty habits of articulation will be firmly established, and a successful surgical result rarely produces immediate and spontaneous improvement in speech, although normal speech may eventually result.

E. A., aged 27 years, was referred for speech therapy with an unrepaired cleft of the palate. She had an obturator which assisted speech but did not provide full control of the nasal outlet of air. Consonant sounds were all defective except [l] [w] [j (y)] and [r]. She used a glottal stop for all plosive consonants and [s] and [ʃ (sh)] were pharyngeal. Other consonants were omitted entirely. Surgery was discussed, but she refused operation at that time. Speech therapy aimed to provide her with speech which was intelligible but which could not be normal. Some progress was made, but many consonant sounds were only normal when she closed her nostrils with her fingers, so increasing the oral pressure. After 18 months speech was good, but accompanied by a slight leak of air which she could not control, and consonant sounds were not completely normal. She then decided to consult a plastic surgeon, and operation was successfully performed on a cleft of the palate which extended nearly to the alveolar ridge. Speech showed some improvement soon after operation, but the full result was not apparent for a further two years, during which time a pharyngeal [s] was slowly but surely eradicated.

A. M., aged 29 years, was admitted for operation for an unrepaired cleft of the soft and one-third of the hard palate. An analysis of her speech and a gramophone recording were made the day before operation. The consonants [l] [w] [j (y)] and [r] were normal. She substituted a weak lateral sound resembling [l] for [s] [ʃ (sh] [tʃ (ch)] and [dʒ (j)], and a glottal stop for all other consonant sounds. Following operation she attended for three months for speech therapy. She had adequate nasopharyngeal closure and normal co-ordinations developed rapidly. Speech was also normal by the end of this period and was maintained in conversational speech.

Ambrose Jolleys (1954) studied clinical records of 254 cases and examined 165 patients operated upon for cleft palate by various surgeons and techniques some years previously. He divided these patients into groups according to the age at operation, and classified the speech results in four groups as follows:

'Bad' speech was mostly unintelligible. 'Fair' speech was intelligible but only with care, and there were many defects of articulation. 'Good' speech indicated minor defects of articulation only, such as a defective [s], and 'excellent' speech was indistinguishable from normal. He found a significant correlation between the speech results and age at operation, those operated upon before two years of age having better speech than those operated upon at a later age, but he found no significant relationship to the type of operation performed. He also found a relationship between the severity of the deformity and speech, and illustrated his findings in the diagrams shown in Figures 77 and 78.

Growth

In recent years attention has been directed to the fact that following operation in infancy there is interference with the growth and development of the maxilla and the alveolus. The most rapid growing period occurs under four or five years of age, by which time five-sixths of the total growth is probably

SPEECH RESULTS IN RELATION TO AGE AT OPERATION AND TYPE OF CLEFT

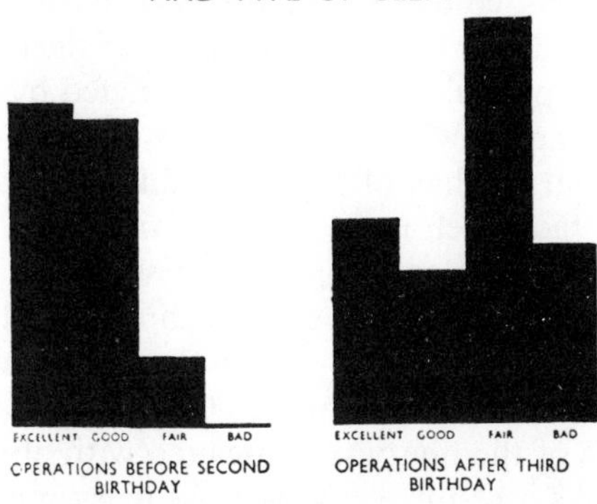

FIG. 77

The speech results in relation to age at operation (*Jolleys* (1954).)

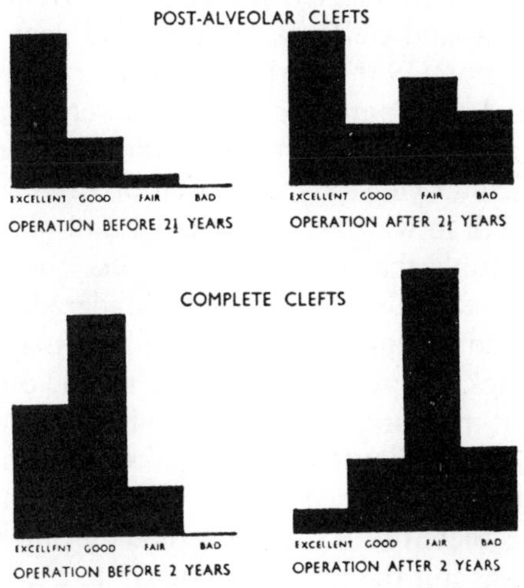

FIG. 78

The speech results in post-alveolar and complete clefts of the palate in relation to age at operation. (*Jolleys* (1954).)

Reprinted from *Brit. J. plast. Surg.* (1954-55), **7**, 229.

completed, although some further development occurs until 19 or 20 years of age. For this reason it has been suggested that surgery should be postponed until six or seven years of age or later, until rapid growth of the maxilla has ceased.

Graber (1950) states that where there has been no repair of the palate growth has continued in the two halves of the palate and has suggested that the growing points of the maxilla may be damaged, or the palatal blood supply restricted by early surgical interference. The growth of the maxilla is then limited and is not proportional to that of the mandible, with resulting malocclusion and facial deformity. It is advised that an obturator should be fitted at an early age to assist speech development (Fig. 79) until such time as operation can be safely attempted.

Growth, however, involves more than that of the palate, and it is found that in the unrepaired cleft there is an increase in the dimensions of the pharynx associated with abnormal width of the skull. As a result of the normal tension exerted by the united muscles, such growth is usually controlled, but where this is absent there is abnormal increase in the size of the pharynx, especially from side to side. Wardill (1928) carried out measurements on normal and cleft palate skulls and demonstrated this deformity. Peyton (1931) carried out similar measurements on living skulls and also found a greater transverse diameter of the upper jaw or maxilla. Later repair of the palate may therefore be more difficult, whilst early operation may prevent such abnormal growth in width of the maxilla and pharynx.

It is also possible that palatal growth may be stimulated by union of the palatal muscles rather than hindered. Jolleys (1954) believes that acting singly the muscle fibres may fail to grow because they lack the pull of the muscle on the other side. He also carried out measurements and found that although growth of the maxilla may be limited in the repaired cleft in the horizontal plane there is continued full development in the vertical direction. He therefore considered that the interference with development was not the result of damage to the blood supply, nor to the growing points of the maxilla, but that growth was restricted by fibrous tissue which may result from operation. The problem is therefore one of surgical technique, which must be designed to unite the two halves of the palate without tension, and with the formation of minimal scar tissue, so that the normal processes of growth may be stimulated rather than hindered.

As a result, therefore, of apposition and union of the bilateral muscles of the soft palate, the muscular forces exerted may approach normal in direction and strength, and growth of the hard and soft palates may be assisted whilst abnormal increase in the size of the pharynx is prevented. Such stimulation of growth will be most effective in early infancy before the period of rapid development is past, and may produce little advantage after four or five years of age.

Although the most important factor concerned in the subsequent development of normal speech is probably the technique employed and the skill of the surgeon, it is also probable that early operation assists not only the normal development of speech but also the more normal growth of the mouth and pharynx.

POST-OPERATIVE MANAGEMENT AND TREATMENT

Post-operative treatment of the cleft palate patient may require not only the efforts of the surgeon but also the co-operation of the orthodontist and speech therapist, and children should be seen regularly every six months following operation for assessment of progress and observation as to the need for dental or orthodontic treatment, advice concerning the development of speech, or speech therapy.

The children who have been seen by us during the last six years have been submitted to operation usually between one and two years of age. An assessment of their speech development and articulation is made by the speech therapist at the time of each visit to the follow-up clinic. Speech therapy is only undertaken after four years of age if it is thought that normal articulation is unlikely to be achieved spontaneously by five years of age when the child is starting school life.

Tests for Function

Simple tests for the competence of nasopharyngeal closure are carried out as soon as possible. These tests are:

1. Ability to blow with nasopharyngeal closure and no nasal escape of air.
2. Ability to hold air in the mouth under pressure and release it normally through the lips.
3. Ability to articulate normally the sounds in one or two simple first words such as ‘by by’, ‘ta ta’ or ‘Daddy’.

4. More detailed assessment of spontaneous speech is obtained at later visits.

Breath direction

Although normal co-ordinations involving the newly acquired nasopharyngeal sphincter may develop rapidly following operation for sucking and swallowing, breath direction on blowing may continue to be through the nose with the lips closed. This may continue for several months or even longer and may have an adverse effect on the co-ordinations normally required for articulation, even when nasopharyngeal closure is possible.

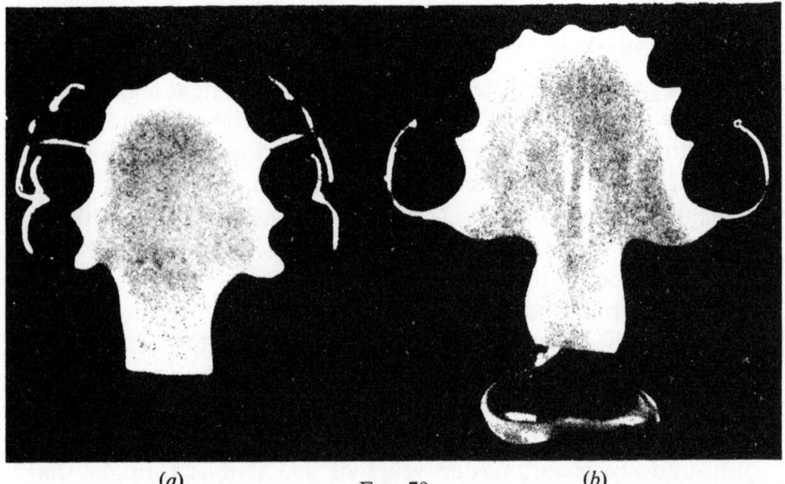

(*a*) FIG. 79 (*b*)

Incomplete and completed speech aids for small children. (*a*) Palatal section extended to the divided uvula; (*b*) Completed speech aid with pharyngeal section.

From Harkins, Cloyd S., & Baker, H. K. (1948). Twenty-five years of Cleft Palate Prosthesis. *J. Speech Hear. Dis.*, **13**, 23.

The mother is then asked to assist the normal direction of breath for blowing by nipping the child's nostrils until he develops the ability to blow through the mouth with the nasopharyngeal sphincter closed. This helps to improve the tongue position in the mouth, as blowing through the nose may be, in part, due to the high position in the mouth of the back of the tongue. The ability to maintain a steady air stream through the mouth on blowing or whistling will also form a basis for the use of the fricative consonants. In the main, however, it establishes the ability to direct air through the sphincter of the lips whilst the nasopharyngeal outlet remains closed. Sucking and blowing through a drinking-straw may also be encouraged, as palatal movement may thereby be assisted.

At a later stage, if use of consonants is defective as speech develops, the mother is advised to practise with the child such sounds as [f] . . . [s . . .] or [ʃ (sh) . . .], or repeated plosive sounds such as [pppp . . .] or [tttt . . .] and so forth, but she is asked not to correct the actual pronunciation of the words the child uses.

If there is an anterior fistula in the hard palate, the development of normal articulation may be hindered, as with insufficient oral pressure for normal consonant sounds the child may substitute defective habits such as the glottal stop or pharyngeal fricative sounds. In some children with such a fistula the consonant sounds [k] and [g] may be normal, thus indicating the existence of an adequate nasopharyngeal sphincter. The orthodontist will then fit a small dental plate as early as is possible, so that the child may have every chance to develop normal speech spontaneously at the optimum time.

Blakeley (1969) has also used obturators when nasopharyngeal closure is inadequate. He found that, at first, there was a marked tendency for the palatopharyngeal muscles to be relaxed around the bulb of the obturator in order to maintain the accustomed hypernasal speech, indicating a subconscious resistance to any change in vocal tone and speech. It was therefore necessary to ensure that the obturator bulb was large enough to prevent even nasal breathing (it was removed at night for comfort), to ensure that speech was hyponasal or denasalised.

Once the child became accustomed to his denasalised manner of speaking, usually within a few days or a week or two, the size of the obturator bulb could be reduced. The child then tried to maintain speech without nasal escape of air by using the palatopharyngeal muscles to form a seal around the obturator bulb. As ability to do this increased, the size of the bulb could be gradually reduced further over a period depending upon the reactions of the individual, in some children to the point at which the obturator was no longer required.

Orthodontic treatment may also assist the more normal development of the alveolus in children with unilateral or bilateral clefts where growth may produce distortion. It may also be necessary to control dentition, and so assist in providing a dental arch and occlusion with reduced abnormality. This may then improve the child's appearance and assist in the ease with which tongue movements for articulation are accomplished. However, during this process of growth, where the muscle, movements and tensions in the tongue and lips are normally balanced there may be little or no obvious deformity of the upper alveolar arch, even in the complete alveolar cleft. Growth has been stimulated by muscle action following union of the lip and palatal muscles and is not restricted by undue muscle pressures in the upper lip if the surgical repair has been successful. Where, however, there has been only minimal pre-operative development of palatal tissues orthodontic treatment in later childhood may be needed to assist the arch formation. There are many problems concerning growth which can be dealt with only by the orthodontist working regularly in close contact with the plastic surgeon and speech therapist.

It is also probable that some of these children will have in addition other developmental disorders of speech which occur in children who have normal palates. As previously described (p. 55) between three and five per cent of children in the normal childhood population have delays in the onset of speech or defects of articulation. For example, the cleft palate child who also has some degree of articulatory dyspraxia will experience greater difficulty in control of the palatopharyngeal muscles and in achieving normal articulation, following successful surgery, than the child with normal ability to reproduce the sounds and sound sequences in words and speech.

When assessing the speech of children following operation for cleft palate from the ages of 12 months at the follow-up clinic three conditions were considered.

(*a*) *Intra-oral air pressure*. That is the competence of the palatopharyngeal sphincter and the presence or absence of a temporary anterior fistula in the hard palate.

(*b*) *Vocal tone and resonance balance*.

(*c*) *Articulation of all speech sounds* as used in conversational speech.

(a) Tests for function, that is the competence of nasopharyngeal closure, have already been described (p. 397).

(b) Vocal tone and resonance. It has been found useful to assess this on a five-point scale. This is a subjective assessment, but does give some indication of the quality of the child's vocal tone. On this scale the grading is as follows:

(1) The normal clear tone of a young child.

(2) Some increase of nasal resonance.

(3) Further increase, but still within the normal range of variation.

(4) Marked nasal resonance but without nasal emission of air.

(5) Nasal emission of air influencing resonance and with weak consonant articulation.

Excessive nasal resonance without nasal escape of air affects mainly vowel sounds and may be due to abnormal pharyngeal contours, subsequent to pharyngoplasties or pharyngeal flap operations. It may also be due to tension in the pharyngeal walls with poor inward movement of the lateral walls. Faulty breath direction, frequently due to a high tongue position in the mouth, will also affect the resonance balance, whilst a long, tight upper lip and malocclusion of the incisor teeth will prevent the use of normal resonance. Environment and habits acquired in infancy before operation also play a part in producing what is recognised as acceptable to any individual.

It has been noticed through regular observation that changes and modifications in resonance occur during growth. The condition is not a static one. There are temporary changes due to nasal catarrh and infections. Growth of adenoid tissues, chiefly between seven and twelve years of age, affects resonance in children with cleft palates as it also does in those with normal palates.

Growth in adolescence again produces changes as the pharynx alters in shape and size. In the boy there is growth in the larynx and in the pharynx in the antero-posterior direction. In the girl the pharynx increases in length in the vertical direction, and again there are normally changes in vocal tone, pitch and resonance.

This assessment can, therefore, only be subjective and liable to changes. It is based on experience, a trained ear and on comparison with what is considered to be within the normal range when compared with children who have normal palates.

(*c*) *Articulation.* An assessment of the speech of patients must always be made finally on their ability to maintain normal articulation in spontaneous conversation at any speed. An analysis of defects of articulation may be made on the repetition of single words, but this is no true criterion of the success of treatment, surgical or otherwise.

In the first few years of life there may be insufficient speech for assessment, but the ability to say 'bye-bye' or 'ta-ta' with normal articulation of the consonants may at least permit a not unfounded optimism. Again many children are too shy to speak freely when revisiting a hospital clinic associated with unpleasant memories, and a true assessment of normal speech may not always be possible before four or five years of age.

It must be remembered that the child born with a cleft palate does not experience the normal basic co-ordinations for sucking and swallowing in infancy, and for the early stages of speech development pre-operatively as for babbling. Some type of compensation will develop and may affect speech development, persisting after successful operation has been performed. The majority of these children, therefore, pass through a period of defective articulation when new co-ordinations are developing spontaneously. This period tends to be more prolonged when operation has been delayed, or in children with severe bilateral or unilateral clefts, other factors being equal.

Intelligence is also a factor which may affect speech development, and mental retardation can cause delay in the use of language, but not necessarily defective articulation although it may affect the ability to change from defective to normal co-ordinations.

Hearing affects the child's ability to use consonant sounds normally, and a congenital hearing loss will affect the development of language and of articulation in proportion to its type and severity. Middle ear hearing loss, occurring intermittently, and usually after speech is developed, may not affect articulation unless it is severe and persistent.

McWilliams and Musgrave (1971) discuss some of the problems encountered in the assessment of cleft palate children. They stress that speech is more than directing the expiratory air stream appropriately for articulation. They also emphasise that children with clefts experience retardation in the early stages of expressive language development in that they do not talk as easily, as well, or as much as normal children. There is a need, they state, to consider intelligence, hearing, emotional factors, dental anomalies and neuromotor ability in addition to velo-pharyngeal valving problems and the adequacy of language function in relation to chronological and mental age.

Lewis (1971) reported the results of intelligence tests of 548 children with cleft lip and/or palate and compared them with those of the normal population. The children ranged in age from 4 to 16 years.

She found no significant difference when the results were analysed according to the type of cleft, but a significant difference between those with an isolated cleft lip and those with a cleft palate, the former having a mean I.Q. equal to that of the normal population. She reported that:

1. The mean I.Q. for the cleft lip and cleft palate children was six points lower than the theoretical I.Q. mean of 100.
2. A significant difference between those with cleft lip and/or cleft palate only and those who, in addition, had an associated congenital anomaly, the latter having a mean I.Q. nine points lower.
3. The mean I.Q. for those with a hearing loss was seven points lower than the mean I.Q.
4. There was no significant difference between the mean I.Q.s for differing types of cleft palate.
5. When siblings were used as a control in 50 children and 50 non-cleft siblings, the I.Q. of the latter was found to be 10 points higher.

She concludes that the survey indicated that multiple causes may account for the difference in intelligence between the cleft palate and the general population, including both congenital and environmental factors.

One must remember, however, that the intelligence test used has a language factor, and that many children with cleft palate have delayed language development which may not be associated with a low intelligence. There are reasons, such as hospitalisation, surgical shock, and emotional trauma, especially for those requiring more than one operation. Other children have limited and inhibited use of speech when they are aware that they are not understood. Hearing problems must aiso be taken into account.

However, the findings in the Newcastle group of children did not show any significant difference in intelligence between the cleft palate children and those in the normal population. This could be related to the successful early surgery which reduces the possibility of hearing loss and permits the natural and normal development of speech, in the majority without any therapy, and before delay in the use of speech is of any significance.

Results of Treatment

In assessing the speech of these children from 12 months of age at a follow-up clinic, the following classification has been found useful:

1. Normal speech, where there is no recognisable defect to a trained ear during spontaneous conversation. The nasopharyngeal sphincter is competent, and there is no trace of nasal escape of air, or of abnormal resonance.
2. Those who have a competent nasopharyngeal sphincter on blowing tests, and on speech, as demonstrated by normal articulation of at least one consonant sound. There may be other persisting defects of articulation and speech may be temporarily unintelligible, but in most of these use of normal speech is a question of time.
3. Those patients who have good clear speech, but with minimal traces of nasopharyngeal incompetence, and abnormal resonance. These are usually patients operated upon in later childhood often as a secondary procedure. Surgery and speech therapy have helped to achieve good speech, but it cannot be classed as completely normal.
4. Those patients in whom surgery has failed to produce a competent nasopharyngeal sphincter. Articulation is defective or may be unintelligible.
5. Those children with other abnormalities of development which bear a direct relationship to speech development such as mental deficiency, or a severe hearing defect.
6. Many children are too young or operation has been too

recent for any assessment of the competence of the nasopharyngeal sphincter or an assessment of speech. We also include here those children in whom the onset of speech is delayed apart from those in Group 5. These children are temporarily placed in this group.

The findings during the assessment and treatment of children operated upon for clefts of the palate will be described for two groups.

1. 360 patients operated upon by one surgeon between 1950 and 1960.
2. 27 patients who were operated upon in infancy between 13 and 18 years ago by other surgeons.

It has been suggested that children may acquire normal speech soon after operation and lose it again as the result of abnormal development of the maxilla, and that nasopharyngeal closure, even if once established, may not necessarily persist. This has not been found by experience, but in an attempt to obtain further evidence, the second group of patients was seen. They had been operated upon between 1937 and 1942, and owing to conditions existing at that time had not been seen regularly following operation. The majority had had no speech therapy.

Assessment of Speech in 360 Patients following Post-operative Treatment

These patients were all operated upon by Braithwaite at the Fleming Memorial Hospital for Sick Children, Newcastle-upon-Tyne, between 1950 and 1960. The method of operation has been fully described by the surgeon in *Text Book of Surgery*, and *Modern Trends in Plastic Surgery* (1963 and 1964).

Of these 360 children, 193 (53.3 %) were boys and 167 (46.7 %) were girls.

Type of Cleft

1. *Clefts of the primary palate* (*lip and premaxilla only*). These children were not included in the survey as this condition rarely affects speech unless associated with a cleft of the palate.

2. *Clefts of the secondary palate, total, subtotal and submucous.* 183 (58.6%) had clefts involving the hard and soft palate, 45 having complete clefts of the secondary palate to the premaxilla.

34 (9.4%) had clefts of the soft palate, three of these having also a partial left-sided cleft of the lip. Eleven children had submucous clefts, one of these was associated with a cleft lip, one with a fistula in the soft palate, and one with an exceptionally wide pharynx.

3. *Clefts of the primary and secondary palate.* 177 (41.4%) or almost half of the children had complete unilateral or bilateral clefts. Of these 82 were left-sided, 37 right-sided, and 58 were bilateral complete clefts.

Speech was assessed in 330 of the 360 children. Sixteen were not available, and 14 had insufficient speech for assessment, two being due to mental defect, one to a severe congenital hearing loss, whilst 11 had insufficient speech being aged 15 to 35 months with an average age of two years.

Intra-oral air pressure. Nasopharyngeal closure was adequate for articulation in 98% of the children. Some children had a small residual anterior fistula but observation has shown that these tend to close spontaneously following the method of operation used.

Vocal tone and resonance

	Group	
Normal range	(1)	64%
	(2)	23%
	(3)	7%
		94%
Excessive nasal resonance	(4)	2%
Nasality with emission of air (only marked in 2%)	(5)	4%

Articulation

Although when assessed 98% had adequate nasopharyngeal closure at the time of the survey a certain proportion were passing through the period when articulation was developing spontaneously towards the normal, as previously described.

The results at the time of the survey were as follows:

Normal	58%
Resolving defects of articulation	
(8% had minimal distortion of (s) only)	24%
Defective articulation due to	
Inadequate nasopharyngeal closure	4%
Inco-ordination of control of N.P. airway	2%
Anterior fistula	3%
Too young to assess	9%

Hearing and intelligence

Intelligence was approximately assessed according to placement in the educational system, and developmental behaviour. Eight children were mentally defective and at least 25 in addition were considered to be of low average intelligence.

Eighty-four per cent of the children had no hearing disability. Four had a congenital hearing loss of inner ear type, one being severely deaf with no speech. Eight had some middle ear hearing loss which was not sufficient to affect speech, while 32 had occasional otorrhoea, otalgia and intermittent hearing loss with colds. In nine children removal of adenoids was essential, following which two had temporary nasopharyngeal inco-ordination, one had a temporary nasal leak, whilst the remainder retained normal nasopharyngeal closure.

Speech therapy

As spontaneous development of articulation towards the normal is now usual following operation upon cleft palate in infancy, the work of the speech therapist has become that of assessment rather than treatment in cases of cleft palate. Speech therapy is required, however, when there are special difficulties and the child has failed to develop normal or near normal articulation by four or five years of age.

Nineteen per cent of the children described required speech therapy for a short period, and ten per cent more extensive treatment. Seventy-one per cent of the children developed normal articulation spontaneously or were in the process of doing so, and up to the time of the survey had had no speech therapy.

Speech and the Extent of the Cleft Palate

The relationship between speech development and the extent of the cleft palate, and also age at operation is described for 117 children operated upon between 1950 and 1955, as described in the first edition of this book.

In this group of 117 children, previously reviewed in 1955, 12 had bilateral clefts of the palate, alveolus and lip, 39 had unilateral alveolar clefts, 64 had post-alveolar clefts, and two had submucous clefts. The relation between speech and the type of cleft is shown in Figure 80.

	Bilateral	Unilateral	Post-alveolar	Submucous	Total
A. Nasopharyngeal closure	10	36	59	2	107
B. Defective intra-oral air pressure	2	3	5	0	10
	12	39	64	2	117
Speech A. Some consonants normal, but insufficient speech for full assessment	3	4	14	0	21
Defective articulation	5	10	16	1	32
Minimal defect of [s] or resonance	1	11	7	1	20
Normal articulation	1	11	22	0	34
B. Defective articulation and anterior fistula	2	1	0	0	3
Defective articulation and incompetent sphincter	0	0	3	0	3
Good speech, but with some nasal escape of air	0	2	2	0	4
	12	39	64	2	117

Fig. 80
Speech and type of cleft in 117 children.

From these figures it will be seen that operation failed to provide adequate conditions for speech in eight per cent of this group of children, in one-fifth of the children with bilateral clefts and in one-twelfth of those with either unilateral or post-alveolar clefts.

Of the 34 children who up to the time of assessment had developed normal articulation, one had a bilateral alveolar cleft, 11 had unilateral alveolar clefts and 22 post-alveolar clefts.

Speech and the Age at Operation

The majority of these children were admitted for operation between one and two years of age. The age at the time of operation was as follows:

Age :	Under 1 yr.	-2 yrs.	-3 yrs.	-4 yrs.	Over 4 yrs.	Total
Number of children	4	77	21	6	9	117

Of the nine patients who were operated upon over four years of age, two had submucous clefts and two were aged 27 and 30 years respectively, but had had no previous operation on the

	Under 2 years	Over 2 years	Total
A. Nasopharyngeal closure	75	32	107
B. Defective intra-oral pressure	6	4	10
	81	36	117
Speech A. Some consonants normal, but insufficient speech for full assessment	17	4	21
Defective articulation	18	14	32
Minimal defects of [s] or of resonance	13	7	20
Normal articulation	27	7	34
B. Defective articulation Anterior fistula	3	0	3
Defective articulation and incompetent sphincter	2	1	3
Good speech, but with some nasal escape of air.	1	3	4
	81	**36**	**117**

Fig. 81
Speech and the age at operation.

palate. The relation between speech and the age of operation will be compared for those operated upon under two years, 81 children, and those over two years, 36 patients (Fig. 81).

Of those operated upon by the type of operation performed on all these children under two years of age, 92 per cent had nasopharyngeal closure, 33 per cent having already obtained normal speech. Of those operated upon over two years of age,

SPEECH RESULTS AND TYPE OF CLEFT AND AGE AT OPERATION

POST ALVEOLAR CLEFTS OF THE PALATE

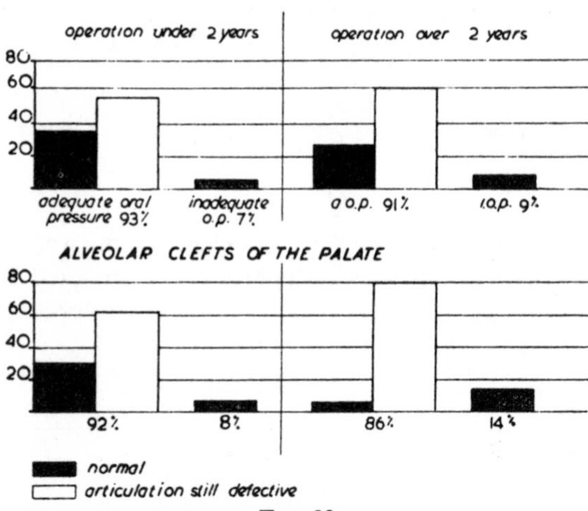

FIG. 82

The relationship between the type of cleft, age at operation, and adequate oral pressure for articulation obtained in a group of 117 children subsequent to operation.

89 per cent had nasopharyngeal closure, 19 per cent having achieved normal speech up to the present time. Although the age at operation may influence the rate at which normal speech is established, it may have little effect on the ultimate speech result. However, some of these children submitted to later operation may not develop normal speech spontaneously owing to the stabilisation of faulty neuromuscular patterns of articulation, and speech therapy may be required.

The relationship between the development of speech and age at operation in alveolar and post-alveolar clefts for this group of children is shown in Figure 82.

In children with *post-alveolar clefts* operated upon under two years of age, 93 per cent had a functional nasopharyngeal sphincter, 36 per cent having normal speech up to the time of assessment. In those operated upon over two years, 91 per cent had nasopharyngeal closure and 27 per cent had acquired normal speech when last seen.

In children with *alveolar clefts*, bilateral or unilateral, 92 per cent of those operated upon under two years had a functional nasopharyngeal sphincter, 30 per cent having so far acquired normal speech, whilst 86 per cent of those not submitted to operation until after two years had nasopharyngeal closure, 7 per cent having so far developed normal speech (Fig. 82).

It must be noted that these results are not final. Many of those with a functional nasopharyngeal sphincter are still under four years of age and should obtain normal speech later, either spontaneously or with therapy.

Post-operative Results in 27 Patients seen between 13 and 18 Years after Operation

Over 100 patients submitted to operation in infancy between the years 1936 and 1942 were recalled, but contact could only be established with 27.

When these patients were reviewed, they were aged 14 to 21 years, the average age being $17\frac{1}{2}$ years. They were all operated upon in infancy by various surgeons using the Wardill technique.

It was found that only two of these 27 patients had severe defects of articulation with lack of control of the nasopharyngeal outlet, one aged 14 years, and one aged 18 years who was mentally defective, and in whom the repair of the palate had broken down.

However, only ten of these patients had developed speech which was completely normal. One had had speech therapy, and one had had therapy for a stammer but not for defects of articulation. In addition, six patients had nasopharyngeal closure and had good but not quite normal speech. Three of these had minor defects of articulation, one had a pharyngeal [s], and two had defects of resonance. Sixteen (59 per cent) of these 27 patients, therefore, had a good functional result, 36 per cent having achieved normal speech.

Nine patients had an incompetent nasopharyngeal sphincter, and in two there was an anterior fistula in the hard palate. In eight of these 11 patients speech was good, but there was very slight nasal escape of air. Of the remaining three, one had a persistent pharyngeal [s], one a lateral [s] and one could not use the sounds [k] and [g], in addition to slight nasal escape of air.

Nasopharyngeal closure and adequate intra-oral air pressure for articulation . 16 (59%)	Defective intra-oral air pressure for articulation 11 (41% *A*. Anterior fistula . 2 *B*. Incompetent sphincter 9
Group I. Normal articulation . 10 Group 2. Good articulation, but not quite normal . . . 6	Group 3. Good speech, but some nasal escape of air . 8 Group 4. Poor speech with defective articulation . 3

Therefore 24 of these 27 patients (88 per cent) had developed useful speech, although only ten (36 per cent) had normal speech, and at the age when these patients were seen it was considered unlikely that there would be any further spontaneous improvement.

The ability to achieve closure in the nasopharynx had therefore been maintained in 16 of these 27 patients, but it is not known whether or not the nine patients with incompetent nasopharyngeal closure had ever achieved this following operation. (For further details see Morley, M. E. (1970), *Cleft Palate and Speech*, Edinburgh: Livingstone.)

Defects of Speech associated with Inability to close the Nasopharyngeal Airway

These can be divided mainly into two groups. There are, *firstly*, defects due to lack of sufficient intra-oral air pressure which result in weakness of consonant articulation with nasal escape of air, or in the substitution of plosive or fricative sounds at a lower level than the normal in the pharynx or larynx, where the requisite air pressure can be effectively obtained and controlled. Sounds such as the glottal stop and pharyngeal [s] are then produced as substitutes for plosive and fricative sounds for which the patient is unable to obtain adequate pressure at the normal point of articulation.

Secondly, there may be defects of resonance. Normal resonance results when various partial tones or harmonics are superimposed on the fundamental laryngeal tone, due to vibrations set up in the various resonance cavities of the chest, pharynx, mouth and head. Changes in the size and shape of some of these cavities in the cleft palate patient will affect resonance and also the possibility of achieving a more normal balance between oral and pharyngeal resonance. Defective habits of resonance associated with abnormal breath direction may not be completely corrected by surgery. The tongue may customarily have occupied too high a position in the mouth in some cleft palate patients, thus directing vocal tone into the nasopharynx rather than through the mouth. Adjustment of the tongue position, with relaxation of the muscles of the oropharyngeal isthmus, may be necessary before more normal resonance is achieved.

An abnormally large pharynx with an incompetent nasopharyngeal sphincter will affect the resonance balance, and where there is scarring and decreased mobility of the pharyngeal muscles following pharyngoplasty, abnormal resonance may be persistent.

Speech Therapy

The essential aims in the treatment of patients with an incompetent nasopharyngeal sphincter are the development of adequate control of the expiratory air stream for articulation and adjustment of resonance so that it approaches what is generally accepted and recognised as within the normal range.

With the advancement of surgical technique, speech therapy is becoming less important in the treatment of many of these patients and involves only those in whom surgery has failed to provide the necessary requirements for normal speech and those who have failed to develop spontaneously the normal coordinations for articulation in spite of all that surgery can do. The most important considerations in treatment are as follows:

1. If nasopharyngeal closure does not develop spontaneously after operation, the patient must be helped to achieve this where possible.

2. This involves the development of control of the nasopharyngeal outlet and normal co-ordination in the use of the nasopharyngeal sphincter with the muscles for phonation and articulation.
3. It may be necessary to adjust the tongue position so as to permit normal breath direction and resonance.
4. It may be necessary to change faulty persistent habits of articulation acquired before the nasopharyngeal sphincter was competent, and to substitute the normal consonant sounds, including the incorporation of these newly acquired patterns of co-ordination and articulation into spontaneous speech.
5. If the nasopharyngeal sphincter remains incompetent and further surgical procedures are not possible, adequate control of the outlet of air through the nasopharynx will be impossible and the therapist must aim to obtain the best articulation which is possible under the existing circumstances.
6. In many patients with cleft palate attempts to use intelligible speech have been accompanied by effort and abnormal tension in the muscles of the larynx, pharynx or oropharyngeal isthmus including the back of the tongue. All exercises must therefore be carried out with minimum effort, especially at first, until the patient is able to relax these former faulty neuromuscular patterns and obtain adequate movements and co-ordinations for articulation.

Blowing games and exercises

These are only useful if they assist in the improvement of breath direction and tongue position. At one time it was thought that forcible repeated blowing exercises might assist the development of pharyngeal muscles and contribute towards nasopharyngeal closure. This may occur to some extent. However, gentle well-directed blowing has been known to improve articulation and resonance when the nasopharyngeal sphincter is not competent, and to assist in its control when closure is possible.

The position of the tongue in the mouth may be abnormal. In infancy it may have occupied a higher position in the mouth, perhaps lying in the cleft in the palate, and in this position it may even have assisted in the process of sucking. If the raised position is maintained during speech, the air stream is directed through the nasopharynx rather than through the mouth. There will then be an excess of nasal, as compared with oral resonance, with little air pressure where it is required for the articulation of plosive and fricative consonant sounds.

Exercises for control of the nasopharyngeal sphincter

Where closure of the nasopharyngeal sphincter is possible but not maintained in speech, the following exercises may be useful:

1. Hold the air under pressure in the mouth and pharynx with the oropharyngeal isthmus open and the tongue low in the mouth. Some patients attempt to maintain air pressure in the mouth by raising the back of the tongue to close the oropharyngeal isthmus. Keeping the mouth closed, let the patient release the air through the nasopharyngeal sphincter, and then reverse the procedure, and maintaining closure in the nasopharynx release the air through the mouth.
2. Ask the patient to hum. Vibrating air is now passing through the nasopharynx and down the nose. Then ask the patient to attempt to interrupt the humming sound by closure of the nasopharyngeal sphincter, his lips also remaining closed, allowing air to be directed into the mouth and causing increased intra-oral pressure with distension of the cheeks.

Exercises for co-ordinating the use of the nasopharyngeal sphincter and articulation

Though the patient may be able to open and close the nasopharyngeal sphincter at will, he may not be able to maintain closure for articulation, and he may have acquired faulty habits of co-ordination, even relaxing the sphincter for articulation. This is more likely to occur in adult patients where nasopharyngeal closure has been inadequate for many years. When asked to hold the air under pressure in the mouth and then say ['pɑ:'] or [p], the patient can maintain the pressure at first but relaxes the nasopharyngeal sphincter before relaxing the sphincter of the lips. The air then escapes through the nasopharynx and there is insufficient pressure for the plosive consonant.

Under such conditions the following exercise may be useful:

1. Let the patient hold air in the mouth under pressure. Prevent the release of this air through the nasal airways by closing the anterior nares by finger pressure if the patient cannot maintain closure of the nasopharyngeal sphincter. Then allow the patient to release the air as for [p]. When he has experienced normal pressure for the articulation of [p], he should attempt to repeat it without closure at the anterior nares.

2. When this can be accomplished easily, a syllable such as [pɑ:] or [ɑ:p] should be substituted for the isolated consonant. A cleft palate patient may find it easier to obtain a consonant in the final position.

3. He must next develop the ability to alternately open and close the nasopharyngeal sphincter with increasing rapidity, gaining the requisite control to direct the air stream through either the nasal or oral outlets at will. Exercises involving alternation of a nasal and its corresponding plosive consonant are used, at first slowly—[m------pɑ:, m------pi:, m------po:,] etc. The nasal consonant is sustained, then nasopharyngeal closure occurs with the interruption of the hum. Air pressure is then built up in the mouth and sustained until the moment when the air is released through the lips for the plosive consonant.

4. When normal co-ordination between the nasopharyngeal sphincter and that of the oral outlet at the lips has been established, the exercises should be practised with repetition of the syllables at speed and with maintenance of normal pressure on the plosive consonants, using [m] with [p] and [b], [n] with [t] and [d], and [ŋ (ng)] with [k] and [g].

5. Later the nasal resonant is omitted, and the various plosive consonant sounds are practised in simple repetitive exercises.

Such exercises are useful in all cases of incompetent nasopharyngeal sphincter whether or not associated with clefts of the palate (see also treatment for articulatory defects in general, p. 261).

Defects of articulation

Patients who have developed speech with an incompetent nasopharyngeal sphincter may have failed to develop normal articulation for plosive and consonant sounds and have substituted pharyngeal or laryngeal plosive or fricative sounds. It is no easy matter for a patient with long-established speech habits of this type to inhibit the muscular contractions which he has used in the pharynx and allow the breath stream to proceed unhindered to the front of the mouth.

Fricative consonants. These sounds may often be best introduced on a basis of gentle blowing. The patient is shown how to produce a gentle and well-directed air stream through the lips followed by a vowel sound. The sound of the issuing breath should resemble [ʍ (wh)]. When co-ordination of this breath stream and vowel sounds is established, various modifications of the position of the articulatory organs can be superimposed on the air stream to change the sound produced to any of the fricative consonants [f] [s] [θ (th)] or [ʃ (sh)].

Plosive consonants. The plosive consonants may often be obtained at first without the intention of the patient. If, while the patient is producing a nasal consonant [m] [n] or [ŋ (ng)], the therapist unexpectedly nips the patient's nostrils with her fingers, the air pressure then directed into the mouth may be automatically released orally with a resultant plosive sound corresponding to the position of the articulatory organs at the time. Thus if [m] is being produced the resultant consonant will be [p] or [b]. This may not happen if the patient attempts to articulate the sound himself, as he may then substitute his former pattern of articulation for the particular sound he is trying to make. The consonant [p] is usually obtained most easily. Air may be held under pressure in the mouth and the therapist may release it by tapping the lower lip, producing intermittent opening and a series of plosive sounds. When the patient has acquired the sensation of one normal plosive sound, as distinct from the glottal stop, others are more easily obtained.

The association of such a consonant sound in the initial and final position with vowel sounds is the next step, and again may be difficult if phonation is associated with relaxation of the nasopharyngeal sphincter rather than with maintenance of closure.

When all consonant sounds can be used easily in simple repetitive syllable exercises as previously described under general principles of treatment, they may be gradually incorporated into spontaneous speech.

Where Nasopharyngeal Closure is not possible

Where patients are unable to obtain adequate control of the outlet of expiratory air through the nasopharynx, good speech may often be achieved, although this cannot be described as normal.

The chief aim is to direct as much of the air stream as possible through the mouth and to lessen that tending to escape through the nose. There must be as little resistance as possible to the passage of air through the mouth due to the position of the tongue, and articulation must be effected with the minimum of effort. The contacts for articulation should then be light for the plosive consonants and offer as little resistance to the air stream for the fricative consonants as is conducive with the production of recognisable articulation.

If these principles are adapted to the individuals' need, useful intelligible speech may be possible. Some patients even achieve this without therapy, as the following case history indicates:

Mrs. W. brings her son to the follow-up clinic, and for speech therapy following operation on his cleft palate. She herself has an unrepaired cleft of the palate extending to the alveolus and she does not wear an obturator. A unilateral cleft of the lip was repaired in infancy.

She speaks quietly and without effort. Her voice has increased nasal resonance with a breathy quality due to nasal escape of air, but her speech is easily intelligible with no serious defect of articulation apart from weakness of the consonant sounds.

With good ability to imitate speech without effort or forcing some patients are able to develop useful speech, and it is probable that this is more easily accomplished where the mouth and nose form one cavity, separated only at the anterior end by the lip and alveolus. Under such conditions speech may be better than when operation has provided a dividing partition, but has failed to provide a nasopharyngeal sphincter which is competent to separate the oral and nasal airways completely for speech.

The family history in the case described is interesting. Mrs. W. had nine children, only the youngest of whom had a cleft palate. The condition also occurred in her father, in his sister and in the son of his brother (Fig. 83).

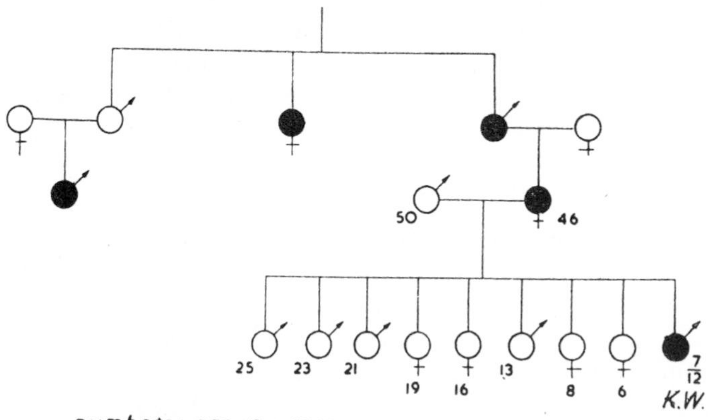

FIG. 83

The inheritance of cleft palate through three generations in the case of K. W. The ages shown relate to the time when K. W. was aged 7 months.

OTHER STRUCTURAL ABNORMALITIES WHICH MAY AFFECT SPEECH

MACROGLOSSIA

Occasionally a case is seen where an exceptionally large tongue interferes with articulation because it cannot be contained easily in the mouth and there is insufficient space for the rapid movements and adjustments required for speech. This may be illustrated by the following case history:

M. H. This little girl was referred at the age of three years two months for an opinion concerning the advisability of speech therapy. The tongue was large and protruded in general about one and a quarter inches. She found it almost impossible to enclose the tongue within the mouth, and so difficult that it normally rested between her teeth and hung down towards her chin. As a result of its position she had developed mal-occlusion of the upper and lower incisors with a severe degree of open bite. She had excellent ability for the imitation of speech and had compensated so well that articulation was easily intelligible, though not normal. At that time no therapy was advised, but she was asked to try whenever possible to hold the tongue within the mouth, the lips being closed. She was an intelligent and co-operative child and was seen at intervals over a period of three years. During this time growth of the tongue did not increase proportionately with that of the mouth so that she was increasingly able to maintain normal closure of the lips. Speech improved correspondingly and without treatment. Had this condition been associated with an articulatory dyspraxia, much greater difficulty would have been experienced in obtaining intelligible articulation.

Tongue-tie

This condition is frequently blamed for defective articulation. It is, however, possible for speech to be normal to the casual ear when there is a severe degree of tongue-tie.

One child, aged three and a half years, had such a short fraenum linguae attached so near the tongue tip that the tongue could not be protruded beyond the lower incisor teeth. She had excellent speech, however, with clear articulation. The consonant [r] was weak, but apart from this there was no noticeable defect. Operation was eventually carried out for cosmetic reasons.

A rather older boy aged six years had a similar condition. His articulation was also clear and intelligible. In this case the mucous membrane of the upper surface of the tongue became slightly raised in a small, longitudinal fin-like projection which he used for the articulation of the tongue-tip alveolar consonant sounds.

It is therefore probable that where defective articulation persists in association with a short fraenum some other factor also exists. It may be that there is an associated articulatory dyspraxia, or in some cases the muscles of the tongue, such as the genioglossus or other intrinsic muscles of the tongue, are also involved. The defective articulation associated with clumsy movements of the tongue then persists after the fraenum has been divided.

Stretching exercises for the fraenum may sometimes be useful. The child may be encouraged to remove with his tongue tip chocolate which has been warmed and smeared across the upper lip. This can best be carried out before a mirror, so that the child can watch the success of his efforts. At first, so that he may not become unduly discouraged, he should attempt to reach only the margin of the upper lip, or what is only just beyond his reach. A variety of such tongue movements may be devised to improve the mobility of the tongue tip, and exercises associated with articulation may also be used as required.

Dental Abnormalities

Mal-occlusion of the teeth may contribute towards defective articulation, but in the majority of children the tongue is capable of such mobility and compensatory adjustment that even in severe cases of open bite, inferior or superior protrusion, articulation may be normal. If there is an associated articulatory dyspraxia or dysarthria, the deformity of the jaws may render defects of articulation more likely and improvement in articulation more difficult, but generally speaking it is recognised that mal-occlusion itself, unless very severe, causes little interference with the ability to develop and use normal articulation.

Van Thal (1951) examined 180 children who were attending a dental hospital for orthodontic treatment. She found normal speech in ten cases, a slight error in the use of [s] in 40, a gross defect of articulation in 55 and a minor defect in 69. In six there was a disorder of speech such as stammering or dysphonia which did not affect articulation. Although 55 had a serious defect and 109 a minor defect of speech, Van Thal states that control tests on children with normal dental formation also show a high incidence of minor defects of articulation, and that there is 'sufficient evidence available to prove that adaptability and skill in the use of the tongue compensates for many dental malformations'. She also believes that faulty dentition may influence but does not necessarily cause defects of articulation, and considers that the cause 'lies rather in the faulty innervation of the lingual muscles'. This condition may be what we have described as articulatory dyspraxia or isolated dysarthria.

Abnormal occlusion, such as open bite, does not necessarily affect articulation, but it certainly requires ability on the part of the child to compensate for the condition. The air pressure required in the mouth for the articulation of say (t) and (d) is maintained in a closed cavity between the upper surface of the blade of the tongue and the palate. The lateral borders of the tongue are flexible and adjust to the upper lateral teeth and alveolar arch in order to prevent lateral leakage of air, the anterior part of the tongue tip being in contact with the upper incisors. The air is then released by a rapid and tiny movement of the tongue tip for the production of the sound. For the consonant (s) the position is similar, but the air is allowed to escape through a small anterior groove in the tongue in a continuous stream. Any lateral escape of air, as when the tongue tip makes firm contact with the incisor teeth or anterior palate, will produce the familiar defective lateral (s).

When the upper incisors protrude over the lower, it is still essential for the tongue tip to make contact with the central upper incisor teeth for (t) and (d), and to approach the internal aspect of these incisor teeth for (s). The tongue therefore will lie over and protrude anteriorly to the lower incisor teeth. This has sometimes been described as 'tongue thrust', but in many children it is merely the essential compensation for the abnormal occlusion in order to produce what to them is auditorily a normal sound.

Nevertheless, a true tongue thrust, or a compensatory habit as just described may, through pressure on the upper anterior incisor teeth render orthodontic treatment difficult and may counteract the treatment of the orthodontist.

Tonsils and Adenoids

Defective articulation may occur following operation for removal of tonsils and adenoids in children, who may temporarily have an incompetent nasopharyngeal sphincter when speech was previously normal. This condition has been described earlier in this chapter. The enlargement of the tonsils and adenoids does not in itself, however, cause a true defect of articulation. The child with enlarged adenoids and inability to breathe through the nose may be unable to use the nasal consonants [m] [n] and [ŋ (ng)], and 'Mummy' may become 'Bubby'. Vowel resonance may also be distorted and nasal resonance decreased. Tonsils which are very large may cause some interference with tongue movements, and speech may resemble that of a child talking with a large sweet in his mouth. If the defective articulation is the result of a true developmental disorder of speech, removal of tonsils and adenoids will cause no improvement in such articulation.

An exception arises when the enlarged adenoids have given rise to a hearing loss which is sufficiently severe to hinder the development of normal speech and the imitation of articulation. It is, however, rare for such a hearing loss, the result of middle ear conditions, to be sufficiently severe and persistent as to affect speech development, and it usually occurs later in childhood when normal speech has already been established.

Where there is deterioration in speech following such operation, it may be due to a transient absence of normal palatal movement. Full movement of the soft palate may have been impossible for a considerable time owing to a large adenoid mass, after removal of which the normal range of palatal movement may not immediately be re-established. In some there may be a more persistent disability, and speech therapy may be required to assist the use of the nasopharyngeal sphincter for speech.

In some children with unsuspected developmental dysarthria, removal of tonsils and adenoids to improve the speech may cause further deterioration. Movement of the soft palate may have been limited due to some degree of palatal paresis. In such cases the adenoid pad may have been compensating for the inadequate palatal movement. When this is removed nasopharyngeal closure is more difficult than before and the speech defect more obvious.

Treatment follows that already described, and mainly involves the adjustment to any structural abnormality which cannot be changed and assistance in the development and use of normal patterns of articulation using the principles of treatment as outlined in Chapter XV.

It cannot be overstressed that in work with children with

cleft palate, team work is essential. The surgeon, paediatrician, otologist, orthodontist, prosthodontist and speech therapist can secure the optimum conditions for the treatment of these children when working in close co-operation. Westlake and Rutherford (1966) have also had experience of such team work and discuss many points of view on varying aspects of speech pathology in relation to cleft palate to stimulate and encourage further investigation and research.

However, in my own personal experience and observations in other countries as well as at home, it is probable that the most important variable in the attainment of adequate speech is surgical success at an early age, preferably before the end of the first year and before abnormal neuromuscular and sensorimotor patterns of phonological development are stabilised.

REFERENCES

Ardran, G. M., and Kemp, F. H. (1952). The Protection of the Laryngeal Airway during Swallowing. *Brit. J. Radiol.*, **25,** 406.

Ardran, G. M., and Kemp, F. H. (1955). A Radiographic Study of the Tongue in Swallowing. *Dent. Practit.*, **5,** 8.

Blakeley, R. W. (1969). The Rationale for a temporary speech prosthesis in palatal insufficiency. *Brit. J. Dis. Commun. IV*, **2,** 134.

Braithwaite, F. (1963). Cleft Palate. In *Modern Trends in Plastic Surgery.* Ed. T. Gibson. London, Butterworth.

Braithwaite, F. (1964). Cleft Lip and Palate. In *Text Book of Surgery.* Eds. C. Rob and R. Smith. Chap. 5. London, Butterworth.

Calnan, J. S. (1955). Movements of the soft palate. *Brit. J. Plast. Surg.*, **5,** 4. *Speech*, **19,** 14.

Graber, T. M. (1950). Changing Philosophies in Cleft Palate Management. *J. Pediat.*, **37,** 3, 400.

Harkins, C., and Baker, H. K. (1948). Twenty-five years of Cleft Palate Prosthesis. *J. Speech and Hear. Dis.*, **13,** 23.

Hynes, W. (1950). Pharyngoplasty by Muscle Transplantation. *Brit. J. plast. Surg.*, **3,** 2, 128.

Hynes, W. (1954). The Primary Repair of Clefts of the Palate. *Brit. J. plast. Surg.*, **7,** 242.

Jolleys, A. (1954). A Review of Results of Operation on Cleft Palate with reference to Maxillary Growth and Speech. *Brit. J. plast. Surg.*, **7,** 229.

Lewis, R. (1971). Survey of the Intelligence of cleft lip and cleft palate children in Ontario. *Brit. J. Dis. Commun. VI*, **1,** 17.

Lucas Keene, M., and Whillis, J. (1950). *Anatomy for Dental Students.* London, Arnold.

McWilliams, B. J., and Musgrave, A. H. (1971). Diagnosis of speech problems in patients with cleft palate. *Brit. J. Dis. Commun.*, **6,** 26.

Morley, M. E. (1970). *Cleft Palate and Speech.* 7th ed. Edinburgh, Livingstone.

Peyton, W. T. (1931). Dimensions and Growth of the Palate in the Normal Infant and in the Infant with Gross Maldevelopment of the Upper Lip and Palate. *Arch. Surg.*, **22,** 704.

Podvinec, S. (1952). The Physiology and Pathology of the Soft Palate. *J. Laryng.*, **66,** 452.

Van Thal, J. H. (1951). The Relationship between Faults of Dentition and Speech Defects. *Proc. 2nd Int. Cong. Phonet. Sci.* Camb. Univ. Press.

Wardill, W. E. M. (1928). Cleft Palate. *Brit. J. Surg.*, **16,** 61.

Wardill, W. E. M. (1937). Cleft Palate. *Brit. J. Surg.*, **25,** 97.

Westlake, H., and Rutherford, D. (1966). *Cleft Palate.* New York, Prentice Hall.

Whillis, J. (1930). A Note on the Muscles of the Palate and the Superior Constrictor. *J. Anat., Lond.*, **55,** 921.

PART IV
STAMMERING

XVIII. Stammering

INTERFERENCE with the utterance of speech has been recognised and described since the history of civilisation was first recorded. In the English language it has been called stammering or stuttering, the two terms being synonymous, but has less frequently been defined, and those of us who attempt to treat this disorder of speech are working towards alleviation of a symptom without full understanding of the true nature of the condition. Consequently many theories have been suggested and many different forms of therapy devised.

Stammering has been described by various writers as a hesitation in the regular rhythm of speech; interruption of the rhythm of speech with spasms of the speech mechanism, a form of anxiety tension affecting the fluency of speech, and an excessive non-fluency with avoidance reactions. Despert (1943) described it as 'a neuromuscular dysfunction always associated with neurotic manifestations, and with anxiety always present'. She states, however, that the anxiety may be the *result* of stammering rather than the cause, and also that 'early signs of constitutional inadequacy are lacking'. To Hahn (1944) it was the result of an inner psychological condition known as 'dysphemia', which is not defined. According to Wendell Johnson (1951), the suggestion that it is basically a psychoneurosis found no support in research findings, and he described it as 'a type of learned behaviour pattern that is perpetuated and re-inforced by the stutterer's anxiety or fear of its recurrence'. Again, he states that 'stuttering is a form of behaviour that the child inadvertently learns, and that probably any child properly stimulated, frustrated and thrown into conflict in certain specific ways, under the right sort of circumstances, could and would learn to stutter'.

Robert West (1950) stated that 'stuttering, strictly speaking, does not become a speech pathology until the patient learns to fight his speech blocks. Everyone has such blocks, the difference lies in the attitude of the stutterer towards the blocks'. Stammering is not a habit, but, as Van Riper (1947) states, bad habits of postponement, of forcing and of avoiding are built round it. Falck (1969) describes a stutterer as a man who has learned to stutter, and he regards stuttering as 'the behaviour demonstrated when the neuromuscular patterns of normal speech are habitually interfered with due to fear responses which are either in anticipation of, or a reaction to, real or imagined non-fluencies'. He asks, 'can, therefore, "stuttering be unlearned?" '

Much research work has been undertaken which has contributed to a knowledge of the symptom and has investigated many possible causes of stammering. Much knowledge is also gained by the therapist through the experiences of the patients themselves and their reactions to treatment, but we remain in ignorance as to why one individual develops a stammer and another does not. No adequate fundamental difference, neurological, physiological nor psychological, has yet been proved.

Again, we must consider stammering in relation to normal speech, and this is not always fluent. There are many variations in the ease and fluency with which individuals express their thoughts. Is stammering merely the absence of, or interference of, varying degrees with such fluency, or does it differ in nature from the lack of fluency experienced at times by most people?

Experience would suggest that when most speakers hesitate, or repeat, they do not react with any feelings of embarrassment or anxiety, but that the stammerer is unduly aware of this difficulty and seeks to avoid the interruption in fluency, or the words and sounds which he believes are the cause of it. Does the symptom of stammering occur then only as a result of anxiety concerning the speech situation? This might be true to some extent, but would not account for the initial onset of stammering.

Emotional stress, self-consciousness or nervousness may produce varying degrees of inhibition of the thought processes, so that verbal expression is hesitant, but this is not usually associated with any abnormality of muscle tone, or of movements, nor resultant anxiety as occurs in stammering, although basically the cause may be similar.

Later research was concerned with the normal lack of fluency and of hesitations in the speech of young children.

Wendell Johnson (1948) stated that 'research has shown that normal children between the ages of two and five years repeat syllables, or whole words or phrases, on the average 45 times per thousand running words', and he considers that the normal range may extend to over 100 repetitions per thousand words.

These observations have led to the theory that the diagnosis of this normal condition by the parents as stammering may be responsible for its perpetuation, and Johnson (1946) considers that, 'stammering is born in the mind of the parent and not in the mouth of the child'.

Andrews and Harris (1965) carried out an intensive study of stammering, and their monograph attempts to cover five main areas of research into stuttering, namely, incidence and prevalence; aetiology; pathogenesis; course and prognosis and treatment. The study has been carried out on the lines of a survey of 10 and 11 year old children, with some experimental treatment arising directly from the work.

'It would appear to us' they state 'that a stutter starts as the result of the interplay of environmental factors upon a genetic matrix, and the complex and severe symptoms of stuttering develop subsequently as learned responses.'

In the past there was a tendency to regard all stammering as a single condition and to search for a 'cure'. A failure to find this led to much careful research and investigation into the nature of the condition. However, as pointed out by Wyke (1970), we still do not have adequate scientific information upon which an acceptable aetiological theory can be based and from which an agreed therapeutic rationale might be derived. However, Van Riper (1947) recognised three varieties, neurotic, dysphemic and developmental learning. The significance of physiological dysfunctions, biochemical and neurogenic, have been considered, and interference with the development of normal fluency in childhood, leading to learned adverse behaviour, or an underlying neurosis, are still the main lines on which thought and research have proceeded.

Stammering may perhaps be *described* as an interference in the control and co-ordination of those muscles involved in the oral expression of speech, involving abnormalities of muscle tone in one or more of those groups of muscles used for respiration, phonation and articulation, when formulated thought is clear and urgently seeking expression. Having described the symptom, we are still unaware of the full nature of its *cause*.

The Symptom

The following descriptions are indicative of various severe forms of stammering as experienced by patients attending for treatment:

E. B., aged 12 years. Initially he has an outlet of breath without voice. This is followed by a bilabial spasm which prevents utterance for one or two seconds. A few words are then spoken before a repetition of the spasm occurs.

D. L., aged 28 years. Here there is complete inhibition of utterance for 10 to 20 seconds, with no visible sign of effort or spasm. Speech may then be fluent for a few minutes. At times, he is quite unable to say the word he wishes to use. At home with his wife, speech is always fluent.

J. S., aged 17 years. This boy was advised to 'take a deep breath before speaking'. The spasm subsequently took the form of repeated gasping inspirations with elevation of the shoulders, movement of the arms, reddening of the face and neck, followed by the release of a few words.

J. B., aged 26 years. This patient experienced severe spasm of the jaw, neck and tongue muscles. Speech attempts were associated with a wide-open mouth, rapid protrusion and withdrawal of the tongue associated with a respiratory spasm which suggested suffocation. There was tension involving the whole body with backward and forward movements of the feet, almost resembling dancing. The spasm was so violent at times that even the floor shook. This stammer was said to have commenced following an operation in childhood for removal of tonsils and adenoids.

H. B., aged 19 years. The spasm here consisted of a complete block on consonants associated with a prolonged laryngeal tone on inspiration. This sound tended to rise in pitch and resembled a crowing sound. A few words were then spoken on expiration.

Conditions affecting the Stammer Symptom

It is well known that nearly all stammerers can speak normally under certain conditions, as when alone in a room with the door closed, in unison with others, as in the repetition of rhymes and stories or in choral speaking. Stammering is rare during singing, and is often reduced if the usual habits of speaking are modified as in acting, or when whispering, using a higher or lower pitched voice, or even slow speech. Rapid speech, however, may increase the occurrence of stammering.

Again, stammerers vary considerably in the amount of stammering when angry. In some the emotional stress inhibits the flow of speech, whilst others report that it seems to unloose the food gates and speech is fluent and unobstructed.

Variability of the symptom

The stammer may be persistent, varying either in its apparent type and degree from day to day or with circumstances, whilst others speak normally at times but experience severe stammering under certain speech situations. These may be when attempting to read aloud in class, answering questions, or when speaking to those in a superior position, as the teacher in school.

Here it would seem that the personal and social adjustment of the stammerer plays a greater part. Some speak easily with friends and equals, whilst others speak more easily to strangers who are unaware of their disability, or fluently on the stage or in public speaking, but are unable to speak easily in conversational situations.

The type of stammer also varies in different individuals, and in the same individual from time to time. The chief difficulty may be associated, for example, with respiration, or with spasm of the diaphragm, of which the stammerer is conscious but which he is unable to control. There may then be gasping inspiration, or speech on inspiration rather than on expiration.

Or, again, the chief difficulty may be associated with phonation. The vocal cords are normally open for breathing, closed during swallowing and approximated for speech. If their adjustment for speech is not easily maintained, difficulty may be experienced in the initiation of speech, especially on vowel sounds.

More frequently the control of the muscles of articulation, lips, tongue, jaw and palate are involved with varying types of inco-ordination of the required movements, and of their co-ordination with phonation and respiration. Sheehan (1946) found that stammering occurs more frequently on consonants than on vowels in the proportion five to one, but that in all those examined there was some difficulty with both. In 96 per cent of the stammering incidents it was associated with the initial sound of a word, whether vowel or consonant.

Andrews (1971) also describes the wide variations in severity of an individual's stammering and the factors which are thought to produce variability. He mentions speaking when alone, with children or superiors, the adaptation factor, under delayed auditory feedback, when using syllable-timed speech, under operant conditioning, and conditions in the family system at any particular time. All or any of these may affect the severity of stammering in any individual.

Resolution of the symptom

It seems probable from the literature that in nearly half of those who stammer the symptom disappears spontaneously, or at least without treatment. The probable age at which this occurs is not stated, however.

Andrews and Harris (1964) found that in 80 per cent of children who stammered the symptom had remitted by the age of 16 years, through gradual improvements leading to recovery. Such recovery, they believe, as others have also suggested, related to mildness of the disorder and to short duration, whether due to late onset or early recovery. Recovery in adult life does occur spontaneously, or without professional treatment, but is infrequent in the older and severe stammerers.

It is known that in many young children an episode of stammering may last no longer than a few weeks or months. Many children acquire normal speech when leaving school, and in later life there may be abatement of the symptom without specialised treatment. Others are enabled to obtain improved speech through treatment when they were unable to do so alone, whilst, in some, little improvement is achieved even with the help which recognised methods of psychotherapy or speech therapy attempt to provide.

Personality and the symptom

The majority of stammerers do not allow their speech disability to interfere with their ability to lead a normal life. They obtain work and maintain their position; they marry and accept responsibility for themselves and for others. A few avoid situations requiring speech either in social life or at work, as one who deliberately chose to be a bus driver because he thereby avoided the necessity for speech.

It has been stated that some even wish to retain their stammer as an excuse for avoiding social obligations. It would certainly seem that some prefer to use their usual manner of speaking, even if this involves stammering, rather than attempt a manner of speaking which is unfamiliar, even if more fluent. Johnson (1946) states, however, that 'various psychological tests have demonstrated that the majority of stammerers do not wish, either consciously or unconsciously, to stammer'.

Theories concerning the Cause of Stammering

During the last 25 years many theories have been suggested and many investigations carried out in an attempt to discover the nature and cause of stammering. These have included investigation into neurophysiological instability, for example, cerebral dominance; biochemical imbalance; endocrine disorders; heredity; psychoneurotic factors, and so forth. The findings may be summarised as follows:

Cerebral dominance

At one time it was considered that a stammerer was essentially a left-handed individual who had been taught to use his right hand and that this had caused the symptom of stammering. Bryngelson and Rutherford (1937) reported 81 per cent of a group of 127 stammerers with left hand preference who had been taught to use the right hand.

Travis (1931) stated that 'there is a conflict between higher and lower neural levels. The stutterer lacks a dominant gradient of excitation in one cerebral hemisphere of sufficient potentiality to integrate the bilateral structures of speech.' This supposes that there is therefore a neuromuscular dysfunction associated with this lack of a sufficiently dominant lateral gradient, such a gradient being considered essential to the normal integration of speech function.

The cerebral dominance was inferred from a knowledge of the individual's preference for hand and foot, and for the preferred eye in monocular sighting.

Heredity

Studies of the incidence of stammering in relatives of those who stammered led to the assumption that a tendency to stammer may be inherited, but that only if precipitating factors are encountered does the stammer actually occur. Jameson (1955), in a study of the results of treatment in young stammerers, found a history of stammering in near relatives of 36 per cent in a group of 69 children. Kingdon Ward (1941) reported 50 per cent, and Wendell Johnson (1948) 44 per cent as compared with 12 per cent of a group of children with normal speech. Jameson also found in her series that a severe stammer was more commonly associated with a family history of stammering (57 per cent) than a slight stammer (14 per cent).

Rhythm

Tests have been carried out to ascertain if lack of neuromuscular ability to perform rapid and rhythmic movements of the lips, tongue, jaw or fingers was related to stammering, but no evidence has been produced to show that there was any difference in this respect between stammerers and those who have never stammered.

Physiological tests

The results of biochemical tests for endocrine imbalance, and so forth, are conflicting but have failed to produce any evidence of marked deviation from the normal which could account for the symptom of stammering. The findings have been summarised and presented by Hill (1944).

Electroencephalography

Tests were carried out by Jasper (1937), Douglas (1940) and others. They were based on the belief that the percentage time the alpha rhythm was present might be related to what is termed 'cortical excitatory state'. Stimulation which should lead to increased excitatory state should therefore cause a decrease in the percentage time of alpha rhythm present. The findings showed that the percentage time the alpha rhythm was present during silence was usually greater in the non-dominant hemisphere. Stammerers tended to have a higher percentage time of alpha present in the left than in the right occipital areas, and no significant difference was found between the right and left motor areas. Jasper states that this experimentally confirms the difference in central laterality of stammerers and non-stammerers as suggested by the dominance theory, in that there is a higher incidence of absence of left-sided cerebral dominance in stammerers.

Non-fluent speech may certainly occur due to cortical and subcortical lesions, as described by Allan (1970). In particular Allan described the non-fluency related to the extrapyramidal type of dysarthria found in Parkinson's Disease.

Neurogenic stuttering is also described by Canter (1971) who mentions dysarthric stuttering, particularly in patients with acquired cerebellar lesions who evidence ataxic dysarthria. He also describes apraxic stuttering and dysnomic stuttering, a disturbance in word finding.

Wyke (1970) accepts the definition of stammering as *involuntary* repetition, which suggests to him that the disorder is a disturbance of one or more of the reflex mechanisms which are involved in the normal production of speech. He mentions mechanoreceptors located in the mucous membrane lining the respiratory tract, in the capsules of the laryngeal and temporomandibular joints, in the cochlea and in the phonatory, articulatory and respiratory muscles themselves.

He suggests that it might be reasonable to regard stammering as a manifestation of phonatory ataxia resulting from temporal dysfunction in the operations of the voluntary and/or reflex mechanisms that continuously regulate the tone of the phonatory musculature during speech.

This hypothesis awaits investigation in comparative electromyographic and microphonic studies of normal subjects and stammerers.

Whilst testing the threshold for auditory discomfort at 300 Hz prior to testing the effect of auditory masking on speech fluency in adult stammerers, MacCulloch, Eaton and Long (1970) discovered that the stuttering group had a lower threshold of auditory discomfort than the controls. In 1971 they reported on reduced auditory pain threshold in 44 stammering children (MacCulloch and Eaton, 1971). They tested the threshold of pain in 44 children who stammered and in 44 controls, matched for age and school grades and areas. They found a highly significant difference between stutterers and non-stutterers in the threshold of auditory discomfort. For both sexes the threshold of auditory discomfort was significantly lower in the stutterers than in the controls. These findings suggest to them a physiological or pathophysiological difference in the speech systems of stutterers, and that even small abnormalities 'may so disorganise data arriving at the higher centres as seriously to impair the executive speech loop'.

Psychoneurosis

Although some stammerers have symptoms of psychoneurosis, investigations have suggested and it has now been largely accepted that the proportion of these is approximately the same as in the normal population and that the majority of stammerers as a group are more similar to normal individuals in their emotional and social adjustments than they are to those with deep-seated emotional maladjustment. It is also thought that most of the stammerer's personality problems may be attributed to the frustrations and anxieties which are secondary to the stammer symptom.

Fransella (1970) also emphasises that research workers have failed to establish that stutterers have personality or behaviour characteristics which could be described as neurotic. However, Freund (1966) does not believe that stuttering can be entirely understood in terms of learned behaviour. He regards it, in the first phase, as an expectancy neurosis triggered off by many causative factors. Thereafter anticipatory anxiety develops, related and conditioned to varying situations. Many others have stressed the anxiety related to expectancy of stuttering, although not describing it as a neurosis, and Freund does not believe that stuttering can be adequately treated by a purely psychiatric approach. He suggests that the stammer does not cause psychopathological conditions unless they existed previously, but rather that it tends to make apparent weaknesses already existing.

Van Riper (1948, 1963) described expectancy in the stutterer's techniques of postponement and avoidance, and Woolf, writing in 1967, again describes stuttering in terms of struggle, avoidance and expectancy. Bloodstein (1959) found anticipation to be present at all stages of stuttering, and states that without such expectancy it is unlikely that stuttering would occur.

Learned behaviour

Research during the last ten years has led to the most recent theories which support the concept that the stammer occurs inadvertently in the early years of life whilst the neuromuscular patterns of speech are still unstable; that at this stage it differs little from the normal hesitations of childhood until regarded as abnormal by the adults in the child's environment. If the child's speech difficulty becomes associated with emotional reactions on the part of the parents, and these are always more evident where there is a family history, continuing failures are linked with growing fear and humiliation, and even feelings of panic on the part of the child. Attempts to correct the speech increases self-consciousness and may inculcate faulty habits and mannerisms which do not help and indeed may hinder the child in his own attempts to speak. Later speech becomes an act involving more self-consciousness than is normal, with rapid substitution of words for those feared and in some with avoidance of difficult speech situations.

In others, however, the stammer persists in the absence of any noticeable anxiety reactions concerning themselves, their environment, or even their interrupted flow of speech. They may be aware that their speech differs from the normal, but they have accepted it as their way of talking and have felt no need for help. This may occur in the child of school age, where the anxiety is felt chiefly by the parents, who request treatment for their child. In later life it may be realised that such a speech difficulty can be a hindrance in one's career, and advice and treatment may then be sought by the stammerer himself.

Bloodstein (1970) still stresses that, as a clinical disorder, stuttering is mainly a more extreme degree of certain forms of normal non-fluency, and discusses the relationship between speech interruptions of children who are considered to be stutterers and those of children regarded as normal speakers. He suggests that his observations indicate that such behaviour as part-word repetition, word repetition, sound prolongation and forcing, as found in the speech of stuttering and nonstuttering children, represents varying degrees of the same thing.

His experience and investigations have led him to believe that the attitude of stutterers towards their symptom is the major dimension of stuttering. The anxiety, anticipation and expectancy of stuttering, and the stutterer's built-in belief that speaking is difficult, are the chief factors in its persistence. A severe stutterer has little if any experience of the unconscious ease of speech which is common to non-stutterers. He describes (1960) how the stutter develops through five main phases: Phase 1 is characterised by the repetition of small words, increasing with stress situations, but lack of awareness on the part of the child and of emotional involvement. In Phase 2 the stutter has become persistent. It is increased at times of excitement, but the child's speech is not inhibited because of the stutter. Phase 3 is shown by the older schoolchild who has become aware of difficult situations and has developed some means of substitution to avoid feared words and perhaps situations. Phase 4 indicates the fully developed stutter. There is anticipation and fear, and, in some, avoidance of speaking situations, with signs of fear and embarrassment. Phase 5 is reached by the adult stutterer. He may have devised means whereby he can manage his stammer, rather than a real improvement. He himself is aware of his problem but may manage to control his fears, and has developed skills in the avoidance of words and situations which render his problem less obvious to others. A few acquire some conscious control over their stutter, concealing and disguising their tensions, both anticipated and experienced.

From evidence gained from intensive treatment of stammerers Brandon and Harris (1967) suggest that it could be useful to regard stammering as learned behaviour reinforced by its occurrence, thus agreeing with Bloodstein.

Andrews and Harris (1964) reported on an investigation into stammering in 80 children reported to stammer and 80 controls, matched for age, sex and school grading. On the incidence of stammering, they reported 1 per cent in the general school population and 9 per cent in children in schools for the educationally subnormal. They found that factors which correlated with stammering related to the child and to the home. Those relating to the child showed a marked similarity to the criteria for minimal cerebral dysfunction, whilst those relating to the home suggested that the child's disability was a reflection of genetic and environmental influences. Amongst those relating to the child were low intelligence, R/L disorientation and constructional apraxia, poor reading ability, delayed speech development, sociopathy and a history of articulatory defects. Relating to home conditions were mother's poor intelligence, poor school record and poor home life, a broken home and an unsatisfactory father.

They found no evidence that the stammerers were any more emotionally disturbed than normal speakers, although they agree that the theory put forward by Kanner (1957) that the stammer could be the young child's reaction to emotional stress could be substantiated, in that the onset of the stammer could be an expression of current anxiety, and whereas other behavioural symptoms remit, stammering remains.

They suggest that their findings would lead them to propose a psychobiological concept of stammering with predisposing factors, precipitating factors and pathological factors, with reinforcement mechanisms which perpetuate the disorder.

Age of onset. This theory is based largely on the knowledge that the onset of stammering has been found to be rare after the age of seven or eight years. Information concerning the exact age of onset is, however, frequently unreliable. The mother will state the age at which she first became aware of or anxious about her child's difficulty, and the adult the age at which his attention was first directed towards the stammer or when it was first the cause of emotional disturbance. This may have been evoked by parental correction or it may not have occurred until the beginning of school life, or even later during attempts to read aloud, when the teacher or other children drew attention to the abnormal speech.

This variation is shown in two groups of stammerers where an attempt was made to ascertain the age of onset. In 1945 such information was collected in a group of 249 patients who were first seen during school or adult life. Information has already been given (Chapter IV) concerning the age of onset in 37 children who were observed over a period from three and a half to six and a half years of age. These figures are again quoted in comparison with those of the first group and with Jameson's findings (1955) in 64 children who attended for treatment (Fig. 84).

In 85 per cent of the group of 249 patients referred for treatment, stammering was reported before the age of eight years, and in addition the possibility cannot be excluded that in some of the remainder a transient stammer may have occurred in infancy and recurred later in life. Such a temporary period of stammering, if normal speech is attained spontaneously, is rarely remembered.

	Never spoke without stammer	Age in years													
		1–2	–3	–4	–5	–6	–7	–8	–9	–10	–11	–12	–14	20–21	22–23
249 patients	50	2	16	23	20	57	29	14	16	6	4	6	3	2	1
37 children under 8 years of age	—		1	20	12	2	2								
64 children under 14 years of age (Jameson)	—		22	25	10	6	1								

FIG. 84

Age of onset of stammering.

If this theory of learned behaviour can be accepted, it is probable that there is no single cause for the symptom of stammering but that there are various factors which predispose towards the condition, in addition to precipitating factors which cause its onset. Again, other factors are involved in the perpetuation of the symptom.

PREDISPOSING FACTORS

Instability of the neuromuscular mechanism for speech in early life

At the time when the urge to use speech, especially in the intelligent child, is well developed, there is often instability of the neuromuscular mechanism for articulation. It has been found that boys and girls begin to speak at about the same age, but that defects of articulation are more common, and persist longer, in boys than in girls. There are also the normal hesitations and repetitions of words during the development and use of words as described by Johnson. Stammering is more frequent among boys than girls, especially in school and adult life. The proportion of males to females has been found to vary between 1 : 1 and 10 : 1 according to age. In a group of 37 children under six years of age who had a period of stammering during the development of speech the proportion of boys to girls was 2 : 1. Eighteen of these 37 children also had varying degrees of defective articulation. In another group of 190 consecutive patients of all ages referred for treatment the proportion was 167 males and 23 females, or 7 : 1. Is it then reasonable to suggest that in boys there may be a more persistent period of speech instability with a greater tendency to interference with the fluent utterance of speech, perhaps comparable to that which in others is responsible for the difficulty experienced in the development and stabilisation of the normal patterns of articulation?

Again, there may be an inherited tendency towards delay in the stabilisation of the neuromuscular patterns of speech associated with lack of definite right-sided laterality and a dominant left cerebral hemisphere. In Chapter XXI the incidence of cross laterality, ambidexterity and left-sidedness is shown for a group of stammerers. The difference between these and the control group in this respect is not great but is statistically significant. In the family history there is frequently a report of stammering and/or left-handedness, or of a disorder of articulation such as articulatory dyspraxia.

Environmental conditions

These were not found to be a significant factor in the development of speech in the 1000 children reviewed in Chapter II, but changes in the home, or temporary absence of the mother, at times would seem to be associated with at least a transient interruption in the development of speech. A high incidence of speech disorders has also been described amongst children in residential nurseries of children's homes. Unhappy and insecure home surroundings and an inadequate emotional relationship between the child and his parents may contribute toward some interference with the steady and progressive stabilisation of speech and affect the fluency of utterance.

Continuous strain in home or school life, when too high a standard of attainment is set by the parent, may also predispose towards a breakdown in the fluent use of speech. This strain is also present in those children who have some specific learning difficulty in perhaps reading or spelling, or when being pressed to work for a scholarship examination.

The change of hand from left to right is now rarely enforced but feelings of awkwardness and physical discomfort associated with attempts to use the non-preferred hand will cause feelings of inferiority. Fear of punishment for failure to use the more awkward hand may also have been a more probable predisposing cause of a stammer than the actual change of hand. Many predominantly left-handed children learn successfully to write with the right hand without interference with speech, whilst maintaining left-handed preference in other respects.

Physiological conditions

Other predisposing factors may be poor physical condition as the result of malnutrition, poor general health or temporary lack of well-being following an illness. Insufficient sleep or inadequate sleeping accommodation have also been thought to contribute towards a condition in a young child which might predispose towards the development of a stammer.

Precipitating Factors

Sudden shock

It is human nature to attempt to find an explanation and to ascribe the onset of the stammer to some particular incident. Nevertheless, there are sufficient reliable records of the association between some severe shock or fright experienced in childhood with a breakdown in the fluent use of speech to suggest a direct relationship in some children. Some of the incidents related are associated with street accidents, hospitalisation, sudden unexpected absence of the mother, or with illness.

Speech consciousness

Self-consciousness concerning speech may provoke the onset of stammering, as when a child is asked to recite in public, as at a Sunday School Anniversary, or when childish remarks are repeated in his hearing, either with praise or amusement. Although some may respond with pride and satisfaction, others become unduly self-conscious, and speech may be inhibited.

The correction of defective articulation

Attempts to correct the faulty use of articulation in a young child during the development of speech may also lead to frustration and excessive awareness of speech, and resulting interference with its fluent expression.

Imitation

A young child is rarely aware, at least for some time, of the breakdown in the fluency of his speech which is seldom the result of conscious imitation of the stammer of another child. Direct imitation requires the conscious modification of speech, is not associated with any emotional state and is infrequently the cause of a persisting stammer.

Unconscious imitation of the speech of a parent, or other child, may occur, especially where there is an inherited predisposition, or where the child has become aware of the speech difficulties of either parent. However, a parent may stammer, and all the children have normal speech, or one child may stammer severely without influencing the speech of any other member of the family group.

These factors therefore may or may not contribute towards a gradual development of stammering, with increasing hesitation and eventual awareness of the disability. In a few the onset would seem to be more sudden; one adult patient described the onset of his stammer as follows:

> Before I attended school I did not stammer or have any impediment in my speech at all. As a child I was able to speak without the slightest difficulty and was considered quite a wonder when I recited a complete book of nursery rhymes some friend presented me with. My speech was as free and as normal as any other child's.
>
> My earliest recollection of stammering is at the age of about six years. I was at an elementary school, and as was the usual routine, the register was being called. When my name was called, for some reason, I was unable to answer. Unfortunately my memory is not strong enough for me to remember how I reacted, and the teacher

carried on thinking I was absent. At the end she saw I was present, and thinking I had not been paying attention, brought me out to the front of the class. She asked me the reason I had not answered to my name. Again I was unable to reply. She must have sensed something was wrong for she sent me back to my place without further questioning and without punishing me.

From then on I occasionally stammered, though I recall numerous occasions when I read and spoke quite freely, without the least trace of stammering.

In this case there was gradual deterioration from the age of eleven years until adult life.

Onset of stammering in later life is rare, but has been known to occur in association with either personal and emotional inadequacy when facing problems and difficulties in life, or as the result of excessive and unusual strain such as occurred during times of war, and as was experienced by many in the Air Force. It was known that such intense strain could cause a temporary breakdown in the fluent use of speech, recovery being spontaneous after rest. Where the breakdown occurred in those who had experienced a period of stammering in earlier life, however, there was less chance of rapid recovery.

Perpetuating Factors

The chief of these would seem to be the fear and anxiety associated with the stammer symptom itself, whether it be conscious or subconscious. If the normal hesitations of infancy are outgrown without awareness, normal and stable speech will probably be established. If, however, the child becomes aware of and distressed by his inability to express himself as, and when, he wishes through fluent speech, he may react to his difficulty with distress or even panic, a fear of something not understood, comparable to a fear of the dark. The child may then unconsciously adopt an easier manner of speech, or withdraw from speech attempts, or he may use effort to overcome the resistance to utterance which may thereby be strengthened and the pattern perpetuated.

Conscious awareness is rare in young children, but may occur more frequently in the child of high intelligence.

One boy of 16 years remembered saying to his father before three years of age that he could not say the initial sound in the name of a certain town. The father confirmed this, but stated that no one in the family was previously aware of the child's difficulty.

However, awareness of the difficulty is often engendered by parental correction, and although some children develop normal speech in spite of such correction, and even punishment, many develop an increasing anxiety concerning speech. The failure to speak fluently then becomes associated with certain situations or with particular sounds in words.

Jameson (1955) found in her investigation that of 23 children who received little or no correction at home, 70 per cent obtained normal speech. Of 21 children where there was some anxiety and correction at home, 62 per cent obtained normal speech, whilst in ten children where there was persistent home correction only one (10 per cent) obtained normal speech.

Research has demonstrated that anticipation and expectation of stammering is closely associated with its occurrence. A boy aged 19 years once stated that he could not 'say the sound [k]'. When told that he had used it normally during reading aloud 74 per cent of the times it actually occurred in the initial position in a word, he then remarked that he only stammered on it when he saw it coming.

As time continues, the stammerer's attention is frequently divided between the expression of his thoughts and various methods and devices for avoiding what he has learnt to believe he cannot say. There may also be avoidance of situations in which experience has taught him to expect the occurrence of stammering.

So the two chief factors tending towards the perpetuation of the primary neuromuscular inco-ordination would seem to be, *firstly*, the method adopted unconsciously in early life in attempts to overcome the resistance to utterance, involving effort and forcing of the muscles used in speech or even the whole body. *Secondly*, the ever-growing awareness of the symptom resulting in fear and anxiety concerning the use of speech.

The following are brief notes concerning the duration and degree of stammering in some of the 37 children in the 1000 family investigation who had a period of stammering.

20. This child was the youngest in a family of seven, social class 5.

He spoke early, using single words at 10 to 11 months, phrases between 18 and 24 months, and speech was intelligible by three and a half years. At four and a half years he developed a slight but obvious stammer which lasted for about six weeks.

293. This child was the second in a family of two. He was rather late in speaking but used single words between 18 and 24 months, and phrases before two and a half years. He was unintelligible at the age of three years nine months but articulation was normal before the third assessment at six and a half years. A stammer was noticed at the age of 3 years 10 months, occurring chiefly when excited. It never became severe and lasted only three to four months.

73. The onset in this child was at four and a half years. The mother's brother stammered and the child's speech was corrected by the mother. The stammer was obvious and more than hesitant speech. The mother was advised to ignore it, and in spite of the severity of the stammer and the period of correction, speech was normal by five years three months and has remained so. The difficulty in this child lasted for about six months.

9. This boy had an obvious stammer at three and a half years following measles. He had developed intelligible speech by the age of three and a half years although there was some degree of defective articulation when seen at the age of three years nine months. In this child there was slow gradual improvement. At five years there was only an occasional stammer, and speech was normal at the age of six years.

Stammering in a mentally backward child

230. This was a backward child who, after two years in a normal school, was transferred to a school for backward children. He attended a nursery school from the age of three and a half years, where a very severe stammer was noticed. The mother had been advised, not by the staff of the nursery school, to 'make the child repeat each sentence when he stammered'. At this time it was occurring several times a day. For four to five months the stammer was severe, followed by a brief period of almost normal speech. A relapse at about four years lasted two months, to be followed by another period of normal speech until the excitement of Christmas, when he was four and a half years old, resulted in a further relapse. After another two months a slight stammer only remained, which persisted occasionally until he was six and a half years, since when there have been only very slight and infrequent relapses.

Intermittent stammer

464. Hesitant speech was first noticed in this child at about the age of 3 years 4 months for a few weeks. Following a remission, the stammer occurred again on his fourth birthday and was 'bad all day'. The mother said that the child was aware of the difficulty, and when he felt it coming he would whisper to her. At other times he 'chatters a great deal'. After about three months of intermittent and variable degrees of stammering he again spoke normally for a while until he went to school, when a further relapse of short duration occurred. A further temporary relapse of only a few days duration occurred at seven years three months.

634. This child always had normal articulation but had three definite periods of stammering. The first occurred at three and a half years and lasted eight to ten weeks; the second period occurred at five years, when he went to school. The stammer was occasional and slight, occurring chiefly when excited, and it lasted for about one year. Speech was then normal for another six months, but a further period of stammering, still only occasional and occurring when excited, developed again at about six and a half years and persisted until seven years. Speech was then normal again and no further difficulty has been reported since then.

299. In this child some hesitant speech was first noticed about three years five months. The mother explained that he 'could not get his words out'. There was gradual improvement until four years three months when he had a severe attack of whooping cough. Following this, he developed a severe inspiratory spasm which persisted in varying degree, and in spite of speech therapy, from the age of five and a half years. There was some slow improvement, but he had some difficulty, of less severity than formerly, at least every day up to the time of writing when he was nine and a half years of age.

Family history

342. This child had a maternal aunt who stammered. The difficulty was not noticed by the health visitor nor ourselves until the child was aged five years ten months, but the mother then said that the child 'had always stammered'. In this instance the mother often advised the child to 'speak slowly', but the mother herself was somewhat unstable and did not cope well with her home and family. Satisfactory speech was, however, reported at the age of seven years, although she still had recurrent periods of stammering when she was excited. She was transferred from the normal to an open-

air school because of her poor development and general physical condition.

853. This child was the third in the family. The father was said to have stammered until 14 years of age, and an elder brother of the child also had a slight stammer. The onset was at about three and a half years, and the stammer was of short duration, lasting not more than one year. Speech was normal at four and a half years and has remained so.

858. This child developed speech by two and a half years with normal articulation. The stammer was first reported at four years. It occurred in conversational speech only, several times a day, but speech was normal when saying rhymes. The father was said to have a 'slight hesitation', and the child's speech was constantly corrected at home. There was, however, a gradual improvement apart from a short period at five years of age after entering school, when the stammer became temporarily more severe. Speech was normal at the age of six and a half years.

Association with a child who stammered

32. This child began to stammer at three years of age. The mother believed this to be the result of playing with an older boy aged five years who stammered. The initial hesitation cleared up quickly, there was a relapse four months later, but the difficulty had again disappeared by three years seven months. At three years eleven months the child was talking quickly and not very clearly, and the mother was attempting to correct this. No severe stammer resulted, but slight hesitation persisted when excited for about three more months, since when there has been no further relapse.

Correction of the stammer

494. This child was the youngest of six. There was a slight hesitation at three and a half years and an obvious stammer at six and a half years, although speech was normal three months later. In this case the health visitor reported that she heard the father shout at the child, telling him to 'say it like this'.

1033. This child, who began to stammer at four years, was said to have 'copied the boy next door'. The mother said that he 'stopped when corrected' and at four and a half years speech was normal. There is the possibility that this boy had no real difficulty of inco-ordinated speech, but was in fact merely consciously imitating the speech of the other boy, and so could desist when told to do so.

The following are two accounts of stammering as written by adult stammerers, which explain their point of view and describe many of their fears and difficulties.

1. The onset of stammering in this case has already been quoted (p. 445). He continues:

I stayed on at school, for a short period, until I found myself a job. It was here that my stammering proved just how big a handicap it would really be. I had quite a few interviews for jobs, but on each of them my stammering spoilt me and I was turned down. Eventually I found work in a small firm, there only being five people in the whole concern. I was very grateful to my boss for taking me on despite my handicap, and was very happy there. My only bogey was the telephone. From one till two each day, I was left in the shop on my own, while the rest of the staff were at lunch, and soon I dreaded that lunch hour solely for that reason. I had some very anxious moments, and sometimes I left the phone to ring on without bothering to answer it.

Just after leaving school, I joined a boys' club which was run by a group of students. One incident I remember vividly in this club, was when the head was having an interview with each of the lads, trying to get to closer relationship with each of us. When my turn came, I was extremely nervous; why, I do not know, and of course I stammered very badly. I remember only too well how tense I was, how hopeless and foolish I felt. In the end I was obliged to write my answers on a slip of paper, even though he tried his best to make me talk.

My life of stammering has seemed to be in waves, one moment I would be on top of the world talking fairly well, then I would be down and my speech would suffer. Just how low the spirits can sink, only a stammerer can know. During all this my parents still clung to the idea that I should grow out of it, while I myself delved into the public library, in the hopes that I would effect a miraculous cure on myself. The library had not a great many books on the subject, but I read all they had, After reading a book, I would go about grimly determined to stop stammering. For a while I would improve, then some incident would happen, and I would drop back into my usual run. After a while I got tired of trying to overcome this impediment, tired of battling with myself, it all seemed so hopeless. So I drifted on using every dodge a stammerer can use to avoid embarrassing situations. Now I am once again trying to free myself, and this time I think I shall succeed.

Further extracts

I have an extraordinary fear of asking for fares on a tram or bus which I am unable to suppress even now. Even though my speech may be quite good and I am speaking well, if I board a vehicle on which I have to ask for fares, a wave of apprehension sweeps over me. I am quite unable to recall any incident in my childhood which may have caused this fear.

The feeling that fills one during a bad spell of stammering is enough to drive one crazy. A feeling of hopelessness, of helplessness, of uselessness.

Another method of evading speech was to conveniently lose my memory; if I had to pronounce some name, a moment of lost memory gave me a short respite and the word came easier, or else the other person supplied the missing word.

If I impersonate some person, I can nearly always speak quite easily, but it is impossible to be always acting and one soon reverts to one's natural self. I often use this to good effect when describing someone.

Substitution of words is another way out; often when I am talking and sailing along quite nicely, a word crops up on which I feel sure I will stammer. Desperately I rack my brains for a substitute, a word which will express the same meaning but be easier to say. Often before actually trying to say a word I have a substitute already prepared: it is amazing how quickly the mind can produce substitutes after a little practice though often to the detriment of one's grammar.

A stammerer is usually very sensitive and afraid of ridicule. Fear of this often made me remain silent, thus giving people the impression that I was either a snob or a dull dog, while inside of me a raging battle was taking place as to whether I should speak or not.

One of the many heartbreaks that stammering brings is to see lads, whom you knew at school perhaps, lads whom you knew were far inferior to oneself in brains, forging ahead in the world while speech, that most important factor, proves itself as one of the worst handicaps. It all seems so unfair, anger and jealousy creep in . . . Silly? Perhaps it is until one has actually experienced it.

2. Another adult stammerer describes his disability:

Well, feeling in my case is of many different kinds but all based on one thing—helplessness. This helplessness is coupled with short and rapid breathing, sweated forehead and continual twitching of the fingers.

The mind of the speaker, while stammering, is continually centred on what the receiver is thinking. The attitude of the receiver also has a great effect on the feelings of the speaker. For instance, if the person spoken to begins to realise the speaker's predicament and he becomes embarrassed, his attitude has a bad effect on the speaker. Again, if the receiver realises the cause of the faltering and a smile crosses his face, the speaker tries his utmost to translate that smile. Is it a smile of sympathy, a smile of encouragement or a smile of cool derision?

In the course of my work I travel around among 1200 to 1400 men and am never with the same men two consecutive days. This is, I may add, no help to a person who stammers, but I find in other ways an opportunity where I can practise my training to its full extent. The miner is a very understanding man and when I am in the pit I have no fear of talking to any man singly. But, I fear, I fail to be able to speak to them when in a group.

But when I am in the office the tale is somewhat different. If sent a message, the first thing that strikes me is—who will be there to speak to? If it is a person I know I go with great confidence and with very little worry. But if I do not know the person concerned, I nearly always write the message on a piece of scrap paper, and carry it in case of a stammer. I can at any time put the message before the receiver's eyes and read it off without a falter.

At home, speech is practically normal except for a few stops after a night of very little sleep or symptoms of everyday illnesses.

In social life I find the same thing happens as before—I have the fear of a collected number. When at any social function I find it easy to chip in the conversation but I am unable to speak to the whole group for any length of time. As soon as I become conscious that everyone is listening, speech becomes broken and hesitating.

Then there is what I term the fear of a definite answer. By this I mean a question which when answered must have definite wording. For example, what is your name? Where do you live? How old are you? These questions are stumbling blocks to me because whenever asked I immediately become conscious that if I stammer there is no alternative way out.

I have also what I term as pet phrases which I use when a stammer occurs. These phrases are used to try and cover up any fault and are sometimes found very helpful. I have complete confidence in these phrases and never a stammer occurs during their utterance.

REFERENCES

Allan, C. (1970). Treatment of Non-fluent speech resulting from Neurological Disease—Treatment of Dysarthria. *Brit. J. Dis. Commun. V*, i, 3.

Andrews, G. A. and Ingham, R. J. (1971). Stuttering: Considerations in the Evaluation of Treatment. *Brit. J. Dis. Commun. VI*, **2,** 129.

Andrews, G. A. and Harris, M. (1964). *The Syndrome of Stuttering. Clinics in Developmental Medicine*, No. 17. The Spastics Society. London, Heinemann Med. Books, Ltd.

Bloodstein, O. (1958). Stuttering as an Anticipatory Struggle Reaction. In *Stuttering: A Symposium.* Ed. J. Eisenson. New York, Harper.

Bloodstein, O. (1960a). The Development of Stuttering: I. Changes in nine Basic Features. *J. Speech Hear. Dis.*, **25,** 219–237.

Bloodstein, O. (1960b). The Development of Stuttering: II. Developmental Phases. *J. Speech Hear. Dis.*, **25,** 336–376.

Bloodstein, O. (1970). Stuttering and Normal Non-fluency—A Continuity Hypothesis. *Brit. J. Dis. Commun. V*, **1,** 30.

Bryngelson, B., and Rutherford, B. (1937). A Comparative Study of Laterality in Stutterers and Nonstutterers. *J. Speech Dis.*, **3,** 2. Reprinted in *Speech* (1940), **5,** No. 3, 2.

Bryngelson, B. (1940). Treatment of Stuttering in Children. *Speech*, **3,** No. 3, p. 9, No. 4, p. 7.

Canter, G. J. (1971). Observations on Neurogenic Stuttering: A Contribution to Differential Diagnosis. *Brit. J. Dis. Commun. VI*, **2,** 139.

Despert, J. L. (1943). A Therapeutic Approach to the Problem of Stuttering in Children. *Nerv. Child.*, **2,** 2.

Douglas, A. (1940). *A Study of Bilaterally Recorded Encephalograms of Adult Stammerers.* Unpublished dissertation. Iowa.

Falck, F. J. (1969). *Stuttering Learned and Unlearned.* Springfield, Illinois, Thomas.

Fransella, F. (1970). Stuttering not a Symptom but a Way of Life. *Brit. J. Dis. Commun. V*, **1,** 22.

Freund, H. (1966). *Psychopathology and the Problems of Stuttering.* Springfield, Illinois, Charles C. Thomas.

Hahn, E. F. (1944). *Stuttering, Significant Theories and Therapies.* Stanford Univ. Press.

Hill, H. (1944). Stuttering I. Critical Review and Evaluation of Biochemical Investigations. *J. Speech Hear. Dis.*, **9,** 245.

Hill, H. (1944). Stuttering II. Review and Integration of Physiological Data. *J. Speech Hear. Dis.*, **9,** 289.

Jameson, A. M. (1955). Stammering in Children. Some Factors in the Prognosis. *Speech*, **19,** No. 2, p. 60.

Jasper, H. H. (1937). Electrical Signs of Cortical Activity. *Psychol. Bull.*, **34,** 411.

Johnson, Wendell, Brown, S. F., Curtiss, J. F., Edney, J. C., and Keaster, J. (1948). *Speech Handicapped School Children.* New York, Harper.

Johnson, Wendell (1946). *People in Quandaries.* Ch. 17. New York, Harper.

Johnson, Wendell (1951). *Stuttering.* A Lecture to the American Academy of Ophthalmology and Otolaryngology.

Kanner, L. (1957). *Child Psychiatry.* Springfield, Illinois, Charles C. Thomas.

MacCulloch, M. J., Eaton, R., and Long, E. (1970). The Long Term Effect of Auditory Masking on Young Stutterers. *Brit. J. Dis. Commun. V*, **2,** 165.

MacCulloch, M. J., and Eaton, R. (1971). A Note on Reduced Auditory Pain Threshold in 44 Stuttering Children. *Brit. J. Dis. Commun. VI*, **2,** 148.

Sheehan, J. (1946). *A Study of the Phenomena of Stuttering.* Unpublished thesis. Iowa.

Travis, L. (1931). *Speech Pathology.* New York, Appleton.

Van Riper, C. (1947). *Speech Correction: Principles and Methods.* New York, Prentice Hall.

Van Riper, C. (1953). The Treatment of Stuttering. *Speech*, **17,** No. 1, p. 17.

West, Robert (1950). Rehabilitation of Speech. *J. Except. Child.*, March.

Wyke, B. (1970). Neurological Mechanisms in Stammering—An Hypothesis. *Brit. J. Dis. Commun. V*, **1,** 6.

XIX. The Treatment of Stammering

Historically the treatment of stammering has varied and has followed the current beliefs as to its cause. At one time it was thought that a defect in the tongue was the cause, and treatment varied from surgical removal of parts of the tongue to treatment by herbs, or distractions, such as the practice of speaking with a mouthful of pebbles.

When all stammerers were considered to be fundamentally left-handed, the treatment was the establishment of left-handed control for writing and other one-handed activities, but this treatment failed in many patients to assist the fluent use of speech. It probably eased the tension in a child being taught to use his right hand in school, however, and may still have its use in a restricted field.

Hypnosis may produce greater relaxation, and the hypnotic suggestion of easy speech has been known to be maintained for a short while, but in general it has failed to produce a permanent cure. It may also be useful during psychotherapy with the severe stammerer who is unable to speak with sufficient fluency to explain his thoughts and feelings to the psychiatrist.

Psychoanalysis and psychotherapy, with or without the use of drugs such as pentothal, have failed to produce normal speech in many stammerers. Treatment by barbiturates may temporarily alleviate the symptom but prove a hindrance in other respects, and with prostigmin it is said that there is less tension, and the spasm is more easily controlled, but evidence of a complete and final alleviation of the stammer is lacking.

Speech therapy has developed along various specific lines of treatment and in the older child and adult involves active co-operation on the part of the patient. If the stammerer cannot or does not wish to play his part, if unconsciously he has grown to value his stammer as an excuse for avoidance of certain situations, or if he still has unresolved resentment concerning his stammer, and is unable to accept his limitations, speech therapy may fail to help him.

Although speech therapy involves several basic principles of treatment, it must always be designed to meet the needs of each particular individual. Group therapy may be more useful than individual treatment in the young child, whereas in the older child or adult both may be useful.

No rapid improvement is probable in a long-standing case of severe stammer, and a period of two or three years may be required before improvement in the fluent use of speech becomes stabilised sufficiently to meet the tests of everyday life. There are usually many failures and relapses. If it is accepted that stammering is learned behaviour, then the process of changing what has been established must be a gradual process. It involves not only the changing of patterns of speech but also changing adjustments and reactions to situations requiring speech, and learning depends on failures as well as on successes until the new patterns of fluent speech are unconsciously maintained.

In order to assess the value of any form of treatment it is useful to have some means of assessing the severity of the stammer so that improvement may be estimated. This is not easy due to the variability of the degree of stammering, as previously described, and must, to a greater or lesser degree depend upon the subjective opinion of the assessor.

Andrews (1971) describes three problems in assessing stuttering, (*a*) to establish criteria that distinguish between stuttering and normal speech; (*b*) to measure the severity of the disorder and subsequent progress; and (*c*) to evaluate the relation of the final result to normal speech.

Assessment of the Stammer

Brandon and Harris (1967) studied stammering in a number of children and adults and attempted to assess the degree of stammering before and after treatment. Their assessment was based on an analysis of a tape recording of continuous speaking with concurrent observations by the therapist on reactions, tensions and bodily movements. The scale used consisted of four grades: Stammer not heard at interview, Mild stammer (communication not impaired), Moderate, and Severe.

Woolf (1967) described a Perception of Stuttering Inventory (PSI), designed to (*a*) describe comprehensively what the stutterer does when he stutters; (*b*) to broaden the stutterer's understanding of his problem; (*c*) to analyse the patterning or relationships among struggle, avoidance and expectancy; and (*d*) to formulate appropriate goals for therapy and evaluate progress. The PSI assessment has been designed for use with adults and adolescents, and can be used on an individual or group basis. It contains 60 items and is interpretated by means of a profile analysis and by reference to individual items.

Treatment involves:

1. An understanding of the nature of stammering and adjustment of the personal attitude of the stammerer towards his disability.
2. Relaxation therapy.
3. Exercises which help towards the control of the stammer spasm.
4. Discussions concerning individual difficulties and speech situations with suggestions and assignments for practice in meeting these.
5. Group therapy where practice and confidence in the use of speech may be gained.

These five principles of treatment may be briefly described as follows:

1. Adjustment to the Stammer

Many stammerers have a deep-seated fear that they have something seriously wrong with them and that they differ in some essential way from others. These ideas and feelings are the result of their experiences, and particularly of the reactions of others to their speech disorder.

The nature of stammering as we know it is explained, and the fact is stressed that the stammerer has the ability to speak normally but cannot maintain it under all conditions. He is then led to consider stammering in its true perspective as something which is a nuisance in that it delays the expression of thought but that it does not necessarily interfere with living and that many have succeeded with the same handicap.

Again, it is pointed out to him that many who consider themselves as having normally fluent speech, hesitate and even have transient episodes of stammering.

The stammerer is helped to admit and to accept his stammer in as mature and objective a way as is possible and to regard it without fear or emotion. At the same time the unconscious acceptance of the stammer as inevitable must be undermined, and a positive attitude encouraged associated with confidence in his ability to achieve his end.

2. Relaxation Therapy

This has been advocated by some as the only treatment required, and may produce rapid and spontaneous improvement in speech with a general lessening of nervous hypertension. It has been described in detail by Jacobson (1929), and in its relation to the treatment of stammering by Boome and Richardson (1931) and Gifford (1939).

In the first place the practice of relaxation gives rapid recovery from fatigue, both physical and mental, and if practised regularly contributes to a general increase in ease of manner, poise and mental calmness, leading to increased efficiency and confidence in ability to face life without the sense of undue hurry or stress.

There is also developing awareness of undue nervous tension, with growing ability to control it, which contributes towards the control of the actual muscular spasm of the stammer itself.

During relaxation the stammerer may be asked to consider and accept the ideas presented to him in the first part of the treatment, and in some a certain amount of self-analysis may occur, and autosuggestion may also help.

The stammerer also experiences the sensation of easy fluent speech whilst relaxed and learns to associate a general feeling of ease with the act of speaking. Gifford (1939) uses such relaxation as a basis for the development of control of speech through exercises in the experience of stillness, mental stillness and the use of sustained breathy phonation, with loose easy movements of the muscles of articulation. She associates this with emotional stabilisation and re-education of ideas and associations towards speech.

When adequate control of physical tension and a more normal state of muscle tone is achieved, the control of the actual stammer spasm is considered. Although easy, fluent speech has been experienced during relaxation, with perhaps some increase in confidence, the ability to maintain easy speech in everyday life does not necessarily follow spontaneously. It is not expected, nor suggested, that complete relaxation should be maintained during activity. This is, of course, impossible. However, daily practice of relaxation does tend to carry over an increased feeling of ease and reduced tension during speech and general activity. Also, the experience of the ease with which speech can be used tends to increase confidence and to develop a pattern of fluent rhythmic speech without effort which may lead to increasing use of effortless speaking and reduction of stammering.

3. Exercises which help towards the Control of the Stammer Symptom

These may be divided into two groups, being, firstly, those which contribute to the experience of fluent speech under conditions other than general relaxation, and, secondly, those which help him towards direct control at the moment of stammering.

Exercises for articulation have no place in the treatment of stammering except in so far as they convince the stammerer that there are no sounds he is unable to say.

The practice of easy-speaking patterns as described by Kingdon Ward (1941) and Gifford (1939) may be useful and contribute towards control and confidence in the use of speech. Most stammerers want to be given exercises which they feel are a direct approach towards improvement of the symptom, and such exercises provide something concrete which can be practised at home.

The practice of reading aloud and speaking when alone accustoms the stammerer to his own fluent but often unfamiliar use of speech, with normal rhythm and without effort. Its value lies in this, and in its tendency towards the stabilisation of such normal fluent utterance of speech.

Exercises for 'negative practice' have been advised by Bryngelson (1940) and Van Riper (1947) and others. This entails that the stammerer should study in detail every symptom associated with his stammer. He should watch himself in a mirror and observe every abnormal facial or other movement.

He is then asked to imitate accurately, consciously and with voluntary control the stammer as he has observed it in himself. This has been described by Van Riper (1953) as 'the practice of a response for the purpose of breaking the habit of making the response'. The involuntary, undesirable stammer pattern is therefore made voluntary, and becomes something which is subject to control.

Again it is stressed that the stammerer does not gain control by avoiding the stammer, and for this reason Van Riper (1947) aims to help the stammerer to stammer with increasing ease and fluency, but does not suggest that the stammerer should attempt to avoid or prevent the stammer. Habits of avoidance are therefore reversed, and the method of stammering becomes so fluent that the patient ceases to fear its occurrence. Anxiety associated with repression of the symptom is thereby prevented. Again, by so doing, the stammerer is for the time being accepting his own limitations and failures, and attacks rather than avoids his actual stammer spasm and its associated emotional reactions.

Most stammerers find that after stammering on a word they can immediately repeat it without difficulty. Van Riper (1947) has stated that 'the pre-spasm period is full of fear—the spasm period full of struggle or escape, the moment after is where the word can be repeated easily'. He also believes that the struggle is rewarded by the final utterance, and that the satisfaction gained may contribute towards perpetuation of the symptom. He therefore suggests that this satisfaction, derived from the utterance of the word in an abnormal manner, should be denied the patient by what he describes as 'cancelling the block'. Immediately after release of a word through stammering, the stammerer must pause and repeat the word easily before continuing his sentence.

Later the stammerer attempts to gain voluntary control of the spasm before releasing the word.

4. Discussions, Suggestions and Assignments

During each treatment period various problems and situations are discussed, such as those associated with using a telephone, asking for a bus ticket, and others too varied and individual to mention. Suggestions are made and discussed with the patient as to the way in which these difficulties can each be met and overcome in turn. The stammerer is asked to welcome incidents of stammering as opportunities for practising control, and is even asked to make as many opportunities as possible for putting various suggestions into practice.

5. Group Therapy

When the appropriate time is reached, and this varies with each individual, the stammerer attends for therapy in a group where he meets others with whom he can share experiences. Here there are opportunities for practice in an easy speech situation, for discussion and comparison of personal speech problems.

During this period of treatment there is time for the gradual stabilisation of more fluent speech, and of new attitudes and reactions towards situations involving speech. The stammerer ceases more and more to depend on the therapist, and eventually takes the entire responsibility for his own continuing progress.

Results of treatment vary, but in the majority there is at least some alleviation of the symptom. It has persisted frequently for many years, and although in adult life some are enabled to speak without evident stammer, they may retain the momentary sensation of tension of which the listener may be completely unaware. In some this may never be eradicated, but others through time and with increasing self-confidence may lose the memory of their disability and may cease to stammer mentally as well as vocally.

Where treatment commences soon after the stammer symptom is first noticed, a better result can be expected. It is most satisfactory, if by right management, the stammer of a young child is outgrown spontaneously. Children have been known to acquire normal speech and to have no recollection in adult life that they at any time experienced a period of stammering.

Treatment varies, however, with the age of the child, and that used for the pre-school child differs from that of the older child. Improvement is shown by the less frequent occurrence of the stammer, by a decrease in the severity of the spasm, or both, and in increased confidence in dealing with social relationships and with other situations in life.

Others have used intensive group therapy. Brandon and Harris (1967) described in-patient treatment of adults for two-week periods with intensive daily practice using syllable-timed speech. Reading practice was used with, at first, limited speaking, using syllable-timed speech at a rate of approximately 70 syllables to the minute. Later, speaking situations were also provided outside the clinic, including, in the second week, assignments requiring visits to shops, travel agents and so forth.

Fawcus (1970) also approached the treatment of stammering intensively as a form of learned behaviour, using group treatment. She used syllable-timed speech and block modification, as described by Van Riper (1953) and others. She also used assignments designed to reduce anxiety in order to change attitudes towards speech. She feels that such treatment in groups, judging by the results obtained, suggests considerable hope for the future.

Writing in 1971, Andrews discusses the requirements of an ideal method of treatment in that as a result (*a*) speech must be within normal limits after treatment with (*b*) normal non-fluencies, (*c*) that the rate of speech should be under voluntary control and capable of being varied, and that (*d*) pitch, loudness and rhythm should be normal. His observations suggest to him that the present strong interest in physiological theories is justified to account for the onset of stuttering. As there is no evidence that such physiological conditions change with maturity and treatment, treatment might aim to enable a stutterer to become a fluent speaker, if not completely normal, in spite of the persisting neurophysiological conditions. The aim for acceptable treatment might therefore involve the learning of ways of controlling the defect, allowing normal speech to be maintained.

Much has been written concerning the use of delayed auditory feedback (DAF) in the treatment of stammering. Many have suggested that a disturbed auditory feedback loop or a perceptual defect may be implicated in the onset of stammering. Experiments using DAF have shown that normal speech is affected in that it is slowed down and non-fluent, vocal pitch may be raised and errors of articulation may occur.

MacCulloch *et al.* (1970) suggests that DAF induces artificial instability of the speech auditory feedback loop. They suggested that masking low frequency auditory feedback may be preferred to DAF because the former does not affect speed, rhythm nor intonation of speech. Their findings suggested that use of a low frequency masking tone appears to offer therapeutic prospects for the stammerer.

The use of DAF is also described by Van Riper (1970). He discusses the question as to whether or not repetitions and prolongations shown under DAF are similar or identical with stuttering behaviour. Soderberg (1969) and others have shown that the more severe stutterers spoke better under DAF than under normal conditions. Others have noted that the form is changed, the severe reaction being replaced by simple repetitions and prolongations.

Van Riper has used DAF, first to show to the stutterer that other people can be made non-fluent, and secondly to demonstrate to him that his stuttering behaviour can be modified and reduced in severity. He also suggests to the stutterer that he should try to ignore the auditory feedback and concentrate upon the proprioceptive and tactile feedback. He states that it is his impression that such proprioceptive monitoring can be easily transferred from clinical practice to speaking situations in real life, and that the use of DAF as a clinical tool holds some promise.

Neaves (1970) carried out extensive investigations in order to attempt to assess the prognosis of treatment for stammering, based on the assessment of various factors.

She considered four main areas in this prognostic assessment. (1) motor impairment; (2) lateral dominance; (3) intelligence; (4) personality adjustment. She carried out various tests on two groups of children, Group A being 84 children who had responded successfully to treatment, and Group B, 81 children who had failed to respond satisfactorily. Her criteria were that in Group A stammering occurred on not more than 1·5 per cent of words spoken, whilst in Group B, 6 per cent to 30 per cent of the words spoken were indicative of stammering.

Her findings showed a highly significant difference between the two groups on motor impairment, intelligence, personality (self sufficiency/dependancy), speech development, onset of stammer, traumatic experience and familial stammering. Limited significance was found statistically between the two groups in age, lateral dominance, certain personality factors and social class. No significant differences were found in birth history, ordinal position, sinistrality, significant illnesses and twinning.

She concludes that poor neuromuscular co-ordination would appear to be an important factor in stammering, and that this should be considered in treatment.

Wohl (1970) presupposes that certain facts concerning non-fluency have been sufficiently confirmed as to be acceptable as a basis for treatment. These, she states, are (1) that non-fluency comprises several distinct clinical entities which are dysfunctions rather than disorders or symptoms. (2) That auditory feedback and proprioception have been affected as a result of interference during speech activity. (3) That in motor ability, dexterity and lateral dominance the non-fluent speaker does not differ essentially from the normal, and (4) That there is no evidence to prove that they have any particular neurosis or personality disorder apart from that which may result from the dysfunction. She bases treatment on the use of metronome desensitisation by reciprocal inhibition and some training in general relaxation.

Treatment in the Early Stages

This applies chiefly to stammering in the young child before awareness and secondary reactions have become established, and it also includes older children and even adults referred soon after the onset of the stammer symptom.

For many years we have found that no special therapy for the child is required and that wise management at home is usually all that is necessary. Again the advice given varies according to the individual situation and age of the child, but the general principles are as follows:

In the first place there must be a sympathetic and patient attention to the mother's story whilst the child perhaps plays with toys under observation but at the other end of the room. In addition to obtaining information concerning the home background, one must also ascertain the relative relationship of the severity of the stammer and the mother's anxiety. It is important to know how long it is since the stammer was noticed, how frequently it occurs—that is all day, every day, or occasionally—and if the child has shown any awareness of his difficulty.

It is also important to know how the child's difficulty has been managed in the home, and the extent to which he has been corrected or punished.

The advice given aims first of all to alleviate the mother's anxiety and give her some understanding of the nature of stammering in its early stages. The questions of sleeping-accommodation, hours of sleep, eating, play and the relationship of the child to the parents and to other children are also discussed, and where necessary advice is given as to maintaining the general well-being of the child. The child must not be over-protected, but must be treated as other children, discipline being maintained firmly, but calmly.

On the handling of the speech difficulty the mother is asked to refrain from impatience, and a desire to correct, assist or advise the child, and to ensure that his speech is not ridiculed. She is asked to accept the child's hesitant speech as a temporary phase in its development and, as far as is possible avoid any emotional reaction on her part towards it, not an easy thing to achieve.

If the child is already aware of his difficulty and shows signs of fear or of forcing his speech, he must be reassured, as one would deal with any childish fear. A feeling of security and confidence in his relationship to his mother must also be maintained, perhaps by taking the child on her knee for a few minutes to give him the reassurance he may need of her love and care for him, and so ease his excitement and tension.

Although no attention should be drawn to speech at any time, it may reassure the child to repeat nursery rhymes or stories, perhaps in unison with others, if this can be done easily and without stammering. Memories of speech difficulties may then be effaced, and unconscious confidence and experience of fluent speech maintained.

It has usually been found sufficient if the mother returns to report progress at intervals, these varying according to her degree of anxiety and acceptance of the advice given. It is not unusual for her to notice and report improvement within two or three weeks. How far expectancy contributes to this cannot be assessed, but the fact remains that the child's stammer tends gradually to disappear.

Other therapists have regular play groups for such young stammerers and group discussions with the mothers. Knight (1954) has such groups and agrees that it is important to 'make certain that the child is kept free from the fear of speaking. This fear is brought about by the contagion of parental anxiety, which owing to ignorance attaches undue importance to what in these cases is a passing phase in the development of language.' She finds that regular contact between the mothers and children and the therapist ensures the right management at home, and has also found that the best results of treatment are obtained before the stage of perpetuation of the stammer symptom has been reached.

Children aged five to six or seven years, in whom the stammer has persisted for some time, or who began to stammer at a later age and are already attending school, may require group therapy in addition to wise management at home. They are more mature and independent, and in our treatment of these children in groups the mother is not present.

The treatment consists largely in carrying out in a group the advice given to the mother as already described. It is usually found that there is little stammering during free play, or whilst the children in such a group are engaged in various occupations, and such experiences of fluent speech should be encouraged. It does not follow, however, that it will be maintained in speaking situations outside the clinic. Games involving speech are helpful, and the repetition in unison of rhymes and stories. Negative practice may be adapted by encouraging stammering at times, or even deliberate stammering, the therapist and children stammering together and laughing at their abnormal speech. Group relaxation may also be used if adapted to the needs of young children.

The aim of treatment at this age is to permit free speech as far as is possible, and so allow the children to regain unconsciously their experience of, and confidence in, fluent speech. Knight (1954) has said that 'young children never wonder why they have spoken freely, it is enough that they have done so, and because of the respite they gain confidence'.

Treatment of the Older School-age Child

The period from seven or eight years of age to the school-leaving age of 15 or 16 years is for many the age of least response to treatment. The stammer has now become a persistent reaction associated with various school situations, such as reading aloud, replying to the register call, or answering questions. Although many stammerers endure untold miseries of anticipation as a result of their stammer, they often make little attempt, and are perhaps unable, to co-operate in treatment. Many have accepted their disability as their manner of speaking, though not without shame, or even resentment, whilst some appear to be largely unaware of the way in which they stammer, although not unaware of the reaction of other children towards it.

Treatment follows the principles already described, but is modified for the various levels of age and intelligence. It may be mainly group therapy, individual treatment or a combination of both as serves best for each child.

Group relaxation therapy may contribute towards a lessening of tension and form a basis for the experience of easy, fluent speech in unison with others and alone. However the time is actually employed, in speech exercises or games, the principles of reassurance, encouragement of personal self-confidence through achievement, and of confidence in speech through experience are maintained. The child also learns that he is not unique in his disability, and is encouraged by noting improvement in others.

Situations in school frequently aggravate the stammer symptom, and for many this is the time when it is most severe. On leaving school there may be a sudden or gradual improvement in speech. This may be associated with increase in personal confidence in the knowledge of being now a wage earner, but is probably also related to the absence of those feared situations associated with school life to which the stammer had become a conditioned reaction. Some have been known who, at this age, decided they would no longer stammer and with control and persistence were able to achieve their aim without therapy. In others, however, the stammer persists into adult life.

The Part of the Teacher in School

Many children are greatly helped by understanding teachers, but others fail to obtain that assistance in their difficulty. The stammerer may feel inferior and ashamed when he cannot speak normally, and the teacher can do much to encourage confidence and personal self-respect by giving the child responsibility and by maintaining a calm, unhurried and understanding attitude. The teacher's attitude will also influence that of the other children and may thus make the life of the stammerer more bearable.

Some children refrain from giving answers they know well, others may substitute for a feared word and even give what they know is a mistaken answer. Others have reported that they do not attempt to answer because the teacher has been impatient and refused to wait for the child who could not say it quickly.

Reading aloud in school may cause the stammerer to sit in a state of anxiety for an hour or more each morning before the reading lesson, in anticipation of being asked to read before the class.

During the early stages of treatment it is sometimes helpful if the child knows that he will not be asked to read in order to lessen this anxiety and fear. But other children resent being overlooked. It is often helpful if another child is asked to read in unison with the stammerer. He will then experience little or no difficulty, but other children should also read in pairs, so that the stammerer's disability is not made more obvious.

In time, as he gains confidence, he may be able to read alone with fluency and satisfaction. Choral speaking and recitations may also be useful, but elocution or training which draws attention to the manner of speaking may hinder rather than help the stammerer.

In home and school management the child with a stammer must be treated as other children so that he does not experience advantage through his disability. Discipline must be adequate yet with calm insistence rather than angry or excited correction, and he must be encouraged to behave as a normal member of his social group in every way, irrespective of his speech disorder.

SUMMARY

We may therefore summarise these theories concerning stammering and its aetiology as follows:

So far as has been ascertained, the stammerer does not differ essentially from the individuals who do not stammer except that there is a slight but significantly higher incidence of ambidexterity and cross laterality among them than among those who speak fluently. This suggests inadequate left-sided cerebral dominance.

Stammering is not a defect of speech but a disorder of the utterance of speech. All stammerers can speak normally under certain conditions but are unable to maintain fluent speech at all times and in all situations. Although this at first suggests a failure of emotional adjustment, personality tests have failed to prove any basic psychoneurosis, and the anxieties and fears associated with stammering are considered to be largely the result of the stammer symptom and not the cause. Some stammerers show very little if any evidence of even such secondary emotional disturbances, and most lead a normal and useful life in spite of their severe handicap.

The stammer symptom varies from individual to individual and at different times in the same individual. Attempts to speak are associated with muscular hypertonicity and with clonic or tonic spasms of the respiratory, articulatory or phonatory muscle groups. It is probably conditioned by experience, and there is no fixed unchangeable pattern.

Experience again leads to expectation of stammering on certain words or sounds with resultant fear of the spasm which apparently tends towards its recurrence. This may be associated with such secondary symptoms as disturbance of the rhythm of respiration, metabolism, vasomotor imbalance and cardiac arhythmia. All sounds can, however, be articulated easily but cannot always be used easily when part of a speech sequence.

The onset of stammering is rare after the age of seven or eight years and this adds support to the more recent theories that stammering is learned behaviour and that the initial disordered use of speech is associated with the incomplete stabilisation of the neuromuscular co-ordinations required for speech.

Predisposing causes may vary and include increased family

incidence, inadequate left-sided cerebral dominance, temporary ill-health, unhappiness or insecurity. Precipitating factors may be sudden, or the final breakdown in a period of continuous strain. The causes of its persistence may be associated with the adoption of effort in an attempt to overcome the resistance, and growing awareness of the disability.

If the child reacts to interference with the fluency of speech by forceful attempts to speak, he tends to strengthen the resistance, and many of the symptoms we observe are in reality the stammerer's attempt to overcome the resistance to fluent utterance. Growing awareness, however it develops, tends to perpetuate this learned behaviour, associated as it is with increasing fear of its occurrence.

Stammering may occur when there is apparently no emotional stress of any kind, primary or secondary.

It may be possible that the stammerer has developed more than one learned neuromuscular pattern of co-ordinations for speech and at times is unable to use the one which is normal and fluent.

Treatment varies according to the age of the child and involves the adjustment of the stammerer's attitude towards his speech disorder either consciously or unconsciously, relaxation therapy and the experience of easy fluent speech leading to the control of the stammer spasm. It also includes the practice of control in varying situations, and the practice of speech in conversation and in discussions.

The treatment of the pre-school child should be as far as is possible the responsibility of the mother.

The teacher in school may do much to hinder or help the older child with a stammer.

REFERENCES

Allan, C. (1970). Treatment of non-fluent speech resulting from neurological disease—Treatment of Dysarthria. *Brit. J. Dis. Commun.*, **5**, 3.

Andrews, G., and Ingham, R. J. (1971). Stuttering: Considerations in the Evaluation of Treatment. *Brit. J. Dis. Commun.*, *VI*, **2**, 129.

Andrews, G., and Harris, M. (1964). *The Syndrome of Stuttering*. Clinics in Developmental Medicine, No. 17. The Spastics Society. London, Heinemann.

Bloodstein, O. (1958). Stuttering as an anticipatory struggle reaction. In *Stuttering: A Symposium*. Ed. J. Eisenson. New York, Harper.

Bloodstein, O. (1960a). The development of stuttering. I. Changes in nine basic features. *J. Speech Hear. Dis.*, **25,** 219–237.

Bloodstein, O. (1960b). The development of stuttering. II. Developmental phases. *J. Speech Hear. Dis.*, **25,** 336–376.

Bloodstein, O. (1970). Stuttering and normal non-fluency—a continuity hypothesis. *Brit. J. Dis. Commun.*, **5,** 30.

Brandon, S., and Harris, M. (1967). Stammering—An Experimental Treatment Programme using Syllable-timed Speech. *Brit. J. Dis. Commun.*, **1,** 64.

Boome, E. J., and Richardson, M. A. (1931). *The Nature and Treatment of Stammering*. London, Methuen.

Bryngelson, B., and Rutherford, B. (1937). A comparative study of laterality in stutterers and non-stutterers. *J. Speech Dis.*, **3,** 2. Reprinted in *Speech* (1940), **5,** 2.

Bryngelson, B. (1940). Treatment of Stuttering in Children. *Speech*, **3,** 9, and **4,** 7.

Canter, G. J. (1971). Observations on neurogenic stuttering: a contribution to differential diagnosis. *Brit. J. Dis. Commun.*, **6,** 139.

Despert, J. L. (1943). A therapeutic approach to the problem of stuttering in children. *Nerv. Child*, **2,** 2.

Douglas, A. (1940). *A Study of Bilaterally Recorded Encephalograms of Adult Stammerers*. Unpublished Dissertation, Iowa.

Fawcus, M. (1970). Intensive Treatment and Group Therapy Programme for the Child and Adult Stammerer. *Brit. J. Dis. Commun. V*, **1,** 59.

Fransella, F. (1970). Stuttering—not a symptom but a way of life. *Brit. J. Dis. Commun.*, **5,** 22.

Freund, H. (1966). *Psychopathology and the Problems of Stuttering*. Springfield, Ill. Charles C. Thomas.

Gifford, M. (1939). *Correcting Nervous Disorders of Speech*. New York: Prentice Hall.

Hahn, E. F. (1944). *Stuttering, Significant Theories and Therapies*. Stanford Univ. Press.

Hill, H. (1944). Stuttering. I. Critical review and evaluation of biochemical investigations. *J. Speech Hear. Dis.*, **9,** 245.

Hill, H. (1944). Stuttering. II. Review and integration of physiological data. *J. Speech Hear. Dis.*, **9,** 289.

Jacobson, E. (1929). *Progressive Relaxation*. Univ. of Chicago Press.

Jasper, H. H. (1937). Electrical signs of cortical activity. *Psychol. Bull.*, **34,** 411.

Johnson, W., Brown, S. F., Curtis, J. F., Edney, J. C., and Keaster, J. (1948). *Speech Handicapped School Children*. New York, Harper.

Johnson, W. (1946). *People in Quandaries*. Ch. 17. New York, Harper.

Johnson, W. (1951). *Stuttering*. A lecture to the American Academy of Ophthamology and Otolaryngology.

Kanner, L. (1957). *Child Psychiatry*. Springfield, Ill. Charles C. Thomas.

Knight, M. (1954). *Some Thoughts on the Causes and Treatment of Stammering based on a Study of 140 Stammerers*. Unpublished Thesis.

MacCulloch, M. J., Eaton, R., and Long, E. (1970). The Long-term Effect of Auditory Masking on Young Stutterers. *Brit. J. Dis. Commun. V.*, **2,** 165.

MacCulloch, M. J., and Eaton, R. (1971). A Note on Reduced Auditory Pain Theshold in 44 Stuttering Children. *Brit. J. Dis. Commun.*, **6,** 148.

Neaves, A. I. (1970). To Establish a Basis for Prognosis in Stammering. *Brit. J. Dis. Commun.*, **1,** 46.

Sheehan, J. (1946). *A Study of the Phenomena of Stuttering.* Unpublished Thesis, Iowa.

Soderberg, G. (1969). D.A.F. and the Speech of Stutterers. *J. Speech Hear. Dis.*, **34,** 20–29.

Travis, L. (1931). *Speech Pathology.* New York, Appleton.

Van Riper, C. (1947). *Speech Correction: Principles and Methods.* New York, Prentice Hall.

Van Riper, C. (1953). The Treatment of Stuttering. *Speech*, **17,** 17.

Van Riper, C. (1970). The Use of DAF in Stuttering Therapy. *Brit. J. Dis. Commun.*, **1,** 40.

Ward, Kingdon W. (1941). *Stammering.* Hamish Hamilton Medical Books.

West, R. (1950). Rehabilitation of speech. *J. Except. Child.*, March.

Wohl, M. T. (1970). The Treatment of Non-fluent Utterance: A Behavioural Approach. *Brit. J. Dis. Commun.*, **1,** 66.

Woolf, G. (1967). The Assessment of Stuttering as Struggle, Avoidance and Expectancy. *Brit. J. Dis. Commun.*, **2,** 158.

Wyke, B. (1970). Neurological mechanisms in stammering—in hypothesis. *Brit. J. Dis. Commun.*, **5,** 6.

PART V
SPEECH DISORDERS IN TWINS

XX. Disorders of Speech Development in Twins

DEFECTIVE development of speech is found among twins as in other children, but clinical experience has shown that in very few instances is the speech defect similar in both children, and in some pairs of twins the speech of one of the children only is affected. Again one twin may have a minor degree of defective articulation and the other a much more severe disability.

The suggestion has been made that certain disorders of articulation are the result of the close relationship which exists between twins. They are said to be intelligible only to each other or to have an 'idioglossia', or 'language of one's own'. The psychological aspect is stressed, the explanation given being that because between such children there is a strong emotional attachment, they tend to speak in a way which has meaning only for each other and to have little need or desire to develop speech by means of which they are able to communicate with others.

Imitation one of the other may play a part in the use of such defective articulation during the early stages of speech development, especially where there is a true disorder of speech in one of the children. Such an imitative defect would be described as dyslalia. The disability is then temporary and there is usually rapid and spontaneous improvement.

In ten pairs of twins in the 1000 family survey in Newcastle-upon-Tyne, four pairs were boys, four were girls and two were twins of opposite sex.

At three years nine months 12 of these 20 children had normal speech, five had defects of articulation and three were not intelligible. In comparison with the sample group (page 44), 60 per cent of these 20 children who were twins had normal speech compared with 69 per cent in the sample group who had normal or near normal speech. Fifteen per cent of the twins were unintelligible as compared with 11 per cent in the sample group. At nearly five years of age 65 per cent had normal speech compared with 86 per cent in the sample group, whilst two children (ten per cent) were still unintelligible as compared with four per cent in the sample group. At six and a half years only one child had a residual defect of articulation, or five per cent of the group, and this equals that found in the sample group. Four of these children who were twins had attended for speech therapy, however, when between four and six years of age.

Three pairs of twins of the same sex, two pairs being girls and one pair boys, had good fluent speech by the age of two years, whilst another pair of boys had achieved this by two and a half years.

One pair of female twins had similar defects of articulation, or dyslalia, with poor use of language persisting until five years of age.

In one pair of female twins and one pair of male twins speech was dissimilar, and also in one pair of opposite sex. One of the female twins had a more severe defect of articulation than her sister, and it persisted for a longer period. The two boys had somewhat late development of speech, first using words around 18 months and phrases around two years of age. Defective articulation persisted for six months longer in one twin than in the other. In the pair of twins of opposite sex speech developed early, and both were using phrases before the age of 18 months, but whilst the girl had normal articulation, the boy had a period of defective articulation which had cleared by four years of age.

One pair of male twins had a similar and severe dyspraxia with unintelligible speech persisting at five years of age, although speech had commenced at the normal time. An elder sister had had delayed development of speech and later dyslexia. One pair of twins of opposite sex did not use single words until two years of age, with dyslalia persisting until five years.

In addition to these ten pairs of twins, 11 others have been seen during recent years. The speech of these 42 children, 21 pairs of twins, will be summarised (Fig. 85). Fifteen of these pairs were of the same sex and possibly identical, eight being boys and seven girls. Six pairs were fraternal twins of opposite sex. Details concerning the speech of these children are shown in Figure 86.

No.	Sex	Age when seen in years	Type of speech
1 2	M M	3½-8	Normal Normal
3 4	M M	3½-8	Normal Slight transient stammer but normal by 3½ years
5 6	F F	3½-8	Normal Normal
7 8	F F	3½-5	Normal Normal
9 10	F F	3/12-5	Normal Slight transient stammer between 2 9/12-3 years
11 12	M F	3 1/12-8	Normal Normal
13 14	M F	3 1/12-8	Slight lisp until 4 years Normal
15 16	M M	3½-8	Normal Speech development a little late with subsequent dyslalia. Normal at 5 years
17 18	M M	6½-8	Normal Articulatory apraxia
19 20	M M	6½-7	Normal Receptive and executive developmental dysphasia
21 22	M F	4 5/12-5	Articulatory apraxia Normal
23 24	M F	6-9	Normal Articulatory apraxia—unintelligible until 9 years
25 26	M M	4 10/12-5½	Articulatory apraxia—therapy for 10 months Dyslalia—therapy for 3/12—speech then normal
27 28	F F	3½-7	Articulatory apraxia—normal by 8 years. Therapy Dyslalia—normal by 6 years. No therapy
29 30	F F	3 1/12-4 4/12	Articulatory apraxia Normal articulation and a stammer
31 32	M F	4 4/12-4 6/12	Articulatory apraxia—unintelligible till 5 years Minimal dyslalia [k]=[t,] [g]=[d]
33 34	M M	3½-5½	Articulatory apraxia with similar use of consonant sounds

FIG. 85 *(continued overleaf)*

No.	Sex	Age when seen in years	Type of speech
35 36	M M	4 2/12-5	Articulatory apraxia with similar use of consonants
37 38	F F	3½-8	Dyslalia until 4 years Later development of speech with subsequent dyslalia
39 40	F F	4½-10	Developmental executive aphasia with developmental dyslexia and slight occasional stammer in both children
41 42	M	4 5/12-9½	Developmental dysphasia with slight dyslalia and subsequent dyslexia. Both children

FIG. 85

Speech in 21 pairs of twins.

Normal Speech

In seven of these pairs of twins, that is fourteen children, speech development was within the normal limit (Nos. 1 to 14). Five of these pairs were of the same sex, two pairs being boys and three girls. Two pairs were of opposite sex. In two pairs (3 and 4, 9 and 10), one of the twins had a slight and transient stammer, and in a third (13 and 14), one had a slight lisp which did not persist (Figs. 85 and 86).

	Male Twins	Female Twins	Fraternal Twins	Total
Normal speech	2	3	2	7
Defective speech in one twin	3	0	2	5
Defective speech in both twins	3	4	2	9
Total	8	7	6	21 pairs

FIG. 86

Normal and defective speech in twins.

Defective speech development

In five pairs of twins (15 to 24) one child had normal and the other defective speech. Three of these pairs were boys, and two pairs were children of opposite sex.

In nine pairs of twins (25 to 42) both children had some

degree of defective articulation. In four pairs one child had a severe defect of articulation whilst the other had a minimal dyslalia which did not require treatment, or in one case (29 and 30) articulation was normal but there was a stammer.

In the remaining five pairs of children both had a similar defect of speech. Two pairs were boys, two were girls and in one the children were of opposite sex.

Although defective speech development occurred in one or both of the 14 out of 21 pairs of twins, this does not necessarily indicate a higher incidence of defective speech among twins than in the general child population. Children with normal speech are not referred to the speech therapist, and those described here were seen during the 1000 families survey, or were known personally.

Sex and Speech

In the six pairs of male twins with some disorder of speech, defective speech occurred in both children in three pairs, and in only one child in the other three pairs (Fig. 87). Where both

	Male Twins	Female Twins	Fraternal Twins	Total
Similar speech defect in both children	2	1	1	4
Speech defect in both, but dissimilar	1	3	1	5
Speech defect in one twin only	3	0	2	5
Total	6	4	4	14

Fig. 87
Sex and defective speech in twins.

of the twins had defective speech, the defect was similar in two pairs, whilst in the third pair one boy had a severe articulatory apraxia whilst the other had only a minimal dyslalia.

In the other three pairs one child had a severe developmental receptive and executive aphasia (19 and 20), one a severe articulatory dyspraxia with defective articulation persisting at six and a half years (17 and 18) and one had late speech development with a subsequent dyslalia at five years (15 and 16). In each of these three pairs the twin brother had normal speech.

In the four pairs of female twins with defective development of speech, both children had a disorder of speech. In one pair (39 and 40) the defect was similar. There was developmental dysphasia with persisting difficulty in the use of words until at least ten years of age. There was also a tendency to stammer which was never severe, and delay in learning to read.

In the second pair (37 and 38) both children had a dyslalia, but whilst the defect in one was slight, normal speech being established by four years of age, the twin sister had unintelligible speech which lasted until five years.

In another pair (27 and 28) one had an articulatory dyspraxia persisting until eight years of age, whilst her twin sister had a dyslalia and developed normal articulation spontaneously by six years of age. In the fourth pair (29 and 30) one of the twins always had normal articulation but tended to stammer, whilst the sister had a severe articulatory apraxia.

In the four pairs of twins of opposite sex, defective speech development occurred in two pairs whilst in the other two the speech of only one child was affected. In one pair (21 and 22) the girl had normal speech, whilst in the other pair (23 and 24) the boy had normal speech. In each case the twin sibling had a severe articulatory apraxia. In the third pair (41 and 42) the children had a similar difficulty, with developmental dysphasia, a minor degree of dyslalia which resolved spontaneously, and a subsequent dyslexia of similar degree. In the fourth pair (31 and 32) the boy had an articulatory apraxia with unintelligible speech persisting until five and a half years, whilst his twin sister had only a minor difficulty and substituted [t] and [d] for [k] and [g].

Without drawing any definite conclusions as to speech in twins in general, it is clear from those we have seen that a speech disorder is not inevitable, that it may occur in one twin and not in the other, or that twins may each have a speech disorder but of dissimilar type and degree.

PART VI

LATERAL DOMINANCE AND SPEECH

XXI. Lateral Dominance and Speech

DURING clinical experience, information has been gathered concerning lateral preference in patients who stammered and who had various disorders of articulation, and it seemed useful to ascertain whether or not there was any significant difference in laterality between the normal population and children with dysarthria, isolated dysarthria, articulatory apraxia, dyslalia, reading disability and stammering.

In the past mainly between 1935 and 1945, much was published concerning the relationship between disorders of speech and cerebral dominance as indicated by various tests for the preferred hand, eye and foot. The findings were correlated mainly with stammering, and reading disability, and with aphasia as the result of cerebral injury and pathological conditions.

HAND PREFERENCE

The infant shows little evidence of a preferred hand and will use either for grasping or shaking a rattle. Burt (1950) states that soon after the ninth month some preference for right or left may be noticed if effort is required for reaching or grasping. However, the mother usually notices any tendency towards use of the left hand when the child begins to use a spoon around the age of 18 months, and at the time when normally the child is also beginning to use words and develop the use of speech. The development of hand preference is believed to be linked with cerebral development for speech, and in the majority the preferred use of the right hand is developed and maintained throughout life. In others there is delay in the determination of the hand to be used, and the child shows no decided preference for a longer period than is usual. If the child seems to prefer the left hand, the mother may sometimes establish the use of the right hand by repeatedly changing the spoon to that hand, but in others the developing left hand preference is so strong that such attempts are futile. It is then probable that these children will later use a pencil in the same hand and the preferred use of the left hand for skilled acts will persist throughout life.

Such preference is largely determined by heredity, and Russell Brain (1945) states that 'the inheritance of right-handedness as a dominant, and left-handedness as a recessive will explain most, although not all of the facts'. From a survey of various investigators he considers that between 5 to 10 per cent of the population of Britain and America are left handed. Gordon [5] found that 7·2 per cent of elementary schoolchildren were left handed. Burt [3] found 6 per cent of boys were left handed, and 4 per cent of girls and that incidence of left-handedness was higher in backward children (Fig. 88).

	Normal	Backward	Mentally Defective
Boys	6·0	9·6	13·5
Girls	4·0	6·0	10·3
Average	5·0	7·8	11·9

FIG. 88

Incidence of left-handedness in %. (*Burt* (1950).)

It is therefore accepted that most people develop in early childhood a preference for the use of one hand for all single-handed skills as for writing, cutting with a knife or scissors, using a hammer or screw-driver, and so forth. The majority develop a preference for the right hand, but a small proportion have a decided preference for the left hand which persists, often in spite of attempts to establish the use of the right hand.

To some extent, however, such preference is one of degree, as we all use both hands for certain acts, even for such skills as playing the piano or typing, and it is also possible to develop the skill of the non-preferred hand as evidenced by children who are strongly left handed but learn to write with the right hand and eventually prefer it. Others retain the ability to write with either hand. Where there has been cerebral damage, with resulting hemiplegia, even an adult may rapidly learn to write with the non-preferred hand, and the cricketer learns to throw accurately with either hand, but has a preferred hand for bowling and batting.

In some individuals, decided preference never develops as in one girl of 14 years, who wrote with her left hand, and preferred it for using a spoon, scissors and a needle, but threw a ball and played tennis with the right hand. Again another who was right sided for all tests preferred her left hand for the single act of writing.

In some there is a definite feeling of clumsiness in the use of the non-preferred hand which is obvious and difficult to overcome. One child of nine years with brain damage and resulting asymmetrical quadriplegia, with the right side more severely involved, held his pencil more easily in the right hand, but wrote with the left hand. When he did so the writing was firmer and clearer although there was more awkwardness in the actual manipulation of the pencil. The right-handed preference seemed obvious although circumstances had tended towards the use of the stronger left hand.

Foot Preference

Most people show a definite preference for the use of one foot rather than the other in such actions as kicking a ball, stepping up on a chair, or in sliding on ice, when the dominant foot usually leads. Because we use both feet for walking and do not normally develop the use of the feet for fine skills, preference for one or other is often less definite, but the young boy is in little doubt as to which foot is the better for kicking a ball, although the older boy will develop the use of both feet in playing football. In many, however, there is more uncertainty and less definite preference between the two feet than between the hands. There may even be a gradual and unconscious change, as occurred in one boy who at the age of 15 years stated that he used to prefer the right foot, but had recently found that he was using the left more than the right.

Eye Preference

Repeated tests for the preferred or dominant eye have proved that most people have a definite eye preference for monocular sighting, which seldom varies with repeated testing and is established as early as three or four years of age. Because the individual is usually unaware which is the preferred eye it is less likely to be changed by interference, as occurs during education in the use of the hand. It is also possible to ascertain this before practice has influenced to any extent the use of one eye or the other.

Eye preference is not necessarily associated with visual acuity, and in those whose vision is affected the stronger eye may not be the preferred one, as shown by tests, the optically weaker eye being preferred for sighting.

Although Orton (1937) found a graduated series of 'amphiocularity' of varying degrees between the strongly right-eyed and the strongly left-eyed, various other investigators have found that approximately 70 per cent of all individuals prefer the right eye and 30 per cent the left eye, whilst less than one per cent show absence of definite preference.

The Relationship between Hand, Foot and Eye Preference and Cerebral Dominance

The association between a preferred right hand and a dominant left cerebral hemisphere has been generally accepted, and the relationship between laterality and lesions in the cortex affecting speech has been described by many in relation to aphasia. Lateral dominance and its relation to stammering has also been much discussed. At one time it was also believed that left-handed or left-sided preference was associated with dominance of the right cerebral hemisphere.

Humphrey and Zangwill (1952) found that whereas a left-sided brain lesion in the language areas in a right-handed individual is closely correlated with aphasic symptoms, a similar lesion in the right hemisphere in a left-handed individual is not necessarily so. They based their statement on the study of 114 cases of aphasia with unilateral lesions of whom 105 were right handed. In 104 of these right-handed individuals the lesion was in the left hemisphere, and in only one was it in the right hemisphere. Nine were left handed, in five the lesion was in the left hemisphere and in four in the right hemisphere (Fig. 89).

Of ten patients with unilateral lesions in whom left-handedness could be definitely assumed prior to the injury, nine had aphasic symptoms. They occurred in all five of those where the lesion was in the left hemisphere and in four of the five with lesions in the right hemisphere. In this latter group there was less interference with speech and a greater interference with calculation, in space relationships and articulation rather than with integrated use of the symbols of language.

Handedness	Hemisphere of Lesion	
	Left	Right
Right	104	1
Left	5	4
	109	5

FIG. 89
Handedness and hemisphere of lesion in 114 patients with aphasia. (*Humphrey and Zangwill* (1952).)

These ten patients had always considered themselves to be predominantly left handed before their injury, although six had been taught to write with the right hand. Three of these had injuries in the left hemisphere and three in the right. Two had always used the left hand for writing, and two cases of injury in the left hemisphere and at least one (possibly two) with right hemisphere injuries were considered to be ambidextrous (Fig. 90).

Left handed	Hemisphere of Lesion	
	Left	Right
Aphasia	5	4
No aphasic symptoms	0	1
Total	5	5

FIG. 90
Hemisphere of lesion in ten left-handed patients. (*Humphrey and Zangwill* (1952).)

These findings confirm the belief that right-sidedness is associated with left cerebral dominance but suggest that left-handedness may not necessarily be associated with dominance of the hemisphere of the opposite side. It is probable, therefore, that in left-handed patients and in those where there is ambidexterity or cross laterality there may be lack of, or inadequate, cerebral dominance.

Observations by Bauer and Wepman (1955), have confirmed these findings. In 30 patients with unilateral lesions they found 17 who had lesions of the left and 13 with lesions of the right hemisphere. Aphasia was present in eight, seven being right handed and one left handed (Fig. 91).

Hemisphere of Lesion	Handedness	Aphasic Symptoms
Left (17)	Right—12 Left — 5	7 1
Right (13)	Right—9 Left —4	0 1 verbal agnosia 0 1 apraxia of speech and calculation

FIG. 91

(*Bauer and Wepman* (1955).)

By permission of the Editor of the Journal of Speech and Hearing Disorders.

Of the 13 patients with lesions of the right hemisphere, nine were right handed and four left handed. There were no cases of aphasia. In one right-handed man there was a 'verbal agnosia', and in one who was left handed there was 'apraxia of speech and of calculation'.

Of the 17 patients with injuries of the left cerebral hemisphere 12 were right handed, seven of whom showed aphasic symptoms. Five were left handed, one having aphasia.

They conclude that

> cerebral dominance seems unique to the left hemisphere. Those in the population who lack consistent left hemisphere dominance do not appear to have consistent right hemisphere dominance except in rare instances. This would imply that individuals commonly regarded as left handed are more likely to be ambidextrous, and probably should be said to be people in whom lateralisation has not fully developed.

They also suggest that damage to the left hemisphere at birth, or before the development of the speech patterns, may be a possible explanation of aphasic symptoms occurring in association with a lesion of the right cerebral hemisphere.

The relationship between a dominant eye for monocular

sighting and cerebral dominance has never been established. In fact, Brain (1945) states that,

> the eye is not represented in the cerebral cortex as a unit for purposes of visual perception, space perception or ocular movement. The two halves of each retina are represented in different cerebral hemispheres, impulses from each being intermingled with those from the corresponding half of the other retina, so that normally we cannot distinguish what we see with one eye from what we see with the other. The eyes are equally closely linked for purposes of movement and each cerebral hemisphere can only move the two eyes together.

Nevertheless, many children with ambidexterity of hand, foot or eye, or cross laterality, encounter special difficulties in learning to speak and to read, and the incidence of lack of definite preference for the right side (hand, foot and eye) is higher in these children than in the normal population.

Pearce (1953) found the incidence of cross laterality in schoolchildren to be 47 per cent. Of these, 85 per cent experienced difficulty in school. Also, 40 per cent of the children had difficulty or failure in educational attainment, and of these, 70 per cent had some type of cross laterality.

Cerebral Dominance and Disorders of Speech

The relationship between lack of definite preference for the right side and disorders of language development such as stammering, defective articulation and specific reading disability has also been described. Orton (1937) considered that footedness was not so important as eyedness and handedness, although he found that the preferred foot was usually on the same side as the preferred eye and hand. He and others have suggested that eye preference may be determined as a result of hand preference, whilst others believed that the eye preferred or dominant might determine the preferred use of the corresponding hand. He considers that lack of definite dominance for one side or the other constitutes a 'motor intergrading' and is evidence of the absence of a sufficiently strong hereditary tendency to establish preference for one side in all motor acts. Many such children encounter no difficulty in the acquisition and use of spoken or written language, however, although many of those with developmental disorders of speech show evidence of such motor intergrading. He considers that the greatest difficulty is encountered when a tendency to left-sidedness is present but not in sufficient strength to ensure complete unilateral superiority of the right cerebral hemisphere.

Brain (1945) also recognised a relationship between speech disorders and handedness and states that in his view

> the abnormal handedness which so often goes with congenital speech disorders means that incomplete development of the speech pathways has left the child without normal hemisphere dominance on either side—a condition incidentally quite different from 'natural left handedness'.

In Humphrey and Zangwill's study (1952) of ten left-handed adult patients already described, evidence of various types of language disorders occurred in nine. These included disturbances of reading, writing, spelling, calculation, verbal memory or learning ability in addition to dysphasia, both receptive and expressive with difficulties of word finding of varying degrees, and occurred irrespective of the hemisphere which was injured. From their findings in respect of other cases, however, they believe that these various forms of language disorder, except dyscalculia, show a higher incidence in case of injury to the left hemisphere.

Their findings have been tabulated in Figure 92.

Creak (1936) studied the preference for eye and hand in 50 children with reading disability and found that 25 per cent were right sided, 12 per cent left sided and 14 per cent showed evidence of cross laterality, 34 per cent having lack of decided preference for either hand or eye.

Schonell (1946) also describes the association of laterality and reading disability and compares his findings with those of Creak and Monroe in Figure 93. He gives figures concerning eye and hand relationship amongst 73 backward readers and a control group of 75 children. He found almost no evidence of lack of preference for hand and eye, however.

Travis (1931) was concerned with the relationship of laterality and cerebral dominance with stammering which he believed was a neuromuscular dysfunction associated with a lack of a sufficiently dominant lateral gradient, such a gradient being considered essential to the normal integration of speech function.

Hemisphere of injury	Left					Right				
Case No.	1	2	3	4	5	6	7	8	9	10
Site of injury	Temporal lobe	Posterior parieto	Fronto temporal	Fronto parieto	Parietal	Parietal	Posterior parietal	Fronto parietal	Fronto parietal	Parietal
Expression and/or word finding	+	+	+	+	+	+	+	+	+	−
Comprehension	+	−	+	+	+	−	+	+	?	−
Reading	+	+	(+)	+	+	+	+	+	−	−
Writing	+	(+)	+	?	+	?	+	+	−	−
Spelling	+	+	+	+	?	+	−	−	+	−
Calculation	+	−	?	−	−	+	+	+	+	−
Spatial sense	−	−	−	−	−	−	+	+	−	−

+=impaired
−=no evidence of impairment
(+)=probable slight impairment.

FIG. 92

Site of lesion and disturbances of function. (*Humphrey and Zangwill* (1952).)

Laterality	Schonell		Creak Cases 50	Monroe Cases 215
	Normal Pupils 75	Backward Readers 73		
1. R.H.+R.E.	60	43	24	47
2. R.H.+L.E.	25	40	18	35
3. L.H.+L.E.	4	5	12	8
4. L.H.+R.E.	3	8	12	3
5. R.H. either eye	8	3	6	6
6. L.H. either eye	0	1	2	1
7. Either hand Right eye	0	0	16	0
8. Either hand Left eye	0	0	8	0
9. Either hand either eye	0	0	2	0

FIG. 93

Relationship of reading disability to laterality. (*Schonell* (1946).)

Burt (1950) found a higher incidence of stammering in left-handed children than in right-handed children. He states that in right-handed children the incidence of stammering was 1·7 per cent whilst in left-handed children it was 6·5 per cent, also that 3·2 per cent of right-handed children and 11·9 per cent of left-handed children had stammered at some time. He also states that

most frequently neurotic troubles and particularly speech defects are found, not in those who are consistently left handed in all their actions, and left sided with all their limbs, but in those of the so-called mixed type, that is to say in those who are left handed for some tasks and right handed for others, and especially, so it would seem, in those whose dominant eye or foot is on the opposite side to the dominant hand.

In order to investigate the relationship of laterality and disorders of speech in the light of more recent findings concerning the various types of defective articulation already described, information ascertained in patients with speech disorders was compared with the findings in a control group of 661 children and adults.

This control group was composed of the following:

Elementary School, children aged 7 to 12 years .	147
Girls' High School, girls aged 11 to 15 years . .	196
Boys' Grammar School, boys aged 11 to 17 years .	223
University Students and Staff	95
	661

Tests

For the purpose of this investigation simple tests were used as they probably give as reliable a result as some of the more complicated ones. In each case the preferred hand, foot and eye was ascertained.

Many tests have been devised for ascertaining the preferred eye, hand or foot. Our findings have been based on simple tests which were considered to be as reliable as possible for young children, and were as follows:

Eye

The individual is given a card approximately 15 inches square in the centre of which is a small hole $\frac{3}{8}$ inch in diameter. He is then asked to hold it in both hands with arms outstretched and to look through the hole in the card with both eyes at a bright source of light (usually the room light or pocket torch). He has, therefore, no conscious choice of eye, but a spot of light then appears on the preferred eye. If there is doubt, the card can be moved near the face whilst the child continues to look through the hole, and the eye to which the hole is brought is noted. Using a toy telescope has been found unreliable with young children, as they frequently bring it to the non-preferred eye in order that vision with the preferred eye may not be obscured. The spot-light test is best carried out in a partially darkened room.

Hand

The preferred hand was noted for writing, throwing a ball and cutting with a knife or scissors. Where there was evidence of ambidexterity, other additional tests were given.

Foot

The preferred foot for kicking a ball and for stepping up on to a chair was noted. Again, where there was doubt, additional tests were given.

The findings were classified as follows: (1) right hand preferred, (2) left hand preferred, (3) ambidextrous—no definite preference, (4) right eye preferred, (5) left eye preferred, (6) no preference, (7) right foot preferred, (8) left foot preferred, (9) no preference.

From these tests, four groups of individuals were established:

1. Those who were right sided for all unilateral actions.
2. Those who were left sided.
3. Those who had some degree of ambidexterity for eye, hand or foot.
4. Those in whom there was decided preference for eye, hand and foot, but where one of these was opposite to the other two, usually the eye preference being opposite to that for the hand and foot, or cross lateral.

Findings in the Control Group

In the control group we found 86 per cent were right handed, 67 per cent were right eyed and 80 per cent right footed. Six per cent preferred the left hand, 32 per cent the left eye, and nine per cent the left foot. Eight per cent showed variable preference for the use of hand, one per cent for the eye, and 11 per cent used either foot (Appendix, Table XXIX).

Although 86 per cent were right handed only 54 per cent were completely right sided and three per cent left sided. Forty three per cent, therefore, showed lack of definite unilateral preference. In 17 per cent there was ambidexterity in the use of eye, hand or foot, and 26 per cent had cross laterality, having definite preference for the use of eye, hand or foot, but in whom preference for one of these was on the opposite side to that for the other two. In 54 per cent, therefore, the left cerebral hemisphere was probably dominant, whilst in the remainder there was doubt as to which was the dominant one. In three per cent the right cerebral hemisphere may have been dominant, but in 43 per cent unilateral superiority may not have been fully developed (Fig. 94) (Appendix, Table XXX).

Stammering and Lateral Dominance

In a group of 362 stammerers, 288 (80 per cent) were right handed, and 41 (11 per cent) were left handed. This is a higher incidence of left-handedness than in the control group, where it was six per cent (Appendix, Table XXIX).

One hundred and sixty-six (47 per cent) of these stammerers were right sided and probably had left cerebral dominance. Five per cent were left sided and may have had right cerebral dominance. One hundred and seventy-eight (48 per cent) were either ambidextrous or cross lateral. These 178 stammerers may therefore have lacked a dominant lateral gradient (Fig. 94a) (Appendix, Table XXX).

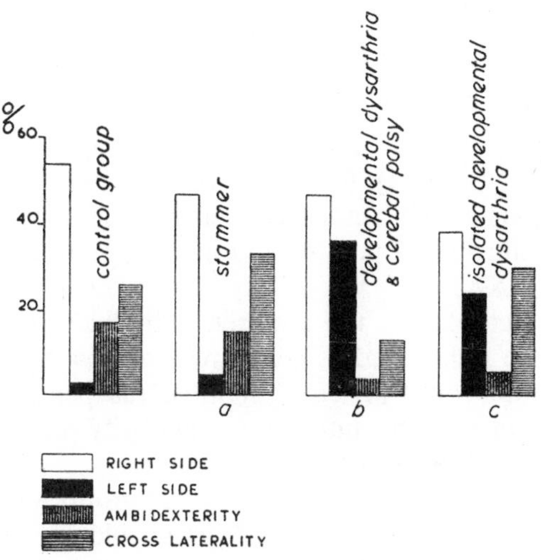

FIG. 94
Preferred sidedness in the control group and in patients with various disorders of speech.

The deficiency of right-handedness, and the deficiency of complete unilateral superiority in stammerers, when compared with the control group, is significant (Appendix, Tables XXXI and XXXII). Nevertheless, these deficiencies are small and the *majority* of these 362 stammerers did not differ in either respect from the control group with normal speech.

DEVELOPMENTAL DYSARTHRIA ASSOCIATED WITH SEVERE OR MINIMAL CEREBRAL PALSY AND LATERAL DOMINANCE

In this group of children with dysarthria there was a much higher incidence of left-sidedness and of left-handedness than in the control group. Forty-seven per cent were left handed and

36 per cent left sided (Fig. 94b) (Appendix, Tables XXIX and XXX).

A statistical analysis of the findings indicated a highly significant increase in left-handedness and left-sidedness in these children with dysarthria, suggesting the development of a dominant right hemisphere following prenatal or neonatal damage to the left cerebral hemisphere (Appendix, Table XXXIII).

Isolated Developmental Dysarthria and Lateral Dominance

These children with an isolated dysarthria but no signs of general motor disability resembled the previous group in that there was again a high incidence of left-handedness (34 per cent) and left-sidedness (24 per cent) (Fig. 94c) (Appendix, Tables XXIX and XXX).

Only 38 per cent of the children with this type of speech disorder were right sided as compared with 54 per cent in the control group, whilst an equal number (38 per cent) showed evidence of incomplete unilateral superiority and were either ambidextrous or cross lateral.

Because the number of children in this group was too small for statistical evaluation, the findings should be treated with some reserve. They suggest, however, an increase in left-sidedness as compared with right-sidedness in children with isolated dysarthria, and on this basis suggest the possibility of a similar, although much less widespread neurological condition, to that found in children with cerebral palsy.

Developmental Aphasia and Lateral Dominance

In a group of 33 children with developmental aphasia 25 (76 per cent) were right handed, three (9 per cent) were left handed and five (15 per cent) had failed to develop a preference for either hand at the time of the examination (Appendix, Tables XXIX and XXX). Forty-two per cent were right sided, however, whilst in 58 per cent there was ambidexterity or cross laterality (Fig. 95b).

Again these figures are too small for statistical analysis,

but they may suggest a delay in the establishment of cerebral dominance, as evidenced by a somewhat higher proportion of ambidexterity associated with delay in the development of speech (Appendix, Table XXXV).

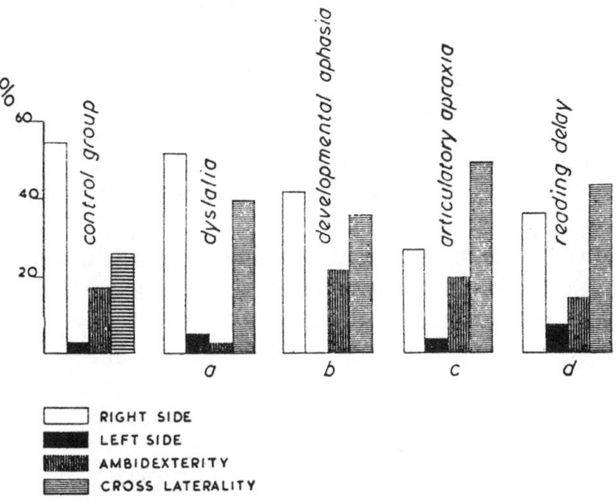

FIG. 95

Preferred sidedness in the control group and in children with delayed speech development or developmental aphasia, dyslalia, developmental apraxia and reading delay.

ARTICULATORY APRAXIA AND LATERAL DOMINANCE

In this group of 67 children with developmental articulatory apraxia there was a high incidence of cross laterality. Only 27 per cent showed a complete right-sided preference, although 61 per cent were right handed. (Appendix, Tables XXIX and XXX). Ambidexterity for eye, hand or foot occurred in 20 per cent and 49 per cent showed cross laterality. Therefore 69 per cent of the children in this group had possibly failed to develop normal hemisphere dominance (Fig. 95c).

Statistically the findings in these children with articulatory apraxia show a highly significant increase in the number of children with absence of a dominant gradient as indicated by a comparison of cross laterality and ambidexterity with right-sidedness (Appendix, Table XXXVI).

Delayed Development of Reading and Lateral Dominance

This group of 14 children who had attended for treatment because of a reading disability was too small for any definite conclusions to be drawn. There was, however, a high proportion of both cross laterality (43 per cent) and ambidexterity (14 per cent) (Appendix, Table XXX). Therefore 57 per cent of these children had failed to develop a definite one-sided preference for unilateral skills, whilst only 36 per cent showed definite right-sided preference as compared with 54 per cent in the control group (Fig. 95d).

In some of these children the reading disability was associated with, or the result of, an articulatory apraxia in earlier life. It is therefore not possible to state whether these findings in this group of children relate to the defect of articulation or to the reading delay or to both.

Dyslalia and Lateral Dominance

The 115 children in this group showed evidence of some increase in cross laterality but a decrease in ambidexterity. The proportion of those with a definite right- or left-sided preference, however, 52 per cent and 5 per cent respectively, was similar to that of the control group (54 per cent and 3 per cent) (Appendix, Tables XXIX and XXX).

Statistical analysis showed that in the relation of right-sidedness to left-sidedness, or right-sidedness to ambidexterity and cross laterality, the findings in this group of children with dyslalia did not differ from those of the control group (Fig. 95a) (Appendix, Table XXXVII).

These findings would therefore support the theory that dyslalia is not organically determined, but that in dysarthria and articulatory apraxia there is probably an organic basis for the disorder of speech, dysarthria being associated with left-sidedness and probably right hemisphere dominance, whilst articulatory apraxia is associated with an increase in the occurrence of cross laterality, and a possible lack of adequate cerebral dominance. In stammering there is a higher incidence of left-handedness, and although this is statistically significant, the majority of stammerers resemble the normal population in respect of lateral dominance.

REFERENCES

Bauer, R. W., and Wepman, J. M. (1955). Lateralisation of Cerebral Function. *J. Speech Hear. Dis.*, **20,** 171.

Brain, W. Russell (1945). Speech and Handedness. *Lancet*, **2,** 837.

Burt, C. (1950). *The Backward Child.* 3rd ed. University of London Press.

Creak, M. (1936). Reading difficulties in Children. *Arch. Dis. Child.*, **6,** 151.

Gordon, H. (1921). *Brain*, **43,** 313.

Humphrey, M. E., and Zangwill, O. L. (1952). Dysphasia in Left-handed Patients with Unilateral Brain Lesions. *J. Neurol. Neurosurg. Psychiat.*, **15,** 184.

Orton, S. T. (1937). *Reading, Writing and Speech Problems in Children.* New York, Norton & Co.

Pearce, R. A. H. (1953). Crossed laterality. A Study of its Significance and Treatment in Ordinary School Life. *Arch. Dis. Child.*, **28,** 247.

Schonell, F. J. (1946). *Backwardness in the Basic Subjects.* 3rd ed. Edinburgh, Oliver and Boyd.

Travis, L. E. (1931). *Speech Pathology.* New York, Appleton.

XXII. Summary and Conclusions

We have seen that the development of normal speech in early childhood is a part of the natural learning process which is dependent on various factors.

There must be adequate hearing with discrimination for, appreciation and recognition of the sounds used in speech.

There must also be comprehension for language and the ability to formulate thoughts, rendering them audible through expressive speech.

This is dependent on the ability to reproduce the sounds of speech accurately, and in the sequences required for intelligible speech.

The movements and co-ordinations of the muscle groups used in articulate speech must also be adequate.

There must be no anatomical condition which would interfere with such movements or render it impossible to obtain the requisite intra-oral air pressure for articulation.

The level of intelligence must be such that there is normal appreciation of spoken language with corresponding growth and development of the thought to be expressed.

Finally, there must be the personal and social adjustment which stimulates the desire to communicate with others through speech.

Defects of Speech

The surprising fact is not that a few have disorders of speech, but rather that the vast majority develop the normal use of speech.

We have described how, when any of these conditions are lacking, or neurological maturation is incomplete or delayed, speech may be delayed in onset, articulation may be abnormal, or there may be interference with the fluent, audible expression of speech. There may also be abnormalities of phonation. Apart from nasalised vocal tone, reference to these has been omitted in the text as such defects are rare in childhood. Dysphonia may result from chronic sinusitis, be a functional condition due to mal-use of the voice, or may be due to growth of papilloma or polyp on the vocal folds. Again, more rarely, it may be the result of an anatomical condition such as fixation of the arytenoid cartilages, when normal vocal tone may be impossible.

The number of children found to have transient defects of speech during the early stages of speech development was unexpectedly high, but whether these were defects of articulation, or interruptions in fluent utterance, there was, in the majority, a spontaneous tendency towards improvement and the use of normal speech. Some children, however, had more severe disorders of speech development with inadequate use of speech persisting into school or later life.

Speech Development and Age and Sex

Contrary again to what we had expected, we found little difference in the ages at which boys and girls first began to speak. Boys, however, experienced greater difficulty than girls in the use of the oral symbols of speech, with defective articulation or unintelligible speech occurring more frequently and persisting to a later age. Defects of articulation were found in twice as many boys as girls at five years of age, and in the proportion of three to two at six and a half years. Unintelligible speech at five years of age was three times as frequent in boys as in girls. Boys also experienced greater difficulty with the fluent use of speech, and we found twice as many boys as girls who had a transient period of stammering.

Position in Family

Again we found that, in general, the age of onset of speech was not related to position in family, that first children were not necessarily backward in this respect, nor that subsequent children always gained through association with an older brother or sister. We found, however, that true disorders of speech, such as developmental aphasia, dysarthria or apraxia, and stammering, were rare in first children. In the family survey there was a highly significant difference between first children and those in other positions in the family in respect of articulation. Of the 365 first children, only nine had severe and persisting defects of articulation and eight had a period of stammering. Again, of the children seen with developmental aphasia and described in Chapter IX (Fig. 42), none were first children, whilst only two of the 12 children described with isolated dysarthria (Fig. 64), and two of the 12 with developmental apraxia (Fig. 65), were first children. It has been suggested that the mother may spend more time in encouraging speech development with the first child, but this theory is not supported by experience. Again, it has been thought that younger children might learn to speak more easily because of close contact with older members of the family, and the mother is often surprised that this is not so, and that the difficulty occurs in the younger children. The reason for this difference between first children and those in other positions in the family remains therefore unknown.

Disorders of Articulation

It has been apparent that there are varying types of defective articulation. Although dyslalia may be a functional condition involving some difficulty in the use of the sounds of speech, it is generally transient with spontaneous improvement towards normal speech, and speech therapy is rarely necessary. We have thought, however, that other defects of articulation were due to a basic, organic condition, even where this is not at first obvious. Articulatory apraxia responds only slowly to treatment in spite of intelligent co-operation on the part of the child, and isolated dysarthria resembles the dysarthria associated with a general motor disability. In this condition a severe or minimal dysarthria, or even normal speech, may be associated with a gross general motor disability, whilst a severe dysarthria may be isolated and not associated with signs of a more widespread cerebral lesion such as spasticity or athetosis. The severity of the dysarthria would therefore seem to bear little relation to the degree of the motor disability, but where this is extensive it is more probable that speech will also be involved.

Our findings suggested that the age of onset of speech was closely related to the general level of intelligence except in those children where there was a hearing defect or a focal or more widespread cerebral lesion, resulting in developmental aphasia or dysarthria. Defects of articulation of varying degrees and stammering were found, however, in children, irrespective of their level of intelligence.

Multiple Disorders

We have also described how a child's speech disability may result from more than one basic condition, as, for example, when a child with a cleft palate or developmental dysarthria has, in addition, a hearing loss or an articulatory apraxia. General mental retardation, and emotional disturbances secondary to or more rarely as a primary cause, may also complicate the picture. Always the condition must be assessed in relation to the child as a whole and not merely as an inability to articulate certain of the phonetic sounds of speech.

Laterality

The relationship of left-handedness, or lack of one-sided preference, to developmental disorders of speech is not fully understood or proved. We noted, however, a high proportion of left-sidedness associated with dysarthria in children with a severe motor disability and also a similar proportion in those with isolated dysarthria. On the other hand, articulatory apraxia was associated with a higher proportion of cross laterality than was found in the control group, whilst there was a relative deficiency or late determination of preference for eye, hand or foot (ambidexterity) in those with delayed onset of speech. In stammerers there was a higher proportion of left-handedness and of cross laterality than in the control group, but the *majority* of stammerers showed right-sided preference, and in this respect did not differ from the normal.

Cleft Palate

The surgical treatment of cleft palate has now become so successful that, if operation is performed in early life, normal speech usually develops without speech therapy. Faulty patterns of articulation often persist for a longer period than is common in childhood, but there is progressive and spontaneous progress towards normal articulation. A few children, even in whom there is adequate nasopharyngeal closure, may have additional difficulties if they have also an apraxia for articulation, or for co-ordination of the movements of the soft palate with those of articulation, dysarthria of neurological origin, or a hearing loss. Speech therapy may then be necessary and it will also be required for older children and adults where faulty patterns of articulation have been well established before operation. In the few where the possibility of nasopharyngeal closure has not been achieved by surgery, speech therapy may again assist the patient towards the use of clear, intelligible speech which, however, will not be normal to the trained ear.

Treatment

The treatment of a patient with a speech disability can never follow precise and definite rules. The speech therapist must first assess, through the history and her examination, the child's need for treatment. Through appropriate questioning, and appreciation of the mother's story, and through careful and critical observation, he or she may be enabled to diagnose the type of speech disorder and assess the need for, and the advisability of, treatment. A full understanding of the speech disorder may not be possible without a medical report, or without subsequent consultation with other specialists concerning any basic conditions which may be the cause of the speech disability, influence treatment, or affect the prognosis. On the other hand the plastic surgeon, for example, will rely on the speech therapist's assessment of the child's speech when considering any further surgical procedure. The speech therapist cannot work satisfactorily in isolation, but is dependent on the co-operation, knowledge and advice of specialists in various medical and surgical fields such as the departments of medicine, neurology, ear, nose and throat, paediatrics, plastic surgery, psychological medicine, psychology, orthodontics, and so forth. Only through such consultations may the true nature of the condition be fully understood to the benefit of the patient, and to the advancement of knowledge of speech pathology.

Treatment, if considered advisable, must then be planned to meet the individual need at each stage of progress. This may be individual or group treatment, or both, simultaneously, or consecutively, or observation at intervals may be indicated to watch progress. In addition to that which aims to improve the actual speech, treatment must also include that of the patient in relation to his speech disorder. This may involve advice to the mother on the handling of the situation in the home, and encouragement of the young child, leading him to increasing self-confidence, independence and happier social relationships. Where the parental attitude to the speech disorder in the home is affecting the child detrimentally, as when there is repeated correction of the defective speech, the mother may gain understanding of the condition from the speech therapist through regular observation of the treatment of her child during visits to the speech therapy department. So she may gradually adjust her ideas and be enabled to co-operate fully. In this way not only can she feel that she is able to share in the treatment of her own child but that it is partly her responsibility, and the child's progress and also the therapist are then helped through regular, useful, daily practice in the home.

The older child with a speech disability may face many difficulties in school life, and although some are able to contend with these, others may be less able to do so. The solution of the problem may not be to remove the child from his difficulties, or even to attempt to remove the environmental difficulties from the child. This may not lie within the field of speech therapy. Rather the therapist should try to so manage relationships with the child during treatment that he is given the support and encouragement which will help him to adjust to his disability, and to gain in personal development by surmounting his difficulties in school or social life.

The aim of speech therapy is to assist those in the community who suffer from a speech disability to acquire normal speech. They may be small in number in comparison with the whole, but to those concerned, and to their relatives, the disability is important and far reaching in its effects. Where normal speech may never be possible due to the severity of some underlying organic condition, the aim must be to render speech as intelligible and as useful as possible.

The need for speech in our civilisation is inescapable, and without adequate means of communication with others the individual so affected must always be at a disadvantage.

APPENDIX

THE AGE OF SPEECH DEVELOPMENT

TABLES I-V

I.—In the Sample Group—114 Children

Age in years	Age in months	Single words	Per-centage	2-3 word phrases	Per-centage	Intelli-gible speech	Per-centage
	6–8	8	7	—	—	—	—
	–10	31	28	1	1	1	1
1	–12	42	38	9	8	6	5
	–14	9	8	6	5	4	4
	–16	4	4	9	8	7	6
	–18	9	8	45	40	36	32
2	–24	6	5	30	27	24	21
	–30	2	2	5	5	9	8
3	–36	—	—	6	5	8	7
	–42	—	—	1	1	4	4
4	–48	—	—	—	—	2	2
	–54	—	—	—	—	5	5
5	–60	—	—	—	—	2	2
6½	–80	—	—	—	—	3	2
Total Assessed		111	100	112	100	111	100

Mean age for the first use of words . . . 11·8 months
Mean age for the first use of phrases . . . 18·6 months
Mean age for intelligible speech . . . 24·1 months for 111 out of 112 (1 not intelligible)

3 children at the age of 6½ years relapsed into unintelligible speech at times of stress.

II.—The Age of Speech Development in 162 Children with Defective Speech

Age in years	Age in months	Single words	Per-centage	2-3 word phrases	Per-centage	Intelli-gible speech	Per-centage
	6–8	8	5	—	—	—	—
	–10	19	12	—	—	—	—
1	–12	43	27	4	3	2	1
	–14	16	10	3	2	0	0
	–16	11	6	13	8	3	2
	–18	36	22	23	14	6	4
2	–24	16	10	44	27	11	6
	–30	9	6	37	22	13	8
3	–36	2	1	21	13	20	12
	–42	2	1	13	8	30	19
4	–48	—	—	—	—	14	9
	–54	—	—	1	0·5	19	12
5	–60	—	—	—	—	7	4
6½	–80	—	—	—	—	31	19
No. Assessed		162	100	159	98	156	96

3 children used no phrases at 6½ years—2 per cent.
In 6 children speech was not intelligible at 6½ years—4 per cent.
The mean age for the first use of words . . . . . . 14·9 months
The mean age for the first use of phrases . . . . . 24·2 months
The mean age for intelligible speech . . . . . . 43·3 months

III.—The Age of Speech Development in 44 Children with unintelligible Speech persisting until 4 years 9 months

Age in years	Age in months	Single words	Per-centage	2-3 word phrases	Per-centage
	6–8	1	2	—	—
	–10	4	10	—	—
1	–12	13	31	—	—
	–14	4	10	1	2
	–16	2	5	2	5
2	–18	10	23	7	16
	–24	4	10	10	23
	–30	3	7	11	26
3	–36	1	2	7	16
	–42	—	—	5	12
4	–48	—	—	—	—
	–54	—	—	—	—
5	–60	—	—	—	—
6½	–80	—	—	—	—
No. assessed		42	100	43	100

In 37 children speech became intelligible between 4 years 9 months and 6½ years. (12 of these children attended for speech therapy).
5 children remained unintelligible at 6½ years.
2 had left the district and could not be assessed at 6½ years.

In these children the mean age for the first use of words was 15·1 months and the mean age for the first use of phrases was 25·5 months.

IV.—The Age of Speech Development in 29 Children who had a Period of Stammering during the Development of Speech

Age in years	Age in months	Single words	Per-centage	2-3 word phrases	Per-centage	Intelli-gible speech	Per-centage
1	7–12	12	41	—	—	—	—
	–18	11	38	4	14	—	—
2	–24	5	17	15	51	8	27·5
	–30	1	4	5	17	5	17
3	–36	—	—	4	14	3	10
	–42	—	—	1	4	4	14
4	–48	—	—	—	—	0	0
	–54	—	—	—	—	8	27·5
5	–60	—	—	—	—	1	4
6½	–80	—	—	—	—	—	—
No. assessed		29	100	29	100	29	100

The mean age for the first use of words was . . . . . 14·5 months
The mean age for the first use of phrases . . . . . 23·5 months
The mean age for intelligible speech . . . . . . 35·3 months

V.—A Comparison between the Ages of Speech Development in four Groups of Children

	The sample group. 114 children	Defective speech group. 162 children	Severe and persistent defects. 44 children	Children who stammered. 29 children
	Mean Age in Months			
First Words	11·8	14·9	15·1	14·5
First Phrases	18·6	24·2	25·5	23·5
Intelligible Speech	24·1	43·3	over 57*	35·3
	Age Range in Months			
First Words	6–30	6–42	6–36	7–30
First Phrases	9–42	11–54+	13–42	13–42
Intelligible. Speech	9–80+	11–80+	60–80+	19–60

* 5 remained not intelligible at 6½ years.

ASSESSMENT OF LANGUAGE ABILITY

TABLES VI-VIII

VI.—In the Sample Group—114 Children

Age in years	No. assessed	Sentences			
		A	B	C	D
3 9/12	110	69 63%	34 31%	6 5%	1 1%
4 9/12	102	90 88%	11 11%	1 1%	0 0 %

Sentences.

A. Fluent and well constructed.
B. Minor defects of language.
C. Incomplete sentences with inversions, etc.
D. Limited, poor use of language.

Age in years	No. assessed	Rhymes			
		A	B	C	D
3 9/12	102	54 53%	38 37%	7 7%	3 3%
4 9/12	100	77 77%	17 17%	5 5%	1 1%

Rhymes.

A. Can say several well, unaided.
B. Needs prompting.
C. Repeats line by line or adds the last word only.
D. Can say no rhymes.

VII.—Assessment of Language Ability in 44 Children with a Severe Defect of Articulation persisting until 4 Years 9 Months

Age in years	No. assessed	Sentences			
		A	B	C	D
3 9/12	40	5 12%	24 60%	10 25%	1 3%
4 9/12	44	19 43%	22 50%	2 4%	1 3%

Sentences.

A. Fluent and well constructed.
B. Minor defects of language.
C. Incomplete sentences with inversions, etc.
D. Limited, poor use of language.

Age in years	No. assessed	Rhymes			
		A	B	C	D
3 9/12	37	9 24%	10 28%	12 32%	6 16%
4 9/12	42	18 43%	12 28%	7 17%	5 12%

Rhymes.

A. Can say several well, unaided.
B. Needs prompting.
C. Repeats line by line or adds the last word only.
D. Can say no rhymes.

VIII.—Assessment of Language Ability in 22 Children who Stammered. (15 of the Group of 37 Children were not assessed)

Age in years	No. assessed	Sentences			
		A	B	C	D
3 9/12	21	6 28%	10 48%	3 14%	2 10%
4 9/12	21	12 57%	9 43%	0 0%	0 0%

Sentences.

A. Fluent and well constructed.
B. Minor defects of language.
C. Incomplete sentences with inversions, etc.
D. Limited, poor use of language.

Age in years	No. assessed	Rhymes			
		A	B	C	D
3 9/12	21	5 24%	7 33%	8 38%	1 5%
4 9/12	18	9 50%	9 50%	0 0%	0 0%

Rhymes.

A. Can say several well, unaided.
B. Needs prompting.
C. Repeats line by line or adds the last word only.
D. Can say no rhymes.

ARTICULATION

TABLES IX-XIII

IX.—In the Sample Group—114 Children, at 3 Age Levels

Age in years	Total assessed	Normal	Defective [th] and/or[r]only I	Intelligible speech, but defects of articulation. II	Unintelligible speech III
3 9/12	113	47 42%	30 27%	23 20%	13 11%
4 9/12	113	73 64%	25 22%	10 9·5%	5 4·5%
6½	113	107 95%	5 4%		1 1%

Of those with normal or intelligible speech at 6½ years 3 relapsed to unintelligible speech at times.

X.—Defective Articulation in 944 Children at 3 Age Levels

Age in years	Total assessed	Intelligible speech, but defects of articulation. II	Unintelligible speech III	Delayed development of language IV
3 9/12	162 17·5%	64 7%	93 10%	5 0·5%
4 9/12	100 11%	53 6%	44 5%	3 0·3%
6½	31 3%	22 2%	6 0·6%	3 0·3%

Defective use of [th] and/or [r] not included.

XI. Defects of Articulation in 37 Children who had a Period of Stammering

Age in years	Normal speech	Intelligible speech, but defects of articulation II	Unintelligible speech III
3 9/12	19 50%	9 25%	9 25%
4 9/12	28 75%	7 19%	2 6%
6½	32 86%	5 14%	0 0%

When compared with the sample group at 3 years 9 months the correlation between stammering and defects of articulation is not significant.

XII.—Incidence of Consonant Defects occurring in 112 Children in the Sample Group showing the number in whom they were defective in the initial Position in Words at 3 Years 9 Months

	Plosives [p] [b] [t] [d] [k] [g]	Fricatives [f] [v] [s] [tʃ] [dʒ]	[θ (th)]	Total	Semi-vowels [l] [w] [j]	[r]	Combinations of consonants.
Voiced Voiceless	11 14	16 45	6 34	33 93	6	39	r+ 42 s+ 16 l+ 3
Total	25	61	40		6	39	61

N.B.—[tʃ (ch)] and [dʒ (j)] were classed as fricatives.
[z] was not assessed.

XIII.—Incidence of Consonant Defects occurring in 162 Children with Defective Articulation showing the number in whom they were Defective in the Initial Position in Words at 3 Years 9 Months

	Plosives [p] [b] [t] [d] [k] [g]	Fricatives [f] [v] [s] [tʃ] [dʒ]	[θ (th)]	Total	Semi-vowels [l] [w] [j]	[r]	Consonant Combinations
Voiced Voiceless	41 83	62 211	22 118	125 412	42	85	r+ 96 s+ 79 l+ 45
Total	124	273	140		42	85	220

N.B.—[tʃ (ch)] and [dʒ (j)] were classed as fricatives.
[z] was not assessed.

THE DEVELOPMENT OF SPEECH AND SEX

TABLES XIV AND XV

XIV.—Sex and the Age of Development of Speech in the Sample Group—114 Children

Boys—55 Girls—59

Age in years	Age in months	Single words		2-3 word phrases		Intelligible speech	
		Boys	Girls	Boys	Girls	Boys	Girls
	6–8	3	5	—	—	—	—
	–10	13	18	—	1	—	1
1	–12	24	18	5	4	3	3
	–14	1	8	2	4	2	2
	–16	2	2	4	5	2	5
	–18	4	5	22	23	17	19
2	–24	5	1	12	18	6	18
	–30	1	1	3	2	5	4
3	–36	—	—	6	0	7	1
	–42	—	—	—	1	4	0
4	–48	—	—	—	—	1	1
	–54	—	—	—	—	3	2
5	–60	—	—	—	—	1	1
6½	–80	—	—	—	—	2	1
Total assessed		53	58	54	58	53	58

1 boy was not intelligible at 6½ years.

	Boys	*Girls*
The mean age for the first use of words was . .	12·0	11·4 months
The mean age for the first use of phrases was . .	19·4	17·9 months
The mean age for the use of intelligible speech was .	26·8	21·7 months

The difference between the ages when words and phrases were first used by boys and girls is not significant.

Boys developed intelligible speech on average at 26·8 months compared with 21·7 months in girls. The difference is 5·1 ± 2·22 months and is highly significant The difference between the sexes appears to be most marked at about the second birthday.

XV.—Sex and the Age of Development of Speech in 162 Children with Defective Articulation

Boys—103 Girls—59

Age in years	Age in months	Single words		2-3 word phrases		Intelligible speech	
		Boys	Girls	Boys	Girls	Boys	Girls
	6–8	6	2	—	—	—	—
	–10	13	6	—	—	—	—
1	–12	26	17	3	1	1	1
	–14	9	7	2	1	0	0
	–16	6	5	7	6	2	1
	–18	25	11	12	11	1	5
2	–24	12	4	29	15	5	6
	–30	4	5	27	10	7	6
3	–36	1	1	13	8	11	9
	–42	1	1	8	5	22	8
4	–48	—	—	—	—	8	6
	–54	—	—	—	—	13	6
5	–60	—	—	—	—	4	3
6½	–80	—	—	1*	2*	22	6
No. assessed		103	59	102	59	102†	57

* 1 boy and 2 girls were not using simple phrases at 6½ years.
† 6 boys still had unintelligible speech at 6½ years.

	Boys	*Girls*
The mean age for the first use of words was . . .	14·5	15·2 months
The mean age for the first use of phrases was . . .	24·7	25·5 months
The mean age for intelligible speech was	45·5	38·2 months

Again these figures fail to indicate any significant difference in the ages at which first words and phrases were used by boys and girls.

The boys in this group developed intelligible speech on average at 45·5 months compared with girls at 38·2 months. The difference is 7·3 ± 2·7 months and again is highly significant.

DEFECTIVE ARTICULATION AND SEX

TABLES XVI-XVIII

XVI.—Sex and Defective Articulation at 3 Age Levels in the Sample Group—114 Children

Boys—55 Girls—59

Group I.—Defective [th] and/or [r] only.
Group II.—Intelligible speech, but with defects of articulation.
Group III.—Unintelligible speech.
Group IV.—Delayed language, articulation not assessed.

Age in years	No. assessed		Normal articulation and I	II	III	IV
3 9/12	Boys	54	33	11	10	0
	Girls	58	44	11	3	0
4 9/12	Boys	54	44	7	3	0
	Girls	59	54	3	2	0
6½	Boys	54	52	1	1	0
	Girls	59	59	0	0	0

The difference between boys and girls in this group in the use of defective articulation when assessed at these ages is not significant.

XVII.—Sex and Defective Articulation in the Whole Group of 944 Children at 3 Age Levels

Boys—490 Girls—454

Age in years	No. assessed	Normal articulation and I No.	%	II No.	%	III No.	%	IV No.	%
3 9/12	Boys 490	387	88·7	36	4	64	7	3	0·3
	Girls 454	395	88·8	28	3	29	3	2	0·2
4 9/12	Boys 490	425	92·9	30	3	34	4	1	0·1
	Girls 454	419	95·8	23	3	10	1	2	0·2
6½	Boys 490	472	98·3	11	1	6	0·6	1	0·1
	Girls 454	441	98·8	11	1	0	0	2	0·2

At 3 9/12 yrs. $x^2=11{\cdot}6$, $n=1$, $P<0{\cdot}01$
At 4 9/12 yrs. $x^2=7{\cdot}1$, $n=1$, $P<0{\cdot}01$

At each age tnere is a highly significant difference between boys and girls in the development of normal articulation.

XVIII.—Defective Articulation and Sex in 44 Children

44 Children, 5·2%, were recorded as having Severe Defects of Articulation with Unintelligible Speech persisting until 4 Years 9 Months.

Sex. 34 boys+10 girls=44

$x^2=13{\cdot}1$, $n=1$, $P<0{\cdot}01$

These figures show a very highly significant difference between boys and girls in this group.

THE DEVELOPMENT OF SPEECH AND POSITION IN FAMILY

TABLE XIX

Position in Family and Age of Development of Speech in the Sample Group—114 Children

Age in months	Single words		2-3 word phrases		Intelligible speech	
	First	Remd.	First	Remd.	First	Remd.
6–8	5	3	—	—	—	—
–10	8	23	—	1	—	1
–12	19	23	3	6	3	3
–14	4	5	2	4	2	2
–16	1	3	3	6	3	4
–18	4	5	17	28	13	23
–24	2	4	15	15	13	11
–30	—	2	0	5	3	6
–36	—	—	2	4	3	5
–42	—	—	—	1	0	4
–48	—	—	—	—	0	2*
–54	—	—	—	—	2	3
–60	—	—	—	—	—	2
–80	—	—	—	—	—	4
No. assessed	43	68	42	70	42	70

* 1 Not intelligible.

	First and only	Remainder
The mean age for the first use of words was . .	11·5	11·9 months
The mean age for the first use of phrases was . .	18·4	18·8 months
The mean age for use of intelligible speech was . .	21·2	26·6 months

These figures show no significant difference in the ages for use of first words and phrases by first children and those in other positions in the family.

First children developed intelligible speech on average at 21·2 months compared with 26·6 months for later children. The difference is 5·38+2·35 months and is highly significant.

N.B.—Due to the small number of children in this group it was only possible to consider two classes of children. As a large proportion were first children the comparison was made between first and only children and those in other positions in the family, that is 44 first children and 70 in other positions.

POSITION IN FAMILY AND DEFECTIVE ARTICULATION

TABLES XX AND XXI

XX.—In the Sample Group—114 Children at 3 Age Levels

	Age in years					
	3 9/12		4 9/12		6½	
	First	Remd.	First	Remd.	First	Remd.
Normal, or defective [th] and/or [r] only	34	43	41	57	44	67
Percentage	79	62	93·5	82·5	100	97
Defective articulation, but intelligible	7	15	3	7	0	1
Percentage	16	22	6·5	10	0	1·5
Unintelligible speech	2	11	0	5	0	1
Percentage	5	16	0	7·5	0	1·5
No. assessed	43	69	44	69	44	69

When the relation between position in family and defective articulation is assessed at 3 9/12 years, the difference is suggestive only, with a relative absence of defects in first children.

At 4 9/12 years the difference is not significant.

XXI.—Position in Family and Defective Articulation in 44 Children

Position in family of 44 children with severe defects of articulation and persistent unintelligible speech until 4 years 9 months.

1	2	3	4	5	6	7+	Position in family
9	17	10	7	0	1	0=44	Number of children

$$x^2 = 9{\cdot}4,\ n = 1,\ P < 0{\cdot}01$$

The position in family according to these figures is highly significant in relation to defective articulation with a relative absence of defects in first children.

SOCIAL STATUS AND THE DEVELOPMENT OF SPEECH

XXII.—Social Status and the Age of Speech Development in the Sample Group—114 Children

Groups 1+2—12 children Group 3—63 children
Groups 4+5+N.C.—39 children

Age in months	Social Group								
	1+2	3	4+5+N.C	1+2	3	4+5+N.C.	1+2	3	4+5+N.C.
	Single words			2-3 word phrases			Intelligible speech		
6–8	1	3	4	—	—	—	—	—	—
–10	3	13	15	—	—	1	—	—	1
–12	5	28	9	1	4	4	1	4	1
–14	0	7	2	1	1	4	1	1	2
–16	0	2	2	2	4	3	2	3	2
–18	2	6	1	4	30	11	3	22	11
–24	1	3	2	2	20	8	1	16	7
–30	—	—	2	0	3	2	1	6	2
–36	—	—	—	2	1	3	1	4	3
–42	—	—	—	—	—	1	0	2	2
–48	—	—	—	—	—	—	1	0	1
–54	—	—	—	—	—	—	0	5	0
–60	—	—	—	—	—	—	1	0	1
–80	—	—	—	—	—	—	—	—	3
Total	12	62	37	12	63	37	12	63	36
No. assessed	111			112			112†		

† 1 child in social groups 4 and 5 was not intelligible at 6½ years.

	Social groups	1+2	3	4+5+N.C.
The mean age for the first use of words was	.	12·0	11·3	11·6 months
The mean age for the first use of phrases was	.	19·2	18·4	18·8 months
The mean age for the use of intelligible speech	.	24·0	22·8	26·5 months

SOCIAL STATUS AND ARTICULATION

TABLES XXIII AND XXIV

XXIII.—Articulation and Social Status in the Sample Group —114 Children at 3 Age Levels

Age in years	No. assessed	Social group	Normal and defects of [th] and/or [r] only	Intelligible speech with defects of articulation	Unintelligible speech
3 9/12	113	1+2	8	2	2
		3	43	15	5
		4+5+N.C.	26	6	6
4 9/12	113	1+2	10	2	0
		3	58	5	0
		4+5+N.C.	30	3	5
6½	113	1+2	12	0	0
		3	62	1	0
		4+5+N.C.	37	0	1

XXIV.—Social Status in 44 Children with Severe Defects of Articulation

Social group	1+2	3	4	5+N.C.	Total
No. of children	4	14	11	15	44
No. expected	4·4	23·5	6·3	9·9	44.1

x^2=9·0, n=1 (1, 2, 3 together v. 4, 5, and N:C. together)
P=<0·01

In this group the difference is highly significant, with a correlation between severe defects of articulation occurring in the social classes 4, 5, and not classed.

OTHER CONDITIONS

TABLE XXV

OTHER ENVIRONMENTAL CONDITIONS AFFECTING THE 44 CHILDREN WITH SEVERE DEFECTS OF ARTICULATION

(*a*) *Maternal Capacity.*	Able to cope.	Not able to cope.	Var. Unc. +N.R.	
	32	6	6	=44
Expected	36	4·3	3·7	
	Not significant			

(*b*) *Deprivation.*	*Recorded.*	*Expected.*
Total children	19	19·9
Details.		
Perm. loss of father	1	2·9
Temp. loss of father	3	3·8
Perm. loss of mother	0	0·5
Temp. loss of mother	1	1·2
Part. loss of mother	3	6·3
Mother working	10	11·8
Parental incapacity	6	5·7
Marital instability	5	6·0

There is no significant difference.

(*c*) *Family Dependency.*	*Recorded.*	*Expected.*	
	12	8·9	Not significant
(*d*) *Neglect.*	12	9·5	Not significant

(*e*) *Miscellaneous.*	*Recorded.*	*Expected.*	*Significant.*
Nursery	8	5·4	—
Enuresis (3)	11	10·1	—
Enuresis (5)	8	3·9	Poisson Graph suggests P about 0·05.
Fits	2	2·6	—
Behaviour disorders	2	2·9	—
Papular urticaria	12	13·8	—
T's & A's	2	3·3	—
Acute otitis	15	8·5	Chi-square=6·5. $n=1$, $P<0{\cdot}02$
Chronic otitis	3	2·7	—
Squint	4	3·0	—
Prematurity	4	1·9	—

THE AGE OF SPEECH DEVELOPMENT IN CHILDREN WITH A GENERAL MOTOR DISABILITY

TABLES XXVI AND XXVII

XXVI.—35 Hospital Patients with Dysarthria and Severe or Minimal Motor Disability

Age in years	Motor Disability			
	Severe 18		Minimal 17	
	Speech		Speech	
	Words	Phrases	Words	Phrases
1–2	2	—	1	1
–3	4	1	3	0
–4	4	2	10	2
–5	4	2	2	6
–6	2	4	1	4
–7	1	3	—	—
–8	1	—	—	—
–9	—	—	—	—
–10	—	2	—	1
–11	—	—	—	—
–12	—	1	—	—
No. assessed	18	15	17	14

XXVII.—32 School Children with Severe Motor Disability and Normal or Defective Speech

Age in years	Normal speech 18		Defective speech 14	
	Words	Phrases	Words	Phrases
1–2	11	8	2	1
–3	3	2	5	2
–4	1	3	5*	3
–5	1	1	1	2
–6	—	1	—	1*
–7	—	—	1	2
–8	—	—	—	—
–9	—	(not	—	1
–10	—	known–1)	—	—
–11	—	—	—	—
–12	—	—	—	1
No. assessed	16	15	14	13

* One child with a partial hearing loss first used words between 3 and 4 years and phrases around 6½ years.

One child used no phrases at the age of 13½ years.

XXVIII.—The Development of Speech and Motor Development in Children with a General Motor Disability

No.	Age in years	Diagnosis	Motor development			Speech development		Articulation
			Sat	Walked with support	Walked	Words first used	Phrases used	
1	2 2/12	Spastic quadriplegia	18/12	—	—	—	—	—
2	2 6/12	Spastic paraplegia	18/12	2+	—	2	—	?
3	2 6/12	Spastic quadriplegia	2	—	—	2	—	?
4	2 8/12	Spastic quadriplegia	—	—	—	—	—	—
5	2 8/12	Spastic quadriplegia	18/12	—	—	18/12	—	not clear
6	2 8/12	Spastic diplegia	—	—	—	14/12	18/12	normal
7	2 11/12	Spastic diplegia	—	—	—	18/12	2½	normal
8	2 11/12	Spastic quadriplegia	15/12	2	—	2	—	defective
9	3 3/12	Spastic quadriplegia	—	—	—	—	—	—
10	3 3/12	Spastic quadriplegia	—	—	—	—	—	—
11	3 6/12	Spastic paraplegia	?	?	2½	15/12	2	normal
12	3 7/12	Spastic quadriplegia	—	—	—	—	—	—
13	3 8/12	Spastic triplegia	3	—	—	3	—	?
14	3 8/12	Spastic diplegia	2 9/12	—	—	—	—	—
15	3 9/12	Spastic quadriplegia	—	—	—	3	—	?
16	3 10/12	Spastic diplegia (slight)	7/12	—	3½	12/12	3	normal
17	3 10/12	Spastic quadriplegia	—	—	—	3	3½	slight dysarthria
18	3 11/12	Spastic quadriplegia	—	—	—	3½	—	?
19	4 1/12	Spastic diplegia	2	—	—	4½	—	?
20	4 3/12	Spastic quadriplegia	4	—	—	2	3½	near normal
21	4 6/12	Spastic hemiplegia	—	—	—	2	3	normal except [r]
22	4 7/12	Spastic diplegia	—	—	—	2	3	normal
23	4 8/12	Spastic quadriplegia	—	—	—	4	4½	? dysarthria
24	4 8/12	Spastic diplegia	18/12	3½	—	4	—	?
25	5 8/12	Spastic quadriplegia	3½	—	—	18/12	2½	normal
26	6	Spastic quadriplegia	—	—	—	5	—	?
27	6 1/12	Spastic quadriplegia	4	4½	—	2	5	dysarthria & dyspraxia
28	6 7/12	Ataxia	?	?	6	2	3	dyspraxia
29	6 11/12	Ataxia	16/12	—	—	2	3	normal

N.B.—In many of these children there was insufficient speech to assess the articulation with certainty.

LATERALITY AND SPEECH DISORDERS

(*TABLES XXX TO XXXVII*)

XXIX.—Lateral Preference in a Control Group and Patients with Disorders of Speech

	Hand						Foot						Eye					
	Right		Left		No pref.		Right		Left		No pref.		Right		Left		No pref.	
	No.	%	No.	%	No.	%	No.	%	No.	%	No.	%	No.	%	No.	%	No.	%
Control group (661)	571	86	39	6	51	8	531	80	58	9	72	11	442	67	213	32	6	1
Stammer (362)	288	80	41	11	33	9	278	77	57	16	27	7	222	61	138	38	2	1
Dysarthria and cerebral palsy (47)	23	49	22	47	2	4	—	—	—	—	—	—	22	47	25	53	0	0
Isolated dysarthria (29)	17	59	10	34	2	7	21	72	8	28	0	0	13	45	16	55	0	0
Developmental aphasia (33)	25	76	3	9	5	15	26	79	5	15	1	6	19	57	12	36	2	6
Articulatory apraxia (67)	41	61	15	22	11	17	44	66	20	30	3	4	38	57	27	40	2	3
Reading delay (14)	10	72	2	14	2	14	11	78	3	22	0	0	8	57	6	43	0	0
Dyslalia (115)	106	91	8	7	1	2	98	85	14	12	3	3	89	77	26	23	0	0

XXX.—Lateral Preference in a Control Group and in Patients with Disorders of Speech

	Right side		Left side		Ambi-dextrous		Cross lateral		Ambi-dextrous +Cross lateral	
	No.	%	No.	%	No.	%	No.	%	No.	%
Control group (661)	356	54	17	3	114	17	174	26	288	43
Stammer (362)	166	47	18	5	56	15	122	33	178	48
Dysarthria and cerebral palsy (47)	22	47	17	36	2	4	6	13	8	17
Isolated dysarthria (29)	11	38	7	24	2	7	9	31	11	38
Developmental aphasia (33)	14	42	0	0	7	22	12	36	19	58
Articulatory apraxia (67)	18	27	3	4	13	20	33	49	46	69
Reading delay (14)	5	36	1	7	2	14	6	43	8	57
Dyslalia (115)	59	52	7	5	3	3	46	40	49	43

XXXI.—Right- and Left-handedness in Stammerers and in the Control Group

	Right hand	Left hand	Ambidextrous+ Cross lateral
Control group (661)	571	39	288
Stammerers (362)	288	41	178

x^2=5·7, n=1, P<0·02–0·01.

Comparing the incidence of right- and left-handedness in stammerers with that in the control group, there is a significant increase in left-handedness in stammerers.

XXXII.—Right-sidedness and the possible absence of a Normal Dominant Gradient in Stammerers and in the Control Group as Indicated by Ambidexterity and Cross Laterality

	Right side	Left side	Ambi-dextrous	Cross lateral	Ambi-dextrous +Cross lateral
Control group (661)	356	17	114	174	288
Stammerers (362)	166	18	56	122	178

$x^2=2{\cdot}7$, $n=1$, $P=$approx. 0·1.

Comparing the incidence of ambidexterity plus cross laterality versus the remainder in stammerers with that in the control group, there is no significant increase in the absence of hemisphere dominance, as defined.

XXXIII.—Right- and Left-sidedness in Children with Developmental Dysarthria and Cerebral Palsy and in the Control Group

	Right side	Left side	Ambi-dextrous	Cross lateral	Ambi-dextrous +Cross lateral
Control group (661)	356	17	114	174	288
Dysarthria (47)	22	17	2	6	8

There is an increased proportion of left-sidedness versus right-sidedness in children with dysarthria when compared with the controls. This is highly significant ($P<0{\cdot}01$).

XXXIV.—Right- and Left-sidedness in Children with Isolated Dysarthria and in the Control Group

	Right side	Left side	Ambi-dextrous	Cross lateral	Ambi-dextrous +Cross lateral
Control group (661)	356	17	114	174	288
Isolated dysarthria (29)	11	7	2	9	11

These figures are too small for x^2 and should be treated with some reserve, but Poisson Graph suggests $P<0{\cdot}01$, i.e. a significant increase in left-sidedness as compared with right-sidedness in these children with dysarthria compared with controls.

XXXV.—Laterality in Children with Developmental Aphasia and in the Control Group

	Right side	Left side	Ambi-dextrous	Cross lateral	Ambi-dextrous +Cross lateral
Control group (661)	356	17	114	174	288
Developmental aphasia (33)	14	0	7	12	19

These figures do not indicate any statistically significant difference between children with developmental aphasia and the controls.

XXXVI.—Right-sidedness compared with Ambidexterity and Cross Laterality in Children with Developmental Articulatory Apraxia compared with the Control Group

	Right side	Left side	Ambi-dextrous	Cross lateral	Ambi-dextrous +Cross lateral
Control group (661)	356	17	114	174	288
Articulatory apraxia (67)	18	3	13	33	46

$x^2=14{\cdot}4$, $n=1$, $P<0{\cdot}01$.

In this group of children there is a highly significant increase in the number showing absence of a dominant gradient (as indicated by ambidexterity or cross laterality) versus the remainder when compared with the controls.

XXXVII.—Dyslalia and Right-sidedness in Relation to:

(*a*) left-sidedness, and (*b*) ambidexterity+cross laterality compared with that of the control group

	Right side	Left side	Ambi-dextrous	Cross lateral	Ambi-dextrous +Cross lateral
Control group (661)	356	17	114	174	288
Dyslalia (115)	59	7	3	46	49

There was no evidence of any significant difference between those children with dyslalia and the control group in either respect.

INDEX OF AUTHORS

INDEX OF SUBJECTS